D1288326

Temporomandibular Disorders
Second Edition

CLINICS IN PHYSICAL THERAPY

EDITORIAL BOARD

Otto D. Payton, Ph.D., **Chairman**
Louis R. Amundsen, Ph.D.
Suzann K. Campbell, Ph.D.
John L. Echternach, Ed.D.

Already Published

Hand Rehabilitation
Christine A. Moran, M.S., R.P.T., guest editor

Sports Physical Therapy
Donna Bernhardt, M.S., R.P.T., A.T.C., guest editor

Pain
John L. Echternach, Ed.D., guest editor

Therapeutic Considerations for the Elderly
Osa Littrup Jackson, Ph.D., guest editor

Physical Therapy Management of Arthritis
Barbara Banwell, M.A., P.T., and Victoria Gall, M.Ed.,
P.T., guest editors

**Physical Therapy of the Cervical and
Thoracic Spine**
Ruth Grant, M.App.Sc., Grad.Dip.Adv.Man.Ther.,
guest editor

**Physical Therapy of the Geriatric Patient,
2nd Ed.**
Osa L. Jackson, Ph.D., R.P.T., guest editor

Physical Therapy for the Cancer Patient
Charles L. McGarvey III, M.S., P.T., guest editor

Gait in Rehabilitation
Gary L. Smidt, Ph.D., guest editor

Physical Therapy of the Hip
John L. Echternach, Ed.D., guest editor

Physical Therapy of the Shoulder, 2nd Ed.
Robert Donatelli, M.A., P.T., guest editor

Pediatric Neurologic Physical Therapy, 2nd Ed.
Suzann K. Campbell, Ph.D., P.T., F.A.P.T.A., guest editor

Physical Therapy Management of Parkinson's Disease
George I. Turnbull, M.A., P.T., guest editor

Pulmonary Management in Physical Therapy
Cynthia Coffin Zadai, M.S., P.T., guest editor

Physical Therapy Assessment in Early Infancy
Irma J. Wilhelm, M.S., P.T., guest editor

Physical Therapy of the Low Back, 2nd Ed.
Lance T. Twomey, Ph.D., and James R. Taylor, M.D.,
Ph.D., guest editors

Forthcoming Volumes in the Series

**Physical Therapy of the Cervical and
Thoracic Spine, 2nd Ed.**
Ruth Grant, M.App.Sc., Grad.Dip.Adv.Man.Ther.,
guest editor

Physical Therapy for Closed Head Injuries
Jacqueline Montgomery, P.T., guest editor

Physical Therapy of the Knee, 2nd Ed.
Robert E. Mangine, M.Ed., P.T., A.T.C., guest editor

Physical Therapy of the Foot and Ankle, 2nd Ed.
Gary C. Hunt, M.A., P.T., O.C.S., and
Thomas G. McPoil, Ph.D., P.T., A.T.C., guest editors

Temporomandibular Disorders

Second Edition

Edited by

Steven L. Kraus, P.T., O.C.S.

Instructor
Division of Physical Therapy
Department of Rehabilitation Medicine
Emory University School of Medicine
Private Practice
Physiotherapy Associates
Atlanta, Georgia

CHURCHILL LIVINGSTONE
New York, Edinburgh, London, Madrid, Melbourne, Tokyo

Library of Congress Cataloging-in-Publication Data

Temporomandibular disorders / edited by Steven L. Kraus. — 2nd ed.
     p. cm. — (Clinics in physical therapy)
    Rev. ed. of: TMJ disorders. 1988.
    Includes bibliographical references and index.
    ISBN 0-443-08924-8
    1. Temporomandibular joint—Diseases. 2. Temporomandibular joint.
I. Kraus, Steven L. II. TMJ disorders. III. Series.
    [DNLM: 1. Temporomandibular Joint Diseases—therapy.
2. Temporomandibular Joint—physiology.   WU 140 T2863 1994]
RK470.T58 1994
617.5′22—dc20
DNLM/DLC
for Library of Congress   94-5632
                                                    CIP

Second edition © Churchill Livingstone Inc. 1994
First edition © Churchill Livingstone Inc. 1988

Distributed in the United Kingdom by Churchill Livingstone, Robert Stevenson
House, 1–3 Baxter's Place, Leith Walk, Edinburgh EH1 3AF, and by associated companies, branches, and representatives throughout the world.

The Publishers have made every effort to trace the copyright holders for
borrowed material. If they have inadvertently overlooked any, they will be
pleased to make the necessary arrangements at the first opportunity.

Acquisitions Editor: *Carol Bader*
Copy Editor: *Paul Bernstein*
Production Supervisor: *Laura Mosberg Cohen*

Printed in the United States of America

First published in 1994   7 6 5 4 3 2 1

To my wife, Pattie, for her love, understanding, and patient support; to my daughter, Emily Jane, who gives me such joy and happiness; and to my parents, Dottie and Kenneth L. Kraus, my inspiration

Contributors

Robert A. Bays, D.D.S.
Associate Professor and Chief, Division of Oral and Maxillofacial Surgery, Department of Surgery, Emory University School of Medicine, Atlanta, Georgia

Peter W. Benoit, D.M.D., Ph.D
Former Associate Professor, Departments of Oral Biology and Oral Medicine, Emory University School of Dentistry; Private Practice, Temporomandibular Disorders and Nondental Pain, Atlanta, Georgia

Susan J. Dreyer, M.D.
Assistant Clinical Professor, Department of Physical Medicine and Rehabilitation, Emory University School of Medicine, Atlanta, Georgia; Associate, Georgia Spine and Sports Physicians, Smyrna, Georgia

Thomas M. Eggleton, M.S., P.T.
Associate Clinical Professor, Department of Dental Medicine and Public Health, University of Southern California School of Dentistry, Los Angeles, California; Faculty Member, Pacific Clinical Research Foundation, San Diego, California; Faculty Consultant, Clinical Research Foundation, San Diego, California, Faculty Member, URSA Foundation, Edmonds, Washington

Robert E. Going, Jr., D.D.S.
Assistant Clinical Professor, Division of Oral and Maxillofacial Surgery, Department of Surgery, Emory University School of Medicine; Private Practice, Oral and Maxillofacial Surgery, Atlanta, Georgia

J. David Haddox, D.D.S., M.D.
Assistant Professor and Director, Division of Pain Medicine, Department of Anesthesiology, Emory University School of Medicine; Director, Center for Pain Medicine, The Emory Clinic, Atlanta, Georgia

Jules R. Hesse, R.P.T., M.T.
Assistant Professor, Department of Craniomandibular Disorders, Academic Center for Dentistry Amsterdam, Amsterdam, the Netherlands

Tom Keith, P.T.
Clinical Instructor, University of Oklahoma School of Physical Therapy, Division of Physical Rehabilitation, University of Oklahoma, Oklahoma City, Oklahoma; Clinical Instructor, Department of Physical Therapy, Langston University, Langston, Oklahoma; Physical Therapist, Physical Therapy Professionals, Oklahoma City, Oklahoma

Steven L. Kraus, P.T., O.C.S.
Instructor, Division of Physical Therapy, Department of Rehabilitation Medicine, Emory University School of Medicine; Private Practice, Physiotherapy Associates, Atlanta, Georgia

Dennis P. Langton, B.S., P.T.
Associate Clinical Professor, Department of Dental Medicine and Public Health, University of Southern California School of Dentistry, Los Angeles, California; Faculty Member, Pacific Clinical Research Foundation, San Diego, California; Faculty Consultant, Clinical Research Foundation, San Diego, California

Eric S. Lawrence, D.D.S.
Director, TMJ and Orthodontic Sections, Division of Dentistry, The Mt. Sinai Medical Center, Cleveland, Ohio; Consultant, Orthodontic and TMJ Dysfunction, Wade Park Veterans Administration Hospital, Cleveland, Ohio; Private Practice, Orthodontics, Orofacial Orthopedics, and TMJ Dysfunction, Mayfield Heights, Ohio

Jonathan P. Lester, M.D.
Assistant Clinical Professor, Department of Physical Medicine and Rehabilitation, Emory University School of Medicine, Atlanta, Georgia; Vice-President, Georgia Spine and Sports Physicians, Smyrna, Georgia

Jeffrey S. Mannheimer, M.A., P.T.
Clinical Assistant Professor, Orofacial Pain and TMD Center, Department of Prosthodontics and Biomaterials, University of Medicine and Dentistry of New Jersey, Newark, New Jersey; Adjunct Assistant Professor, Program in Physical Therapy, Department of Orthopedic Surgery and Rehabilitation, Hahnemann University School of Medicine, Philadelphia, Pennsylvania; President, Delaware Valley Physical Therapy Associates, Lawrenceville, New Jersey

Machiel Naeije, Ph.D. (Physics)
Associate Professor and Chairman, Department of Craniomandibular Disorders, Academic Center for Dentistry Amsterdam, Amsterdam, the Netherlands

Jennifer J. Osborne, P.T.
Physical Therapist, Head, Neck, and TMJ Therapy Center, Denver, Colorado

Samuel J. Razook, D.D.S.
Former Director, TMJ/Facial Pain Clinic, Emory University School of Dentistry; Private Practice, Oral and Maxillofacial Surgery, Atlanta, Georgia

Charles G. Widmer, D.D.S., M.S.
Associate Professor, Department of Oral and Maxillofacial Surgery, College of Dentistry, University of Florida, Gainesville, Florida

Robert E. Windsor, M.D.
Clinical Assistant Professor, Department of Physical Medicine and Rehabilitation, Emory University School of Medicine, Atlanta, Georgia; President, Georgia Spine and Sports Physicians, Smyrna, Georgia

Foreword

The term *temporomandibular disorders (TMDs)* refers to a group of clinical problems that involve the temporomandibular joint (TMJ) or joints, the masticatory musculature, or both. Such disorders are considered to be a subclassification of musculoskeletal disorders and are a major source of nondental pain in the orofacial region. It is estimated that up to 10 percent of the American public has some form of TMD, of whom perhaps 5 percent may seek or need treatment. Furthermore, the quality of life of many affected individuals can be severely impaired by the symptoms associated with these disorders.

The typical complaint of someone with a TMD is facial pain. The pain is usually aggravated by chewing or other jaw function and is frequently accompanied by palpable muscle tenderness, joint soreness, and/or limitation of jaw movement. Since the symptoms and signs of a TMD may be confused with other painful conditions of dental, orofacial, cranial, or cervical origin, the use of reliable and valid diagnostic procedures and criteria are of the utmost importance in arriving at an accurate differential diagnosis. As with similar musculoskeletal disorders, the differential diagnosis of a TMD is based on a critical and unbiased evaluation of the patient's chief complaint, history, and clinical examination, supplemented, when appropriate, with TMJ imaging. The evaluation should be able to differentiate among the presumptive TMD, normal anatomic and functional variations, benign and unimportant conditions, and other disorders whose signs and symptoms may mimic or be similar to those of a TMD. Thus, understanding the role of diagnosis in the care of potential or actual TMD patients is essential to all therapists working in this field. The Second Edition of this book clearly recognizes this need, since it includes new and important information on this subject.

The management of TMDs remains an area of common interest and concern to both dentists and physical therapists. In fact, given that the use of conservative and reversible therapies is more than ever regarded as the standard of care for most patients with a TMD, the overlapping interests of these two professions has been reinforced since the publication of the First Edition of this book. These factors, combined with the many reports of clinical success following the use of physical therapy procedures, compel those clinicians who are interested in the care of TMD patients to study and to understand the role that these procedures may have in the management of such patients. The same understanding is also required of the other conservative and reversible modalities commonly employed in the treatment of TMDs, such as behavioral, pharmacologic, and interocclusal stabilization appliance therapy. As for those therapeutic modalities that are invasive or irreversible, the possible negative consequences of such procedures must obviously be considered along with their presumed efficacy.

A word of caution is in order with regard to all modalities or regimens used or advocated for use in the management of TMDs. It should be recognized by all clinicians that therapeutic success is not scientific proof of cause and effect. This is particularly true with regard to painful musculoskeletal disorders. The reported clinical success of any treatment procedure, however noteworthy and compelling, may be due to naturally recurring cyclical remission of the signs and symptoms, to placebo effects, to specific therapeutic effects, or to some combination of these three factors. One cannot know which phenomenon is operating without reliable and valid scientific evidence based on sound clinical research. Thus, unless such evidence is specifically available, clinicians should be cautious in attempting to interpret the reason that may account for their clinical success or the basic mechanisms underlying that success. This does not imply that treatment should be deferred because objectively-derived efficacy data do not exist. It does imply, however, that the risks, costs, and other possible consequences of any treatment modality or procedure must be compared with the expected positive clinical results, even if the reasons for those results may not be specifically understood.

In view of these important and ever changing clinical and scientific issues, it is noteworthy that Steven Kraus and his collaborators have again been able to produce a very useful and timely contribution to the professional literature. This Second Edition is a worthy update and expansion of the information provided in the First Edition of this book and, as with that earlier edition, is recommended for physical therapists as well as for those dentists and other health professionals who are interested in learning about the diagnosis and treatment of TMDs.

Norman D. Mohl, D.D.S., Ph.D.
Professor
Department of Oral Medicine
School of Dental Medicine
University of Buffalo
Buffalo, New York

Preface

Management of TMD involves a multidisciplinary approach. A discussion of the relevant anatomy and biomechanics provides the necessary understanding of the structure and function of the TMJ. A unified classification system allows clinicians to diagnose TMD using common terminology and criteria. Knowledge of the validity, reliability, and predictive value of diagnostic tests avoids overuse and misinterpretation of test conclusions and, ultimately, misdiagnosis of TMD.

The vast majority of signs and symptoms related to TMD are managed with nonsurgical dental and physical therapy intervention. Nonsurgical care of the TMD patient should be reversible, conservative, and cost-effective. A patient whose signs and symptoms do not respond to a nonsurgical approach may require arthroscopy, arthrotomy, or orthognathic surgery to improve symptoms and function. Rigid criteria will be used to determine those patients who may benefit by the use of a particular surgical option. Pre- and postoperative physical therapy is recommended following either arthroscopy, arthrotomy, or orthognathic surgery to ensure that mandibular activities return to a pain-free and functional state.

Cephalic symptoms and TMJ/mandibular dysfunction are often the result of the altered interaction of multiple functional factors including occlusion, the TMJ muscles, and the muscles of mastication. To adequately analyze these factors, the dynamics of the cervical spine can no longer be ignored. The cervical spine can mimic certain symptoms thought to originate from the TMJ and/or the muscles of mastication. Thus, cervical spine influence upon mandibular function will be examined, and physical therapy and medical roles in the evaluation and management of the cervical spine will be discussed. Finally, psychological and medical management of myofascial pain will be addressed.

Improved clinical knowledge of cephalic symptoms and functional limitations of the TMJ will be of most benefit to the patient. Patient satisfaction depends on a well-integrated team approach. Each team member must recognize the valuable contributions of the other members. Designing an effective treatment plan, based on unified diagnostic criteria and a commitment to the patient's specific needs, will significantly diminish the occurrence of chronic pain and dysfunction.

Steven L. Kraus, P.T., O.C.S.

Contents

1 | Clinical Anatomy of the TMJ Complex

Thomas M. Eggleton
Dennis P. Langton

An anatomist could be considered one who spends a lifetime in the study of anatomy. The authors of this chapter are not anatomists but clinicians who have had the opportunity to study anatomy. As clinicians, we attempt to connect anatomic study with how it can be clinically applied. Therefore, although this chapter is devoted to anatomy, it is presented with a clinical eye and contains statements and opinions concerning the potential clinical significance of the structures being discussed. Some of these statements and opinions are contained within the body of discussion of the individual anatomic element. However, areas of particular "clinical note" are discussed separately and are marked as such. The main focus of this chapter is the TMJ, but those specific adjacent structures that play an important role in the overall combined functions as well as participate in dysfunction of the temporomandibular (TM) complex are also discussed.

This chapter presents the findings from 160 fresh cadaver dissections and observations (105 male and 55 female specimens). The specimens ranged in age from 18 to 89 years, with the average range of 71 to 73 years, and although 60 percent had full or partial dentition, 40 percent were fully edentulous. We preface this presentation with the statement that in each individual specimen, no two sides were the same, and variants were found between specimens according to size, gender, age, occlusal relationships, presumed dysfunction, and pathology. Therefore, the material presented is a best overall representation of both normal anatomy and its clinical significance.

TEMPORAL BONE

The temporal bone (Fig. 1-1A) consists essentially of three parts: the squamosal, tympanic, and petrous portions.[1] A fourth, the mastoid, is generally found fused to the squamosal and petrous portions and, in some texts, is referred to as the petromastoid portion. The squamosal portion is that aspect most visible and palpable. It has been found in our cadaver dissections that the squama is rather thin and, in some cases, nearly translucent. Superiorly, the squamosal portion forms the temporal parietal suture with the parietal bone. Anteriorly, it has its suture junction with the sphenoid. Together these constitute the squamosal suture.[1,2] Along the inferior border of the squamosal portion is found the zygomatic process. Lying at the posterior end along the inferior border of the zygomatic process is the articular portion of the mandibular or glenoid fossa.[1,3] The most posterior portion of the temporal bone, fused to the squama, is the mastoid process. In fresh cadaver dissection, the junction between the mastoid, parietal, and occipital bones is much different from the beveled squamosal suture, and in many instances, the suture between mastoid and squama was still present, making the mastoid a separate portion.[4]

The main interior body of the temporal bone is the petrous portion (Fig. 1-1B), otherwise known as the pars petrosa parim, or the pyramid.[1] It is an expanded inferior portion of the temporal bone that is wedged between the sphenoid and occipital bones at the base of the skull. The tympanic portion of the temporal bone (Fig. 1-1A) is described as a curved plate of bone lying inferior to the squama and anterior to the mastoid.[1-3] Of note in the temporal bone is the petrotympanic fissure posteriorly in the fossa. Fresh cadaver dissection by Dr. Terry Tanaka has traced connective tissue fascia from the mandibular fossa through the petrotympanic fissure extending into the area of the tympanic membrane.[5] This is an area for further study in the quest to find the connection between ear phenomenon and TMDs as has been suggested.

Clinical Note: The tissue described passing through the petrotympanic fissure to the components of the ear is not palpable either laterally or through the external auditory meatus as the tissues move in a posterior direction through the fissure and enter in the medial one-half of the fissure.

MANDIBULAR FOSSA

The mandibular or glenoid fossa (Fig. 1-2A) has an articular portion that extends anteriorly to the articular tubercle, on the lateral border of the zygomatic process, and eminentia articularis, an articular ridge extending medially from the articular tubercle to the medial fossa wall (for the purpose of this chapter, the articular tubercle and eminentia articularis both are termed *eminentia articularis* unless specific reference is required).[4,6,7] The mandibular fossa continues posteriorly to the squamotympanic and petrotympanic fissures.[1,4] The division between the squamosal and tympanic portions of the mandibular fossa is the squamotympanic fissure. Wedged into the fissure is

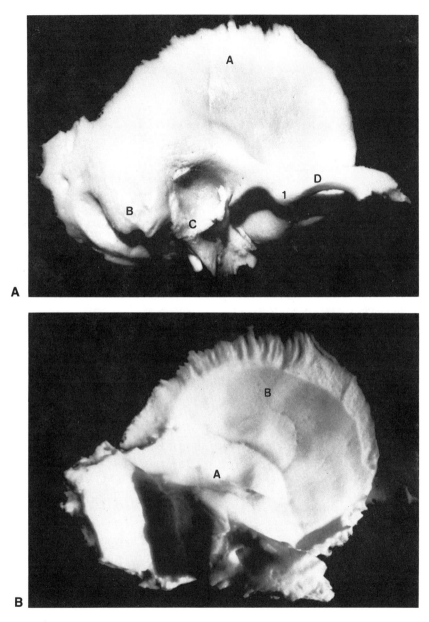

Fig. 1-1. Right temporal bone. (A) Lateral perspective. Squamous portion *(A)*, mastoid process *(B)*, tympanic portion *(C)*, zygomatic process *(D)*, articular tubercle *(1)*. (B) Medial perspective. Petrous portion *(A)*, squamous portion *(B)*.

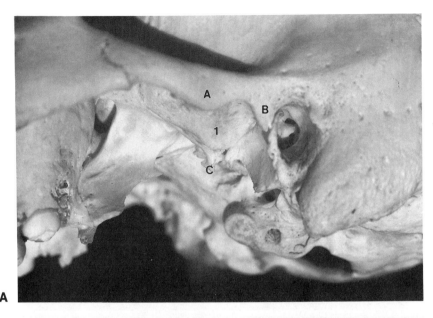

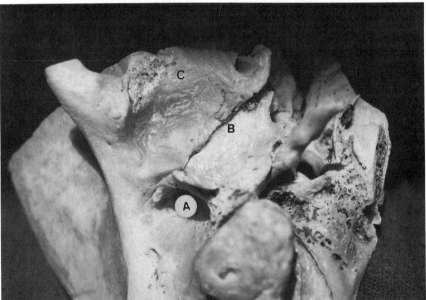

Fig. 1-2. Left mandibular fossa. **(A)** Lateral and slightly inferior view. Articular tubercle *(A)*, eminentia articularis *(1)*, postglenoid tubercle *(B)*, spine of the sphenoid bone *(C)*. **(B)** Inferior view. External auditory meatus *(A)*, juncture of petrotympanic fissure and temporosphenoidal suture *(B)*, eminentia articularis *(C)*.

the edge of the tegmen tympani of the petrous portion, which forms the petrotympanic fissure. For the purpose of this chapter, the more common term *petrotympanic fissure* is used to describe the two fissures. A nonarticular portion extends from the petrotympanic fissure inferiorly about one-fourth of the length of the exposed tympanic portion. A small conical eminence, the postglenoid process, is found at the posterior end at the lateral border. The articular portion of the mandibular fossa is generally considered to be a concave surface extending from the petrotympanic fissure to the apex of the articular tubercle or eminentia articularis. The highest point in the concavity in the squamosal portion making up the anterior, medial, and posterior borders of the fossa is the roof. The roof of the fossa is quite thin and easily pierced when aggressively probed.[4,8] It has been found in fresh specimens that the medial border of the mandibular fossa is also slightly convex as one moves inferiorly along the fossa wall.

When viewed inferiorly (Fig. 1-2B), there is a slight medial rotation of the fossa surface from the coronal plane.[4] This rotation is to match the rotational angle of the mandibular condyle. Dynamically, the shape, depth, and surface smoothness play an important role in the relationship of the fossa to the mandibular condyle and disc as the condyle tracks or moves along its path during the opening and closing cycles.[4]

Clinical Notes: (1) With anteriorly and medially displaced discs, the disc material physically resides in the medial and anterior compartment of the fossa. With this change in disc, fossa, and condyle relationships, you will find a shift in the load that pushes the condyle to the posterior portion of the fossa. In the dissections, osteophytes have been noted along the posterior fossa wall in some specimens in which the disc was anteriorly displaced. (2) An abnormally steep angle of descent between the roof of the fossa and eminentia articularis, creating an extremely deep fossa, has been found. When passively attempting anterior movement of the mandible in these specimens, resistance from the anterior fossa was noted. (3) As mentioned, the roof of the fossa is quite thin. This would suggest caution with passive vertical loading of the mandible if a vertical osteophyte on the condyle is suspected.

MANDIBULAR CONDYLE

When looking at the condyle, it is difficult to examine the structure as it is often portrayed two-dimensionally. One must view the condyle from a three-dimensional perspective. From the superior view (Fig. 1-3A), the condyle is observed, its articular surface being found slightly elliptical to crescent-shaped and measuring about twice as long medial to lateral as it is anterior to posterior. The angle of the condyle when intersected is generally about 20° of medial rotation. Rotation of the condylar head takes the poles out of the coronal relationship, and therefore when viewed laterally, one should assume that the medial pole is actually positioned slightly posterior to the lateral pole.[4,6–8] The

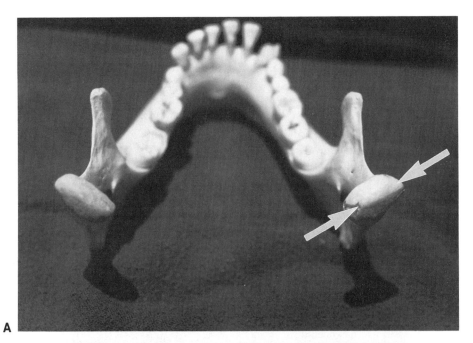

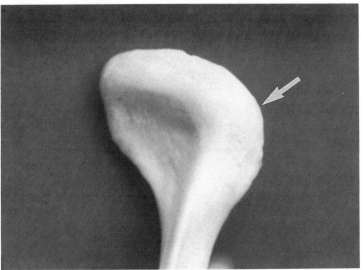

Fig. 1-3. Mandibular condyles. **(A)** Superior and slightly posterior view. The crescent shape of the articular surface is observed. Note the orientation of the individual poles *(arrows)*. **(B)** Anterior view of left mandibular condyle. Erosion of the lateral pole noted *(arrow)*. *(Figure continues.)*

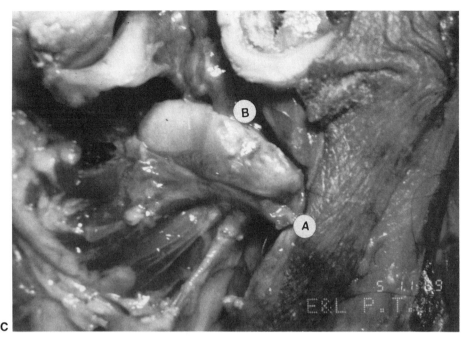

Fig. 1-3. *(Continued).* **(C)** Superior and slight anterior view of a left mandibular condyle. The condyle has been disarticulated laterally and externally rotated. Note pitting of the lateral pole *(A)* and superior lateral surface *(B).*

lateral view also notes that the condyle is convex both anteroposteriorly and mediolaterally.[6]

Clinical Notes: (1) A wide variety of condylar shapes has been found in dry specimens and in our fresh cadaver dissection. Variances are found between two sides and at different chronologic ages. Although bilateral condylar erosion is commonly found, especially in edentulous specimens, lateral pole erosion (Fig. 1-3B) is the most common.[4,6] Other joints have been found to have either vertical or anterior osteophytes. Many anterior osteophytes commonly described as beaking or lipping when viewed from tomography appear on dissection to be a bony extension of the insertion of the superior and inferior tendinous attachment of the lateral pterygoid, possibly caused by excessive pull or load.

Of interest in fresh cadavers has been the appearance of pitted areas of apparent large-scale bone loss on the articular surface of the condyle (Fig. 1-3C), yielding evidence of an ischemic reaction akin to avascular necrosis. However, the presence of avascular necrosis has not been histologically verified in any of our specimens. These pitted areas were found on specimens with and without the appearance of anterior disc displacement. In microscopic dissection performed by Dr. Tanaka, vessels in the posterior surface of the condyle were noted, which would suggest a collateral circulation to the condyle. Whether such a collateral circulation exists normally or as a result of adaptation is not clear and is an area for further investigation.

CORONOID PROCESS

The coronoid process (Fig. 1-4) is a thin, triangular-shaped formation anterior to the condylar head on the mandibular ramus. The apex of the coronoid is generally equal to that of the apex of the articular condyle.

Clinical Note: Increases in the height of the coronoid are often noted, possibly caused by hypertrophy of the temporalis as the temporalis, particularly the anterior portion, was up to 1 cm thick in some of the specimens in which the coronoid process was elevated. Edentulous specimens often have a higher coronoid process. However, degeneration of the condyle and reduced condylar height commonly noted in the specimens may contribute to that appearance.

STYLOID PROCESS

The styloid process (Fig. 1-5A) is an extension of the petrous portion of the temporal bone[1] emerging through a sheath formed by the tympanic portion. It projects inferiorly, anteriorly, and slightly medially and is found posterior to the angle of the mandible.

Clinical Note: Elongation of the styloid process can occur through me-

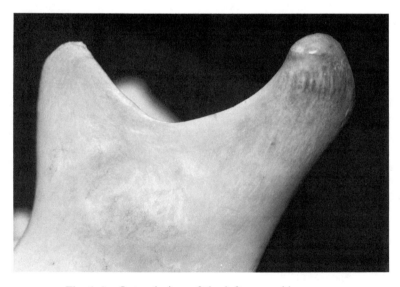

Fig. 1-4. Lateral view of the left coronoid process.

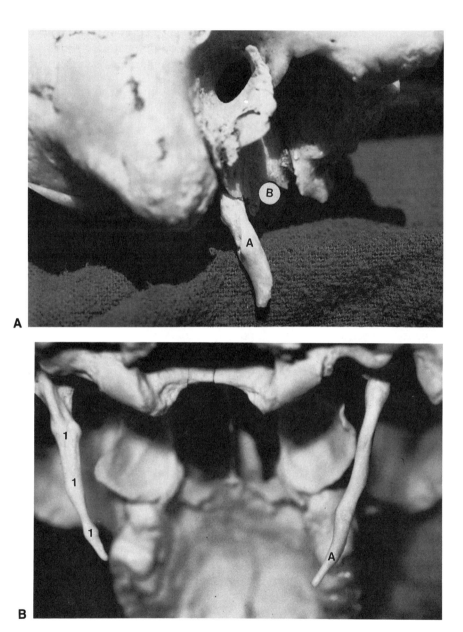

Fig. 1-5. **(A)** Lateral view of right styloid process. The process *(A)* emerges through a sheath of the tympanic portion *(B)*. **(B)** Elongation of the styloid process *(A)*. Note the many growth centers *(1)*.

chanical effects placed on the styloid via the stylomandibular ligament and the styloglossus, stylohyoid, and stylopharyngeus muscles. As these structures generally pass inferiorly and medially to their distal attachments, extensive elongation may move the styloid medially. Elongation of the styloid anteriorly and medially (Fig. 1-5B) can limit cervical function in the area of sidebending and rotation where the styloid actually approximates the paracervical structures (Eagle's syndrome).

SPHENOID BONE

The sphenoid bone (Fig. 1-6) consists essentially of a body located centrally with two greater wings and two lesser wings, both projected laterally. The pterygoid plates are found extending inferiorly.[1] The lateral surface of the greater wing, along with the squamosal portion of the temporal bone, forms the floor for the temporalis muscle. The lateral sphenoidal spine approximates the most inferomedial portion of the mandibular fossa.[1–4] The attachment of the sphenomandibular ligament is found in the area of the lateral spine. Passing ventrally along the lateral sphenoidal spine is the chorda tympani as it exits in close approximation to the auriculotemporal nerve. The lateral sphenoidal spine also serves as part of the attachment of the tensor paliti.[4] The greater wing constitutes the posterolateral wall of the orbit while the inferior and lateral surface forms the pterygoid plate and the hamulus.

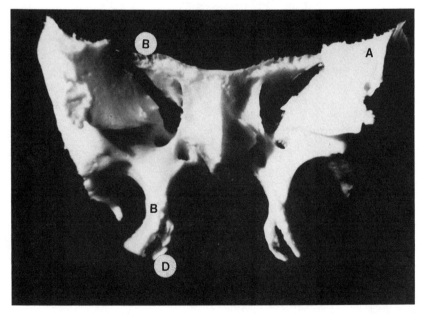

Fig. 1-6. Sphenoid bone viewed anteriorly. Greater wing *(A)*, lesser wing *(B)*, pterygoid plate *(C)*, hamulus *(D)*.

Clinical Note: The chorda tympani is mostly afferent in nature and registers taste for the anterior part of the tongue. The auriculotemporal nerve is mostly afferent and is part of the posterior trunk of the mandibular nerve. It supplies the skin of the tragus of the ear, the skin of the external acoustic meatus, and at times the tympanic membrane, the TMJ, and the skin of the temporal region. Its innervation into the TMJ is discussed in more detail in the section on innervation. The tensor paliti (tensor veli palatini) is also discussed in a later section.

ARTICULAR SURFACE

The articular surface constitutes the mandibular fossa and the condyle itself. The articular surface of the mandibular fossa consists of bundles of fibrocartilage of mostly collagen fibers that are oriented both parallel and obliquely and extend from the petrotympanic fissure and most superior-anterior part of the apex of the postglenoid tubercle to the apex (crest) of the eminentia articularis and articular tubercle.[4,6-8] The anterior aspect of the eminentia articularis has also been found to have fibrocartilage covering it.

The condylar head has fibrocartilage covering the superior two-thirds and is bounded anteriorly by the fovea. In both the mandibular fossa and condyle, the fibrocartilage is found to be thickest in the functional areas where weight-bearing or loading occurs. In the mandibular fossa, this thickening is found on the posterior slope of the eminentia articularis, and on the condylar head, it is found to be thickest on the anterior slope. In both areas just mentioned, the articular cartilage is also thicker medially than laterally. On the fossa roof where there is little or no weightbearing, it is found to be the thinnest. Normally, the fibrocartilage is avascular without nerve or lymphatic systems.

Clinical Note: Although the anterior and medial surfaces of the condyle contain thicker articular cartilage, indicating that the greatest amount of wear and tear takes place there, the lateral pole is the area most commonly noted as being eroded. Because the lateral pole itself does not appear to articulate generally with the fossa, the erosion could be related more to activity of the articular disc and lateral collateral ligament during function rather than to actual wear and tear of the articular surfaces against each other.

ARTICULAR DISC

The articular disc of the TMJ (Fig. 1-7A) is found to be a biconcave fibrocartilage structure.[1,4,6-9] Vascularization and innervation is found in the anterior and posterior attachments of the disc, with a greater degree found posteriorly.[4,68] The disc itself is nonvascular and noninnervated in the middle region.

The disc is comprised of two bands and an intermediate zone. The posterior band is the larger of the two bands and, combined with the anterior band,

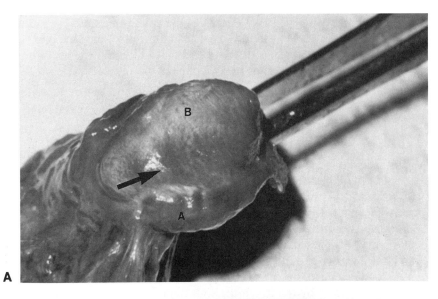

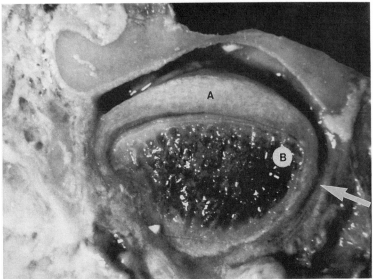

Fig. 1-7.   **(A)** Left TM disc. The anterior band *(A)* is separated from the larger posterior band *(B)* by the intermediate zone *(arrow).* **(B)** Anteroposterior view of a right TMJ, coronal section at midcondylar depth. Note that the disc *(A)* rests slightly more toward the medial pole *(B)* as medial collateral ligament *(arrow)* attaches to it. *(Figure continues.)*

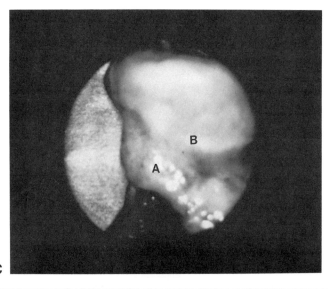

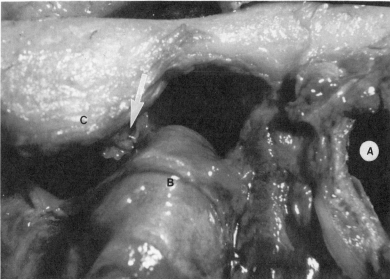

Fig. 1-7. *(Continued.)* (**C**) Magnified view of a left TM disc positioned anteriorly on the condyle. The epimysium *(A)* is identified attached to the anterior band *(B)*. (**D**) Lateral view of a left TMJ. Orientation is made with the external auditory meatus *(A)*, the mandibular condyle and disc *(B)*, and the eminentia articularis *(C)*. A vascularized adhesion *(arrow)* extends from the posterior band to the posterior eminence wall.

creates the biconcave appearance. Functionally, the disc encompasses a condyle much as a loose-fitting cap would, fitting over the head. In fresh cadaver dissection viewed anteriorly (Fig. 1-7B), the disc is generally noted to rest slightly medially and is thicker in the medial portion. The fibrocartilage is very adaptable to the varied shapes of the condyle and to its relation to the condyle and fossa during function. Attachment of the disc to the condylar head is by collateral ligaments attaching to the medial and lateral poles of the condyle. The disc is held anteriorly by the anterior attachment apparatus referred to as the epimysium (Fig. 1-7C). This epimysium commingles with fibers of the joint capsule where both attach to the condyle.[4,8]

Clinical Notes: (1) With compression, water is evacuated out of the fibrocartilage into the synovial fluid. In some instances, this may assist in its lubrication.[10] However, over long periods such as seen with parafunction, this may result in adaptive disc deformity, which creates joint sounds. The changes will appear on tomography as disc space narrowing. (2) With long-term compression of the disc in an anterior and medial position in the fossa, such as seen in disc displacement, the disc can become adhered to the fossa (Fig. 1-7D).[10] Articular adhesions have become significant as many surgeries are performed to release adhesions between disc and fossa.[4,11,12]

RETRODISCAL TISSUE (POSTERIOR ATTACHMENTS)

The retrodiscal tissue (Fig. 1-8A) is made up of connective tissue extending posteriorly from the posterior band of the articular disc and forming two lamina of dense connective tissue (bilaminar zone). There is a loose alveolar central layer, which is more highly vascularized and well innervated.[6,8] The superior lamina passes posteriorly and vertically to attach on the superior fossa medial to the postglenoid spine.[4,8] The inferior lamina moves posteriorly and interiorly to attach to the posterior condyle inferior to the articular surface. Observations from dissections note the inferior lamina attachment to extend along as much as one-third of the length of the neck of the condyle. When viewed with magnetic resonance images (MRIs) taken in succession with the mouth in 4-mm increments of opening (dynamic MRI), this tissue can be seen to fill with blood on opening and empty with closure, acting as an arteriovenous (AV) pump to supply nutrients to the retrodiscal tissues.

Part of the synovial membrane is found in the superior surface of the retrodiscal tissue. This pumping mechanism during opening and closure acts to produce the synovial fluid important for lubrication and nutrition of the articular surface. With an articular disc displacement, there may be an increase in the tension on the joint capsule and synovial membrane via the retrodiscal tissue. If this should occur, changes in lubricity as well as synovial fluid pressures may impair function and could possibly lead to degenerative joint changes.

Clinical Note: In fresh cadaver specimens, the posterior attachment apparatus does not achieve full elongation, even when the mandible is passively

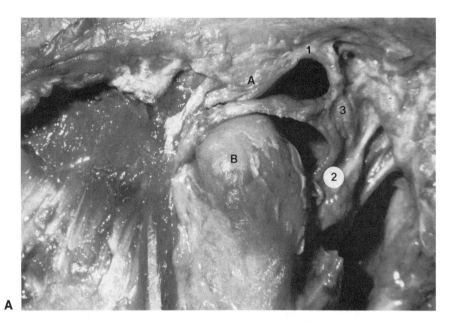

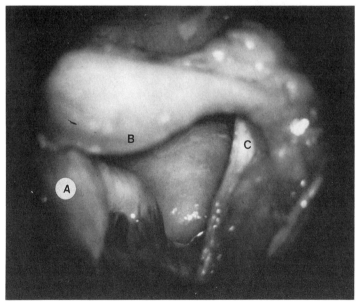

Fig. 1-8. (A) Lateral view of a left TMJ, noting the posterior attachment apparatus. Orientation is made with the eminentia articularis *(A)* and condyle *(B)*. Upper lamina *(1)* and lower lamina *(2)* of the posterior attachments of the disc. Note the alveolar central layer *(3)*. (B) Magnified lateral view of a left TMJ. The condyle and disc *(A)* have moved beyond the crest of the eminentia articularis *(B)* to a fully open position. The upper lamina *(C)* of the bilaminar zone is identified with its attachment at the 1-o'clock position.

brought to greater than full opening (Fig. 1-8B).[4,6,8,13] Although there is some ability of the posterior connective tissue to recoil or shorten because of the elastic properties, it would appear doubtful that it would move a disc posteriorly when stretched when observations show no such stretching occurs. Also, in specimens with anteriorly displaced discs, the retrodiscal tissue did not appear stretched.[12] Therefore, use of mobilization that moves the condyle away from the disc to allow the posterior attachments to "recapture" the disc would not appear to be effective.

JOINT CAPSULE

The fibrous joint capsule (Fig. 1-9) has its posterosuperior attachment to the fossa at the area of the squamotympanic fissure medially and the petro-tympanic fissure laterally. The inferior attachment is to the neck of the condyle at the attachment of the inferior lamina of the retrodiscal tissue.[4,8] Anteriorly, the capsule is supported by its bony attachment along the anterior aspect of the eminentia articularis and the anterior attachment apparatus of the disc. Medially and laterally, the capsule is attached superiorly to the superior border of the mandibular fossa and inferiorly to the neck of the mandible. Laterally, it is thickened for the attachment of the TM ligament and lateral collateral ligaments. In fresh cadaver dissection using microscopic dissection, the TM

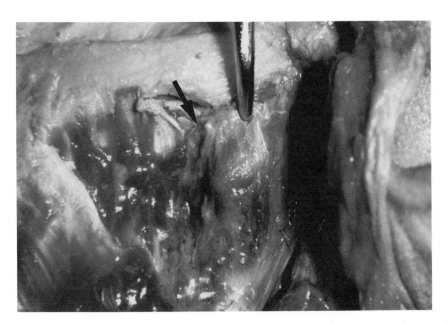

Fig. 1-9. Lateral view of a left TMJ. The probe is resting at the upper attachment of the joint capsule. Anteriorly are the deep fibers of the masseter *(arrow)* attaching into the capsule.

ligament joint capsule and lateral collateral ligament can be distinguished into distinct elements. In fresh cadaver dissection performed in a medial to lateral approach, the medial joint capsule extends along the base of the fossa along its medial portion to the area of the spine of the sphenoid.[4]

The capsule is loose superiorly and taut inferiorly. The anterior capsule with attachment arrangement allows for considerable anterior movement of the contents.[4,8] In passive motion of the joint in fresh material, inward invagination of the anterior capsule is observed with posterior movement of the condyle.

FASCIA

The greatest distribution of fascia found in our dissection is temporal fascia (Fig. 1-10). Various texts have described the temporal fascia extending from the temporal area along but not ending at the zygoma, continuing to the angle of the mandible, and following the border and lower margin of the mandible.[1,2,14] In various dissections, we have found this description to be consistent, where one fascial sheet starts in the temporal area, moving beyond the zygoma to the mandible. Its varied thickness is found depending on the basic morphology of the specimen. Furthermore, we have found temporal fascia binding deep within the temporal suture and having an attachment in this area.

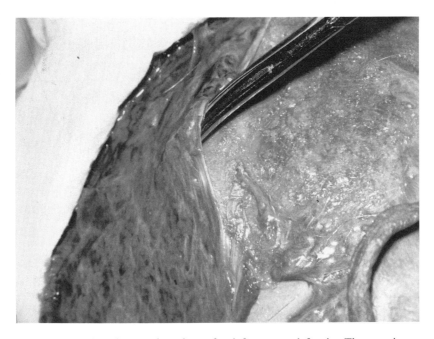

Fig. 1-10. Lateral and posterior view of a left temporal fascia. The specimen was hydrated before dissection to allow the multilayered fascial bands (over probe) to be more visible moving in different directions at each layer.

LIGAMENTS

TM Ligament

The TM ligament (Fig. 1-11) arises from two heads. The anterior portion attaches at the zygomatic portion of the temporal bone anterior to and encompassing the articular tubercle. The fibers move obliquely posteriorly and inferiorly to attach on the lateral and posterior surface of the neck of the mandible. The posterior portion attaches to the zygomatic portion of the temporal bone posterior to the articular tubercle and moves posteriorly and very slightly inferiorly to attach on the mandible with the middle and posterior portion on the capsule.[4]

Clinical Note: This arrangement allows for the TM ligament to assist in mandibular dynamics by resisting inferior movement of the mandible during initial opening and assisting in the transition to and from rotational glide to translatoric glide during the various stages of opening and closure.[4]

Collateral Ligaments

The collateral ligaments are called such because they attach the disc to the two poles of the mandibular condyle.[14,15] In the stricter sense, these ligaments are not truly collateral in they are not transected by the same coronal

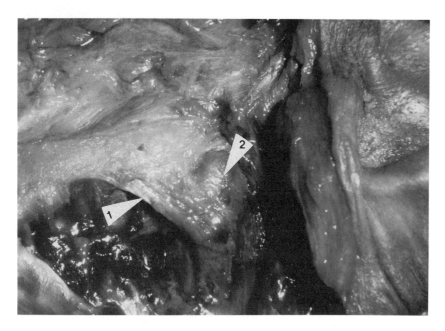

Fig. 1-11.   Lateral view of a left TM ligament. Anterior fibers *(arrow 1)* and posterior fibers *(arrow 2)* in the closed-mouth position.

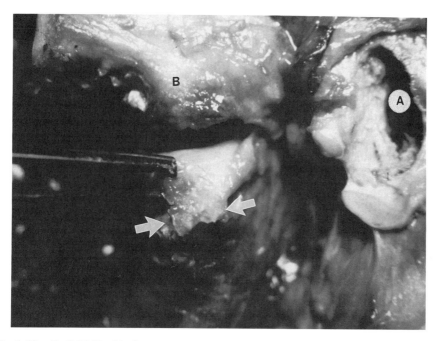

Fig. 1-12. Left TMJ with the external auditory meatus *(A)* and the eminentia articularis *(B)*. The disc is held by the forceps. The broad lateral collateral ligament is noted (between the *arrows*).

plane because of the rotation of the condyles in the coronal plane mentioned previously. The lateral collateral ligament (Fig. 1-12) on fresh material is broad superiorly where it attaches to the disc and narrows as it passes inferiorly to its attachment on the inferior aspect of the lateral pole. It is generally thin, and its thickness varies, possibly because of its function in mastication. On several specimens, the lateral collateral ligament is so thin as to be difficult to discern from joint capsule material. Its lax and broad nature appear to allow the lateral collateral ligament to act in a capacity of control and guidance of motion during mandibular function.[4]

The medial collateral ligament (Fig. 1-13) is much thicker and less broad than the lateral collateral ligament. It attaches to the medial margin of the disc in a convergence with anterior and posterior bands and then passes inferiorly to attach to the inferior surface of the medial pole of the condyle. It resides in a more posterior coronal plane than the lateral collateral ligament. This band is tenacious with greater tightness and less freedom of movement than noted with the lateral collateral ligament and appears more for bracing and limitation of movement.[4,5,8] In fresh cadaver dissections from the anterior and anteromedial perspective, fibers of the lateral pterygoid have been found commingling with joint capsule and possibly medial collateral ligament as the pterygoid wraps around the medial condylar neck.[4]

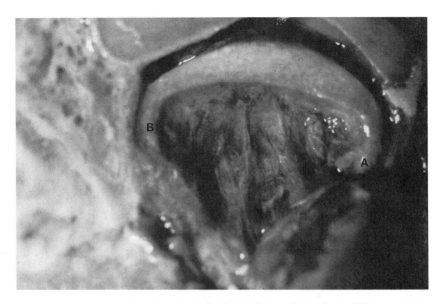

Fig. 1-13. Anteroposterior view of a left TMJ. The medial collateral ligament *(A)* and lateral collateral ligament *(B)* are identified in this midjoint cut.

Clinical Note: In specimens with lateral pole erosion, the lateral collateral ligament was found to be thinner and more lax. The lateral collateral ligament attaches to the inferior aspect of the lateral pole regardless of the condition of the lateral pole itself. Passive joint movement in specimens with thin and lax-appearing lateral collateral ligaments notes an inward depression or pleat appearing in the superior aspect of the ligament and capsule with motion from opening to closure.

Tanaka Ligament

The Tanaka ligament (Fig. 1-14) was first described by Dr. Terry Tanaka in the 1980s as a medial fasciculus from the medial collateral ligament extending medially and slightly anteriorly to attach to the medial fossa wall just posterior to the area of the myofascial attachment of the superior fibers of the lateral pterygoid muscle to the epimysium of the disc, which will be described later, and an area described as the oblique protuberance.[4,8] Further microanatomy dissection indicates that it is more likely to be a separate and distinct ligament.[5] The position of the Tanaka ligament would appear to act to give an increased medial bracing or tether to the articular disc as is moves anteriorly and posteriorly. Therefore, movement of the disc during mandibular opening would occur in an arcuate fashion, with more movement taking place in the lateral aspect of the joint than in the medial.

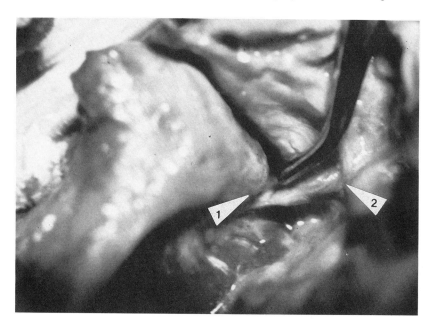

Fig. 1-14. Posterior view of a left mandibular condyle. The probe identifies the Tanaka ligament extending from the medial pole *(arrow 1)* to the medial fossa wall *(arrow 2).*

Clinical Note: The action of the collateral ligaments and the Tanaka ligament just described, along with the rotation of the condyle in the coronal plane mentioned previously, would appear to direct anterior motion of the articular disc in an anterior and medial direction. It would also appear that the lateral collateral ligament would act to control the degree of medial motion of the articular disc with opening and to initiate posterior lateral movement of the articular disc with closure. If the lateral collateral ligament were too lax, it would not initiate such movement with closure. This could contribute to an explanation as to disc displacement from an anatomic basis.

Sphenomandibular Ligament

The sphenomandibular ligament (Fig. 1-15) is a thin flat band residing just medial to the TMJ capsule. It is attached to apex and lateral surface of the sphenoid spine. It descends, moving slightly anteriorly between the pterygoids, to attach near the lingua of the mandibular foramen.[1-3]

Clinical Note: The position of the sphenomandibular ligament would serve to resist vertical descent and anterior translation of the mandible. The sphenomandibular ligament could therefore assist normal function by stopping vertical movement during initial opening as the mandible descends from the pull

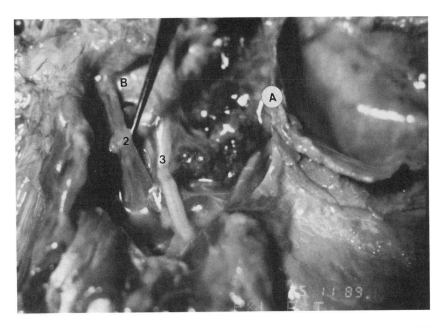

Fig. 1-15. Medial view of a left TMJ. Orientation is made with the posterior orbit of the eye *(A)* and the medial mandibular condyle *(B)*. Sphenomandibular ligament (*2*, over probe) and auriculotemporal nerve *(3)* moving across the sphenomandibular ligament.

of the suprahyoids. Because the ligament passes inferiorly and anteriorly, it would also restrict anterior movement of the mandible. However, because the sphenomandibular ligament attaches below the mandibular condyle, it would not restrict condylar translation if the center of rotation of the mandible shifted from the area of the neck of the condyle to the area of the attachment of the sphenomandibular ligament near the mandibular foramen. Rotation about this attachment would yield translatoric glide of the condyle.[4]

Stylomandibular Ligament

The stylomandibular ligament (Fig. 1-16) is more a fascial band, with superior attachment to the apex of the styloid process. It extends inferiorly and anteriorly to the posteromedial border of the mandible between the attachment of the masseter and medial pterygoid at the angle of the mandible.[1-3]

Clinical Note: (1) The position of the stylomandibular ligament would serve to restrict vertical and anterior movements of the mandible. However, in passive motion testing of several fresh specimens, the stylomandibular ligament did not become at all taut regardless of the opening distance; in fact, the ligament actually becomes more lax. The inferior attachment of the stylomandibular ligament is below that of the sphenomandibular ligament. If the center of rotation of the mandible changes during opening, as mentioned in the clinical note for the sphenomandibular ligament, the angle of the mandibular ramus will then move posteriorly, thus increasing laxity of the stylomandibular ligament.[4] (2) We have observed stylomandibular ligament tautness when the mandible is brought directly forward (protrusion). It would appear that if the mandible moves anteriorly before the rotational phase about the condylar neck is completed, a stretch would take place on both the sphenomandibular and stylomandibular ligaments. Also, parafunction, in particular bruxing, would also tend to stretch the stylomandibular ligament. This in turn could have some bearing on elongation of the styloid process and is an interesting subject of further investigation.

Discomalleolar Ligament

A discomalleolar ligament has been noted in the literature as an extension of the posterosuperior border of the posterior band of the articular disc passing through the petrotympanic fissure connecting to the anterior process of the malice.[1] It has been suggested that the superior lamina of retrodiscal tissue is also a remnant of this ligament. Our dissections have shown that, for the most part, the superior border of the posterior band attaches above the petrotympanic and squamotympanic fissures rather than at the fissures. Microanatomy dissections by Dr. Tanaka have shown an extension of connective tissue

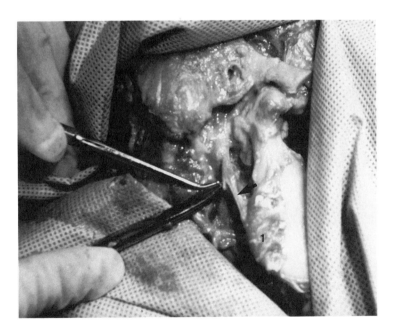

Fig. 1-16.   Stylomandibular ligament *(arrow)* viewed laterally. Orientation is made with the styloid process (probe) and the angle of the ramus of the mandible *(1)*.

through the petrotympanic fissure extending to the tympanic membrane.[5] Our observations through dissection have not yet revealed any functional implications because, as we stated before, we have not observed the posterior attachment reaching full elongation during even the most extreme of passive opening of the specimens. Also, we have not found any clear conclusions in the literature as to any significance of this attachment or the relationship between ear phenomenon and TMD. But the presence of this structure does give rise to questions as to whether there is such a relationship found here, and this is a subject for continued investigation.

INNERVATION

The principal innervation of the TMJ is the auriculotemporal nerve. The auriculotemporal nerve is a branch of the posterior trunk of the mandibular nerve, a division of the trigeminal nerve. It arises from the posterior trunk just after it exits from the foramen ovale.[1,2] It then passes posteriorly along with the superior fibers of the lateral pterygoid to the lateral border of the sphenomandibular ligament (Fig. 1-15) just between the ligament and the condylar neck. It moves upward, parallel to the sphenomandibular ligament, for a centimeter or so and crosses posteriorly around the lateral aspect of the joint and ascends to the temporal area following the superficial temporal vessels. It has been found in our dissections to give off two or three branches inferiorly that proceed upward to divide into the many small branches that center around the joint capsule posteriorly, medially, and laterally.

The masseteric nerve, from the anterior trunk of the mandibular nerve, also sends a filament to the TMJ capsule medially and anteriorly. The posterior deep temporal nerve, from the anterior trunk of the mandibular nerve, also supplies filaments to the anterior aspect of the joint.[1,15]

MUSCULATURE

Many texts describe the insertion and origin of musculature including the function of the muscles of mastication. With review, these texts reveal a slight but noticeable difference. Contributing to these differences in muscle may be the facial types and growth that affect the size, shape, and pull angle of the muscle. The force that a muscle can generate is dependent on the mass of the contractile tissue in relation to its angle of pull and distance from its fulcrum or lever arm. In dealing with muscle palpation, most texts use either artist conceptions or external palpation experience from which to base descriptions of muscle locations. It has been our experience that many muscles once thought palpable were indeed not able to be accurately identified even when the skin had been removed. We have also noted that in working with fresh material, without the induction of preservatives, the individual muscles are myofascially attached to one another and cannot merely be pulled aside to palpate that which is underneath, as is described in some texts.

Temporalis

The temporalis (Fig. 1-17A) is a large fan-shaped muscle that has its origin from the entire temporal fossa extending superiorly and posteriorly to the temporal line of the parietal bone and inferiorly to the posterior root of the temporal bone and anteriorly to the lateral border of the frontal bone and lateral surface of the greater wing of the sphenoid.[1-3] Its insertion is along the coronoid process extending to the anterior border of the ramus to just posterior to the third molar. The muscle is covered by a multilayered fascia.[1,4] The deep temporalis also has fibers attaching into the superior and anterior articular capsule[4,8] (Fig. 1-17B). We have consistently found that many superficial fibers of the temporalis indirectly attached to the deep fibers of the masseter muscle.[1,2,14] We have also found that the deep temporalis is distinguished separately from the superficial in its origins. The shape and thickness of the muscle depend on development and facial type. Normally, temporalis is thin posteriorly, between 1 and 2 mm, and thick anteriorly, as much as 10 mm.[6,8,16] The tendon of the temporalis is quite thick and broad, 2 to 3 cm, and is palpable above the zygoma extending superiorly approximately 3 to 4 cm. The anterior and inferior insertion of the temporalis can be palpated intraorally along the ramus of the mandible. All the fibers of the temporalis contribute to the function of mandibular elevation for closure and particularly for positioning of the condyle at the end of closure and in compression after closure. Biting in an edge-to-edge position or tearing food will use the anterior and middle bellies. Parafunction, particularly clenching, activates the entire muscle, particularly the anterior fibers.

Clinical Note: The fibers extending to the anterior capsule of the TMJ may act to give an anterior and upward pull to the joint capsule during closure to provide a tethering of the anterior capsule during closure.

Masseter

The masseter (Fig. 1-18A) is a quadrilateral muscle consisting of three superimposed layers blending into superficial and deep bellies.[17,18] The superior attachment in the superficial portion is in the approximate anterior two-thirds of the lower border of the zygomatic arch. Its fibers pass downward and backward to the inferior angle attachment of the lateral aspect of the ramus of the mandible. The middle layer rises from the steep surface of the interior $\frac{2}{3}$ of the zygomatic arch attachment passing inferiorly into the middle ramus of the mandible. The deep masseter (Fig. 1-18B) is more difficult to locate, as it is covered by the superficial masseter and parotid glands. The deep masseter attachments come from the temporal portion of the zygomatic arch as its origin with its insertion to the superior half of the lateral body of the ramus of the mandible. Fibers of the deep masseter have been consistently traced to the anterior joint capsule (Fig. 1-18C) in our fresh cadaver dissection. The masseter has a very broad tendon on both deep and superficial bellies that can extend nearly the entire length of the muscle.

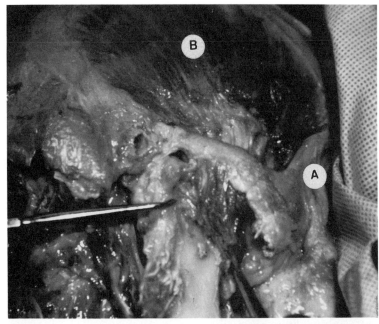

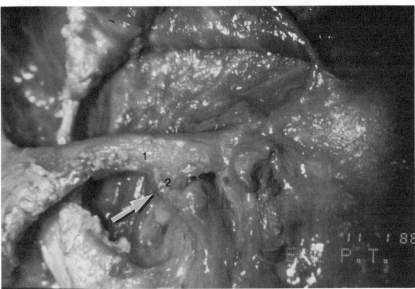

Fig. 1-17. (**A**) Lateral view of a right temporalis muscle. Orientation is made with the orbit of the eye *(A)* and the belly of temporalis *(B)*. (**B**) Lateral view of a left temporalis muscle. The fibers of the deep temporalis *(arrow)* emerge from under the zygomatic arch *(1)* to insert into the joint capsule *(2)*.

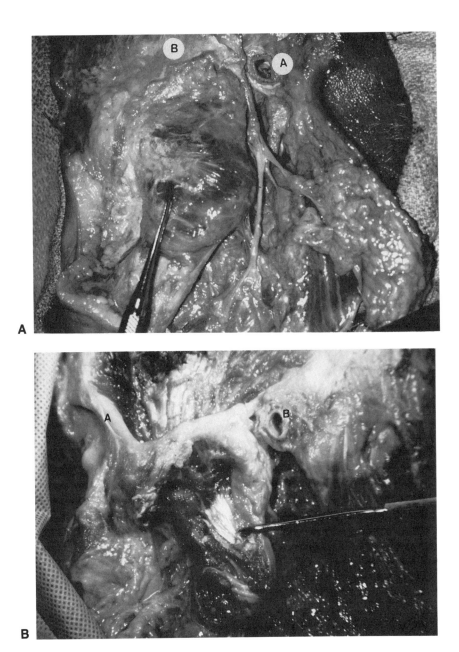

Fig. 1-18. (A) Lateral view of a left masseter muscle. Orientation is made with the external auditory meatus *(A)* and zygoma *(B)*. The quadrilateral shape of the muscle is noted. (B) Orientation is made with the orbit of the eye *(A)* and the external auditory meatus *(B)*. The tendon of the deep masseter is indicated (probe). *(Figure continues.)*

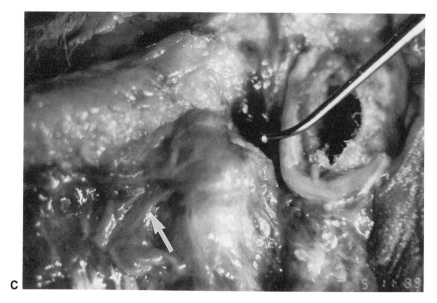

C

Fig. 1-18. *(Continued.)* **(C)** Lateral view of the TMJ. The fibers of the deep masseter attaching to the joint capsule are indicated *(arrow)*.

Clinical Note: The fibers of the deep masseter extending to the anterior capsule of the TMJ may act to tether the capsule anteriorly during closure of the mandible.

Medial Pterygoid

The medial pterygoid (Fig. 1-19) lies on the medial aspect of the mandible in and about the angle. It is a quadrilateral muscle passing upward and diagonally attaching to the pterygoid plate and part of the palatine bone.[17] The anterior belly of the medial pterygoid is found to have a large, strong tendinous lamina. Functionally, it helps to protract and elevate the mandible. Because its upward and anterior pull opposes the upward and posterior pull of masseter and temporalis, it will also assist in decelerating the condyle as it moves posteriorly during closure and in facilitating rotation movements of the mandible at the end of closure.

Clinical Notes: (1) Parafunction in a laterotrusive, side-to-side movement will result in hypertrophy. (2) With the broad tendon extending along much of the anterior belly of the medial pterygoid, one should be particularly suspect of a tendinitis as well as myositis when palpating the area.

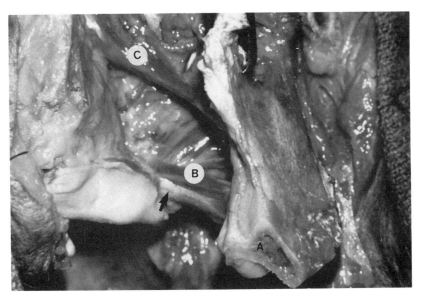

Fig. 1-19.   Anterior view of a left medial pterygoid muscle. The anterior mandible has been removed (cut site *A*), and the remaining segment is laterally rotated. The lower fibers of the medial pterygoid near its attachment to the pterygoid plate *(B)* separating it from the upper fibers *(C)*. Note the tendinous extension of the anterior belly *(arrow)* from the mandible to the pterygoid plate.

Lateral Pterygoid

Lateral pterygoid muscle (Fig. 1-20A) is composed of superior fibers and inferior fibers. The superior fibers (Fig. 1-20B) have their origination in the infratemporal fossa found on the greater wing of the sphenoid (posterior lateral orbit of the eye).[1,2] The inferior fibers have their origination from the lateral surface of the lateral pterygoid plate. Both the superior and inferior fibers of the lateral pterygoid insert into the medial one-half of the condylar neck extending medially to include some of the posterior portion of the condylar neck.[1,8] The upper one-third of the superior fibers appear to have a myofascial attachment to the epimysium and capsule (Fig. 1-20C) of the TMJ.[19] From a medial to lateral approach in fresh cadaver dissection, the sling appearance of the superior fibers of the lateral pterygoid is well demonstrated[15,17] (Fig. 1-20B). Neither the superior nor inferior fibers of the lateral pterygoid can be palpated extra- or intraorally.

The function of the inferior fibers of the lateral pterygoid is for protrusion with or without opening. The slinglike attachment of the superior fibers of the lateral pterygoid acts as a stabilizing force to brace the anterior and medial joint capsule and the articular disc while the condyle moves into full opening.

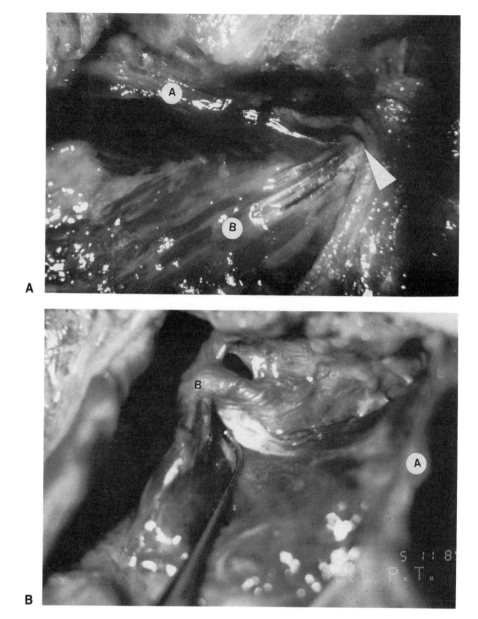

Fig. 1-20. **(A)** Lateral view of a left lateral pterygoid muscle. The upper fibers *(A)*, inferior fibers *(B)*, condylar insertion *(arrow)*. **(B)** Medial view of a left TMJ. Orientation is made with the lateral orbit *(A)* and medial pole of the condyle with disc *(B)*. The probe indicates the tendon of the superior fibers of the lateral pterygoid. *(Figure continues.)*

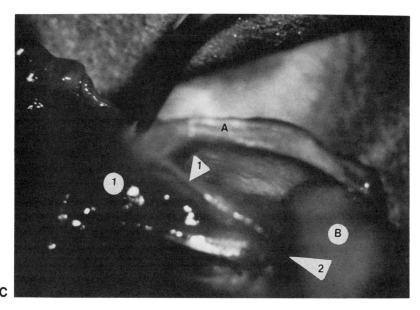

Fig. 1-20. *(Continued.)* **(C)** Magnified lateral view of a left TM disc *(A)* and condyle *(B)*. The probe grasps the anterior band, and the superior fibers of the lateral pterygoid *(1)* pass along the epimysium *(arrow 1)* with a myofascial-type attachment. They then proceed to their tendinous attachment in the condylar neck *(arrow 2)*.

The superior fibers of the lateral pterygoid are active on closure, and the myofascial attachment allows it to tether the joint capsule in a superior direction, lifting the disc out from its position in the anteroinferior and anteromedial recess of the joint. This tether would prevent invagination of the joint capsule, which occurs with the rapid posterior movement of the condyle during closure.[4] Invagination has been observed on our fresh specimens during passive range of motion (ROM) and there is no action of the muscles as well in dissection videotapes by Dr. Tanaka.[8] The superior fibers of the lateral pterygoid also act directly to decelerate the posterior and superior movement of the condyle during closure.

Clinical Note: From dissection observations, it appears that movement of the disc does not occur with muscle function. Movement of the disc occurs via the shape of the disc, condyle ad fossa relationship, attachment by the collateral ligaments, and the synovial fluid acting on the disc as it moves posteriorly and anteriorly during opening and closure. It is our conclusion that the superior fibers of the lateral pterygoid act to decelerate and prevent invagination of the joint capsule with closure of the mandible and therefore play no active part in anterior disc displacement. This assimilates the same action as the articularis genu in the knee, which prevents an entrapment of joint capsule as the patella moves vertically during extension.

Tensor Tympani

The tensor tympani is contained in the tympanic cavity superior to the auditory tube. It originates from the greater wing of the sphenoid at the posterolateral margin and the adjoining auditory tube and inserts to the handle of the malleus.[1,2] The tensor tympani acts to pull the malleus (and tympanic membrane) medially and inferiorly.

Tensor Veli Palantini

The tensor veli palatini (tensor paliti) originates from the scaphoid process of the medial pterygoid plate, the lateral margin of the auditory tube, and the apex of the sphenoid spine. It inserts into the palatine aponeurosis and the palatine bone.[1,14] The tensor veli palatini acts singly to pull the soft palate to the same side and dually to flatten the palatine arch.

Hyoids

Suprahyoids

The digastric (Fig. 1-21) is a straplike muscle composed of an anterior and posterior belly with a tendinous portion found between. The posterior belly originates from the mastoid process, and the anterior belly has its origination

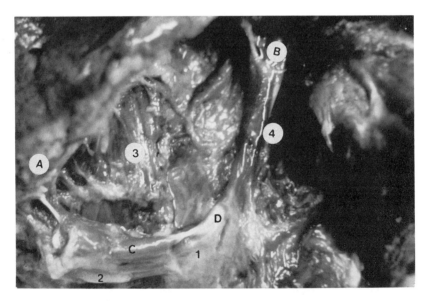

Fig. 1-21. The left digastric muscle is visible running under the mandible *(A)* with the posterior belly *(B)* and the anterior belly *(C)* connected by the tendon *(D)* and sheath *(1)* and hyoid bone *(2)*. Mylohyoid *(3)* and stylohyoid *(4)* are demonstrated.

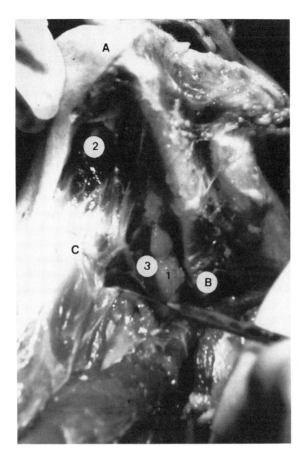

Fig. 1-22. Submandibular area. Orientation is made with the anterior chin *(A)*, the angle of the ramus of the mandible *(B)*, and the hyoid bone *(C)*. Submandibular gland *(1)*, geniohyoid *(2)*, and anterior digastric *(3)*.

along the body of the mandible. The tendon sling is bound to the horn of the hyoid by a connective tissue sheath.[1,2]

The mylohyoid (Fig. 1-21), a bipennate muscle, is superior and deep to the anterior belly of the digastric and is palpable on the muscle floor of the lateral oral cavity or inferiorly from under the chin. Its attachments are along the mylohyoid line of the mandible and body of the hyoid bone near its lower border.[1,14] The two sides converge in a fibrous line that attaches to the symphysis menti of the hyoid bone. Sometimes the mylohyoid is fused with the anterior belly of the digastric.

The geniohyoid muscle (Fig. 1-22) lies deep to the mylohyoid, has its origins from the inferior mental spine of the inner surface of the symphysis menti, and is found external to the medial portion of the mylohyoid.[1] It inserts into the body of the hyoid bone.

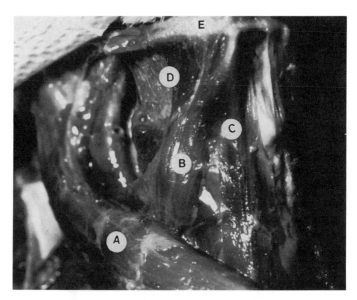

Fig. 1-23. Right lateral subhyoid area. The sternocleidomastoid *(A)* has been moved laterally to expose the omohyoid *(B)*, the sternohyoid *(C)*, and the thyrohyoid *(D)* as they attach to the inferior hyoid bone *(E)*.

The stylohyoid muscle (Fig. 1-21) arises from the posterior surface of the styloid process along with the stylomandibular ligament, passes downward and forward, and inserts into the body of the hyoid bone just above the omohyoid.[1,2,14] It forms part of the tendinous sling of the digastric muscle.

Infrahyoids

The infrahyoids include the sternohyoid, the thyrohyoid, and the omohyoid muscles. The omohyoid (Fig. 1-23), like the digastric, is a strap muscle that consists of two bellies joined by an intermediate tendon. The inferior head originates along the superior-posterior ridge of the clavicle. The superior belly is attached to the lower body of the hyoid.[1,14] The inferior head passes superiorly and medially, and the superior head passes inferiorly and very slightly laterally, descending in front of the carotid sheath. The two bellies meet just anterior to the scalenus anterior and are held by a fibrous sling attached to the clavicle and first rib.

Clinical Note: In nearly all the fresh anatomic dissections in which the full neck was present, the omohyoid and the sternocleidomastoid (SCM) were found to shield accurate palpation of the scalenus anterior even when the SCM was moved anteriorly and medially.

The sternohyoid (Fig. 1-23) is a strap muscle that attaches from the posterior and medial surface of the clavicle and the manubrium of the sternum passing superiorly and medially to the lower body of the hyoid medial to the omohyoid.[1,14]

The thyrohyoid (Fig. 1-23) is a quadrilateral muscle attaching from the superior border of the thyroid passing superiorly and laterally to the lower body of the hyoid inferior to the horn.

When acting in concert, the infrahyoids contract to stabilize the hyoid bone for the suprahyoids to open the mouth.

Suboccipitals

The suboccipital muscles consist of six muscles, four situated posteriorly and two anteriorly. Posteriorly are the rectus capitis posterior major and minor, the oblique capitis inferior, and oblique capitis superior. Anteriorly are the rectus capitis anterior and rectus capitis lateralis.

Rectus Capitis Posterior Major

Rectus capitis posterior major is a triangular-shaped muscle (Fig. 1-24), broader superiorly, attaching inferiorly to the apex of the spinous process of axis and superiorly to the occiput along the lateral one-half of the inferior nuchal line.[1]

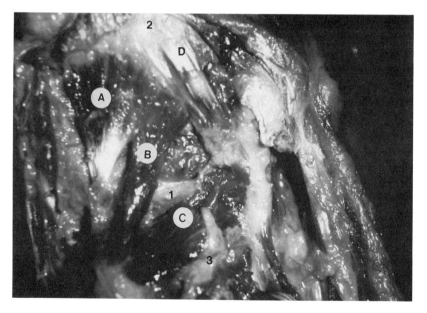

Fig. 1-24. Right suboccipital area. Orientation is made with the posterior arch of C1 *(1)* and external occipital protuberance *(2)*. The rectus capitis posterior minor *(A)*, rectus capitis posterior major *(B)*, inferior oblique *(C)*, and superior oblique *(D)* are identified. Note the emergence of the greater occipital nerve from under the inferior oblique and proceeding superiorly *(3)*.

Rectus Capitis Posterior Minor

The rectus capitis posterior minor is a triangular-shaped muscle (Fig. 1-24), broader superiorly, attaching inferiorly to the lateral tubercle of the posterior arch of atlas and superiorly to the occiput along the medial one-half of the inferior nuchal line.[1,14]

Oblique Capitis Inferior

The oblique capitis inferior is a straplike muscle (Fig. 1-24) with its inferior attachment to the lateral spinous process and lateral border of the axis and superior attachment of the posterior aspect of the lateral one-half of the transverse process of atlas.[1,2,14]

Oblique Capitis Superior

The oblique capitis superior is a straplike muscle (Fig. 1-24) with its inferior attachment to the posterosuperior aspect of the lateral one-third of the transverse process of atlas in conjunction with the superior attachment of the inferior oblique.[1,14] Its superior attachment is the most lateral portion of the inferior nuchal line of the occiput superior to the rectus major and deep to the semispinalis capitis.

Rectus Capitis Anterior

The rectus capitis anterior is a quadrilateral-shaped muscle (Fig. 1-25), broader superiorly, attaching inferiorly to the anterior lateral mass of the atlas and superiorly to the base of the occiput just anterior and lateral to the foramen magnum and occipital condyle.[1,14]

Rectus Capitis Lateralis

The lateralis and anterior are sometimes depicted as existing together (Fig. 1-25). In fresh dissection, however, they can be distinctly identified. The lateralis has its inferior attachment to the anterior border of the transverse process of atlas and its superior attachment along the jugular process of the occiput just posterior to the jugular foramen.

Clinical Note: The suboccipital muscles are generally noted to support the head on the neck and little else. These six muscles, however, play a major role in cervical function and dysfunction. The suboccipital muscle group act both collectively and individually to initiate, stabilize, and control the actions and reactions of atlas and axis when movement of the occiput takes place. These

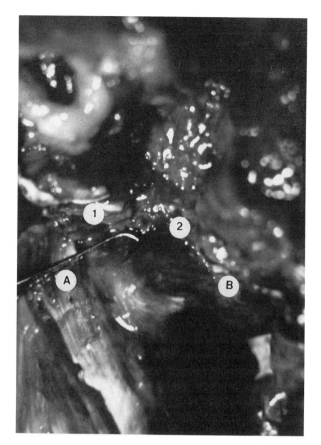

Fig. 1-25. Left upper anterior cervical region. Orientation is made with the superior attachment of longus coli *(A)* and anterior transverse process of C1 *(B)*. The rectus capitis anterior *(1)* to the left of the probe, rectus capitis lateralis *(2)* to the right of the probe.

muscles are those that control the gliding motions of atlas on axis and coordinate the change of rotation between atlas and axis in extremes of range.

The inferior oblique and the trapezius and semispinalis capitis are sites where the greater occipital nerve either wraps around, as is the case with the inferior oblique (Fig. 1-25), or pierces through. These areas may be areas where the greater occipital nerve could be entrapped.

Paracervicals

Although there are a multitude of paracervical muscles in four layers both anteriorly and posteriorly, this chapter focuses on two of those paracervicals. The upper trapezius and SCM are of particular clinical interest in the cervical relationships in treatment of the TMJ.

Trapezius

The upper fibers of the trapezius (Fig. 1-26) are generally noted to attach to an area from the occipital protuberance and the lateral borders of the nuchal ligament.[1,2,14] Most fresh specimens that we have dissected, the fibers of the upper trapezius attached at the nuchal ligament only to the C4 level. It is also noted that the superior fibers of the upper trapezius are generally quite thin and often removed with the fascia. The inferior attachment of the upper trapezius is the superior one-fourth of the spine of the scapula, the entire medial rim of the acromion, and lateral one-half of the clavicle.

Sternocleidomastoid

The SCM (Fig. 1-27) attaches inferiorly by two heads. The sternal head attaches to the rim of the manubrium to the crest of the sternoclavicular fossa. The clavicular head attaches to the medial one-third of the superior border of the clavicle.[1,14] The two heads meet at the level of C6 to form a broad, thick, strap-type muscle. The superior attachment is by short but strong tendon into the entire lateral surface of the mastoid and to the lateral extreme of the nuchal line superficial to the attachment of the splenius capitis.

Clinical Note: The inferior attachments of SCM, along with those of the

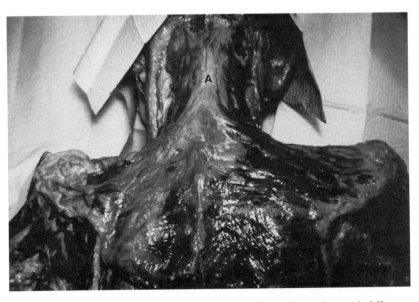

Fig. 1-26. Trapezius muscle. Note the upper attachment into the nuchal ligament at the midcervical area *(A)*.

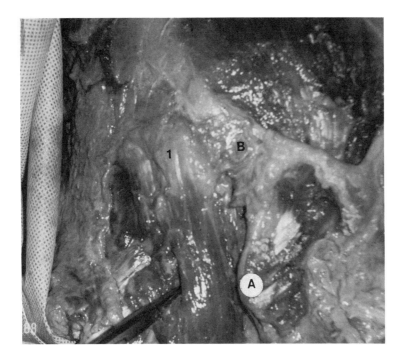

Fig. 1-27. Right SCM. Orientation by the angle of the mandible *(A)* and external auditory meatus *(B)*. Note the broad nature of the muscle (probe) and the large tendon attachment to mastoid *(1)*.

omohyoid, obscure the scalenus anterior from accurate palpation. The superior portion of SCM also obscures any palpation of the posterior belly of digastric.

CONCLUSION

In conclusion, the study of clinical anatomy presented in this chapter is designed to provide the clinician with another tool to assist in the evaluation and treatment of dysfunction. It is of vital importance that the clinician understand fully that which is to be treated for the treatment to be effectively made.

ACKNOWLEDGMENTS

We appreciate the forbearance of our wives, children, and staff in our anatomic research. It is though their understanding and encouragement that we have been able to continue. We would especially like to thank Dr. Terry Tanaka for his patience with our many questions and for the questions that he has created for us.

REFERENCES

1. Gray H: Anatomy of the Human Body. 35th Ed. WB Saunders, Philadelphia, 1973
2. Anderson JE: Grant's Atlas of Anatomy. 8th Ed. Williams & Wilkins, Baltimore, 1983
3. Rohen JW, Yokochi C: Color Atlas of Anatomy. Igaku-Shoin, New York, 1983
4. Langton DP, Eggleton TM: Functional Anatomy of the Temporomandibular Joint Complex. IFORC Publications, 1992
5. Tanaka TT: TMJ microanatomy: an anatomical approach to current controversies. Instructional Video, Clinical Research Foundation, Chula Vista, CA, 1992
6. Tanaka TT: Dissection of the head, neck, and temporomandibular joint. Instructional Video, Clinical Research Foundation, Chula Vista, CA, 1986
7. Dolwick FM: TMJ Internal Derangements of the Temporomandibular Joint. Radiology and Research Foundation, 1983
8. Tanaka TT: Advanced dissection of the temporomandibular joint. Instructional Video, Clinical Research Foundation, Chula Vista, CA, 1988
9. Bourbon BM: Anatomy and biomechanics of the TMJ. p. 15. In Kraus SL (ed): TMJ Disorders: Management of the Craniomandibular Complex. Churchill Livingstone, New York, 1988
10. Moffett B: Anatomy and physiology of the temporomandibular joint and mechanics of growth and remodeling of the temporomandibular joint. In: Lecture Syllabus: The Anteriorly Displaced Disc: How It Becomes Displaced and How It Is Treated. Clinical Research Foundation, Chula Vista, CA, September, 1988
11. Moses J: Arthroscopy of the temporomandibular joint. Instructional Video, Stryker Corporation
12. Merrill R: Oral and Maxillofacial Surgery Clinics of North America. Vol. 1.1. WB Saunders, Philadelphia, 1989
13. Kircos LT, Ortendahl DA, Mark AS, Arakawa M: Magnetic resonance imaging of the TMJ disc in asymptomatic volunteers. J Oral Maxillofac Surg 45:852, 1987
14. Romanes GJ: Cunningham's Manual of Practical Anatomy. Vol. 3. Oxford University Press, New York, 1968
15. Kaplan AS, Assael LA: Temporomandibular Disorders: Diagnosis and Treatment. WB Saunders, Philadelphia, 1992
16. Adams R: Diseases of Muscle. Harper & Row, Philadelphia, 1975
17. Christiansen EL, Roberts D, Kopp S, Thompson JR: Patient assisted evaluation of variation in length and angulation of the lateral pterygoid and variations in angulation of the medial pterygoid: mandibular mechanics implication. J Prosthet Dent 60:616, 1988
18. Grieve GP: Modern Manual Therapy for the Vertebral Column. Churchill Livingstone, New York, 1986
19. Neff P: TMJ, Occlusion and Function. Georgetown University School of Dentistry, Washington, DC, 1975

SUGGESTED READING

Myers LJ: Newly described muscle attachments to the anterior band of the articular disc of the temporomandibular joint. J Am Dent Assoc 117:437, 1988

2 | Biomechanics of the TMJ

Jules R. Hesse
Machiel Naeije

When studying the function of the masticatory system, detailed information is needed about the related anatomic structures, as described in the previous chapter. This highly specialized locomotive system has the important daily tasks of breaking of food (i.e., chewing), swallowing, and speaking. The great versatility and variety of combined functions of this system, when compared with other locomotive systems of the body, are unique. For instance, the high velocity and fine coordination of the mandible during speech accentuate the great mobility and low stiffness of both TMJs.

Understanding joint function means understanding the anatomic design of the different joint structures, the neuromuscular control, the movements taking place in all planes, and the forces (i.e., muscle, gravity, and inertia) acting on that particular articulation. The function and pathofunction of synovial joints have received much attention in the orthopaedic and rheumatology literature. Observation and analysis of joint motion are the specific focus of interest of bioengineers, where in vivo and in vitro experiments are used to reconstruct and simulate various loading conditions in daily life.

Although the TMJ features most of the synovial joint principles, it is necessary to recognize its specific mechanics and neuromotor function. It is therefore also necessary to adapt and modify the methods of investigation that have been used to other orthopaedic fields to study the specific functions of the masticatory system. Yet little has been reported on these matters in the dental, medical, or physiotherapy literature.

This chapter reviews some important biomechanical aspects of synovial joint function in general, as well as its application and clinical relevance to the masticatory system. The different forces acting on the masticatory system in varied situations, such as during symmetric and asymmetric biting, and the importance of a balanced dental support are discussed as well.

BASIC STRUCTURE AND FUNCTION
OF SYNOVIAL JOINTS

Human joints are most often classified according to the type of motion that occurs. Here only the movable joints or diarthroses are discussed. Diarthroses include most of the joints of the body and are characterized by the presence of a joint cavity filled with synovial fluid, an articular cartilage covering the bone, and an intracapsular lining—the synovial membrane (Fig. 2-1).

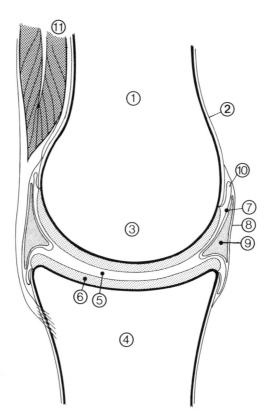

Fig. 2-1. Schematic presentation of a synovial joint: *(1)* bone shaft; *(2)* periosteum; *(3)* condyle (convex); *(4)* condyle (concave); *(5)* joint cavity; *(6)* cartilage; *(7)* synovial membrane; *(8)* fibrous membrane/capsule; *(9)* intra-articular fat pad; *(10)* synovial bursa; *(11)* muscle with tendon entering the joint capsule and bone. (From Hesse and Hansson,[17] with permission.)

Synovial joints in general are characterized by wide ranges of almost frictionless movements. The synovial membrane is mainly smooth in appearance but displays villi and folds in the joint recesses. The cartilage and the intra-articular disc are not covered by the synovial membrane. The outer fibrous layer (i.e., joint capsule), particularly those enforced by ligaments and tendons, can act as an important mechanical constraint. The length and thickness of the restraining capsule and associated ligaments are generally considered the main contributing factors to the passive stability of the joint. Despite these constraints, sufficient functional angular and translatory joint movements can take place. The anatomic design of the joint (structures) and the arrangement of muscles, ligaments, and tendons determine the direction and extent of a roll-glide movement.

The configuration of the articular fossa, condylar head, and an intra-articular disc (if present) are considered to play a joint stabilizing role as well. In human cadaver studies, Hsieh and Walker[1] found that knee joint stability under no loading conditions depends mostly on capsular and ligamentous support, whereas under compressive loads, the conformity of the articulating surfaces appears to be of greater importance in maintaining a stable joint position. Generally, joints that have highly incongruent joint partners are provided with discs for stabilization and force distribution purposes.

An extreme of a joint range that combines an optimum congruency of joint surfaces and a tautened capsule and ligaments is called a "close-packed" joint position.[2] In this position, the joint has optimum stability, which can be preserved by little or no muscle action. The knee joint, fully extended, is a good example of a close-packed position. Away from this position, the joint partners may become less congruent, and the capsule, ligaments, and tendons relax. The joint partners become "loose-packed," thereby displaying an increasing joint mobility. A maximum loose-packed position is considered the optimum starting point for passive examination of a joint by means of manual joint-play techniques.[2]

CARTILAGE, DISC, AND SYNOVIAL FLUID

Cartilage

Cartilage, although fibrous in structure, possesses a nonporous, very springy, smooth surface. In the surface layers, collagen bundles are oriented predominantly parallel to the surface; in the deeper zone, they are more or less perpendicular to the articular surface and to the subchondral bone; in the intermediate zone, they are at intermediate angles. Macroscopic inspection reveals a white and smooth, shiny surface, which may turn somewhat yellow with age.[3] However, electron microscopic scanning has demonstrated irregular depressions of the surface.[4] The elasticity and distensibility of cartilage is derived from the large quantities of water bound by proteoglycan molecules.

Cartilage may be considered as a thin elastic overlay on a rigid substrate and has a limited capacity to withstand stresses. The loading of biologic tissues and their response presuppose the understanding of two important biomechanical features (i.e., stress and strain). Stress is the load per unit area that develops on a plane surface within a structure in response to externally applied loads; in the metric system, it is often expressed as N/cm^2 or N/m^2. The contact area of opposing joint partners increases due to deformation, as opposed to the contact area of rigid surfaces[5] (Fig. 2-2).

This temporary deformation is advantageous, because it enables the system to withstand higher forces per square centimeter (N/cm^2). High-velocity loading causes stiffer behavior of the cartilage when compared with the lesser stiffness found at slow loading rates. Articular cartilage is therefore considered an excellent shock absorber. This is an important viscoelastic property of articular cartilage. Particularly, fibrocartilage is supposed to withstand higher forces across the joint surfaces because it contains a higher proportion of fibers than hyaline cartilage.[6]

The deformation that occurs at a point in a structure under loading is called strain. Relative lengthening (or shortening) of a structure under loading may be expressed in a so-called load–deformation curve (similar to stress–strain curve) and is often used in experimental settings for the testing of biomaterials. The primary part of the curve exhibits a very elastic portion of the curve; the so-called toe portion (Fig. 2-3). Loads in the elastic deformation region of the curve do not cause permanent deformation. Applied loads beyond this region cause permanent deformation (i.e., plastic deformation) and the breakdown of the ultrastructure of cartilage. The stiffness of the material is then represented by the slope of the linear portion of the curve, where a constant deformation occurs with increased or decreased loading.

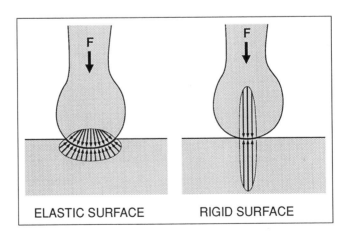

Fig. 2-2.   Schematic presentation of two equal applied loads *(F)* and the distribution of reaction forces *(arrows)* on an elastic and a rigid surface.

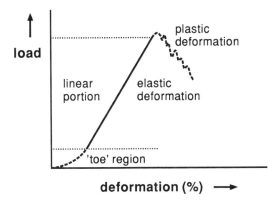

Fig. 2-3.   Schematic presentation of a load/deformation curve.

Clinical Relevance of Fibrocartilage

During mastication and forceful biting, the condyle–disc complex is "balancing" on the slippery posterior slope of the articular eminence. Synergistic actions of the masticatory muscles are now predominantly responsible for the stabilization of the TMJ. Shear forces as reactions to the displacement under loading will cause elastic deformation of the cartilaginous structures. It may be assumed that the higher proportion of dense collagen fibers in the TMJ fibrocartilage is better capable of withstanding the forces and shear (i.e., a loading mode in which a load is applied parallel to the surface of the structure, causing internal angular deformation) reactions occurring during mastication, as opposed to those forces and reactions occurring during perpendicular loading of a fully extended knee joint.[7]

Deformation and breakdown of the ultrastructure of the TMJ fibrocartilage can occur as a result of inflammatory or degenerative diseases. Although degenerative changes are generally found more frequently in the elderly, severe degenerative TMJ changes were observed in young autopsy material.[8] However, in clinical practice, serious radiographic changes are also observed in young TMJ patients. Repetitive loading of the TMJ, such as during parafunctional activities such as grinding is often suggested to be responsible for degenerative TMJ disorders. Although several studies in the field of bioengineering indicate that the degeneration or wear of joints is bound up with the mechanical properties of cartilage,[5] hereto no clinical and experimental evidence exists concerning these matters regarding the breakdown of the fibrocartilage of the TMJ.

Disc

Some of the synovial joints have complete or incomplete fibrocartilaginous, discoid partitions known as menisci or disci. These structures are not constant in some areas (e.g., in the acromioclavicular joint), whereas they are highly developed and well defined in the knee, TMJ, and sternoclavicular joints.[3] The TMJ disc is a wedge-shaped structure that fills the discongruous joint partners (i.e., the condyle, temporal fossa/articular eminence) perfectly and can easily deform under loading and during movement. The collagen fibers of the superficial layers of the anterior and posterior bands as well as the middle band run in an anteroposterior (AP) direction. In the central region of the anterior and posterior bands, the fibers are oriented in a random fashion. This orientation of fibers allows the disc to withstand a variety of forces (tensile and compressive) in different directions.[4]

The intra-articular disc of the TMJ has been given the following functions (modified from reference 9):

1. Partitioning the complex condylar movement into functional components (i.e., two separate synovial joint cavities)
2. Lubricating mechanism (distribution of synovial fluid)
3. Stabilizing the condyle by filling the space between the incongruous articulating surfaces
4. Cushioning the loading of the joint at point of contact (shock absorption)
5. Reducing physical wear (i.e., the removal of material from solid surfaces by mechanical action) and strain (i.e., deformation of a body divided by its original length) on joint surfaces
6. Helping to regulate movements (i.e., passive guidance) of the condyle across the temporal fossa and articular eminence
7. Preserving the shape of the condyle[10,11]

Three decades ago, Hjortsjö[12] described a joint with large rotations and translations across the joint surfaces as an "accentuated grinding joint." He suggested that the disc is a necessary structure to separate the two shear reactions (i.e., between the condyle and the temporal bone) into different compartments to minimize wear. Wear can be divided into two components: interfacial wear caused by the interaction of the bearing surfaces, and fatigue wear caused by the deformation of the contacting bodies.[13] With interfacial wear, the removal of material (e.g., cartilaginous tissue) by either adhesion or abrasion is the result of the interaction of the bearing surfaces. Failure may also occur because of the repetitive stresses across the bearing surfaces. Although the magnitude of the applied stresses may be much less than the material's ultimate strength, failure will eventually occur if stresses are applied often enough; this phenomenon is described as fatigue failure.[13]

The distortion of the disc during heavy loading helps to diminish the indentation of the articular surfaces of the condyle and temporal bone. This allows the condyle–disc complex sufficient movement over the temporal bone without distorting and damaging the surfaces.[14] As opposed to the stabilizing function of the disc, Osborn[14] described the disc as "destabilizing" (i.e., improving the mobility of) the TMJ.

Clinical Relevance of the Intra-Articular Disc

The TMJ disc has been an important focus of interest in TMJ research since the early publications of Costen.[15] This intra-articular disc is held responsible for the most frequently occurring joint sounds (i.e., clicking/popping) in a TMJ population as well as in a nonpatient population. Epidemiologic studies have found clicking to be present on average in 60 percent of the healthy population.[16] A nonpainful clicking TMJ that causes no lasting mechanical impediments in jaw function is generally not treated, other than with home care instructions. If this clicking is disturbing to the patient, reversible and simple treatment is recommended.

The question arises whether we would be better off to function without the disc because it so often interferes with daily TMJ functions. Surgical removal of the disc (i.e., discectomy) in patients with chronic displacement of the disc without reduction or severe internal derangement of the TMJ may greatly improve the mobility and function of the joint at first. However, little long-term information is available concerning the condition of the human TMJ without the articular disc in time. Several authors reporting on animal (e.g., rabbit and rat) experiments in the past,[10] and more recently,[11] have postulated that the articular disc preserves the shape of the condyle. Extremely unusual shapes were found to change with time in rats with removed disc, when compared with control rats. These findings correspond with the earlier postulations of Hjortsjö[12] describing the TMJ as "an accentuated grinding joint." Further studies are needed to clarify the presence of the TMJ disc under physiologic and pathologic conditions.

In a TMJ patient population with an acute disc displacement without reduction, this condition will generally cause considerable limitation of jaw movement as well as joint pain. However, pain is not always present in more chronic stages of this disorder. It is in most chronic cases that joint pains gradually subside but that the limitation of jaw movements remains to some extent. Even though the clinician is often aware of the impossibility of reducing the disc by means of manipulation, manual TMJ mobilization techniques are recommended to improve the mobility of the joint. Restoring symmetry of the TMJ movements is an important goal in the treatment of TMDs.[17] Attempting to restore "previous" TMJ anatomy in a patient may be considered a questionable treatment procedure. Treatments to "recapture" discs or to "prophylactically" interfere with possible progressions should be critically evaluated.[18]

Synovial Fluid

The basic concepts of lubrication, familiar to engineers, have been applied in human joints and, to some extent, have been found lacking in that they could not explain the low friction and the general performance of the human joint when viewed as a bearing. The function of bearings and lubricants has been the focus of interest of engineers for many years. Improvement of the quality of bearings and lubricants has been shown to be advantageous to their general performance and life-span. Living tissues have the intrinsic properties of renewal, restoration, and durability, which give them much greater lubricating capacity than a machine or any artificial tissue.[19]

One of the most important features of synovial joints is the presence of a joint nourishing and lubricating fluid called synovia, or synovial fluid. The word *synovia* was first employed by Paracelsus in 1541, who used this term to describe a fluid that nourishes all tissues. Synovial fluid can be considered as a watery solution with a "viscosity index improver."[5] The long-chain hyaluronic acid is held responsible for the low viscosity (i.e., the resistance of a fluid to flowing) of synovial fluid.[20] However, today other important features of synovia are recognized, particularly its lubricating function and physical behavior. During the past decades, many attempts have been made to understand the lubricating principle underlying the behavior of normal and diseased joints. Gaining insight into pathologic processes of various joint diseases still remains an important goal of particularly bioengineers and rheumatologists.

Healthy joints contain only a small amount of synovial fluid, as only a thin film of fluid covers the surfaces of cartilage and synovium within the joint space. Different mechanical aspects of this fluid can be recognized. The synovial fluid becomes highly cohesive (i.e., "clinging together") during loading but also during unloading. Synovial fluid is found to be adhesive (i.e., "sticking to") relative to cartilage, thereby saturating the cartilage. The synovial fluid is partially squeezed out of the porous layer during loading, known as wheeping lubrication, prohibiting contact between the opposing surfaces. To be any use to a joint, low friction must not only occur while the cartilage is fully saturated with synovial fluid, but also when it is fully squeezed empty. During little or no loading, glycoproteins are supposedly blinding to the cartilage surface to prevent the surfaces from making contact. This process is known as boundary lubrication.[21] This hydrodynamic or fluid film lubrication is able to achieve extremely low values of friction in healthy joints.[22]

Inflammation of the synovial fluid and the inner lining of the capsule (i.e., synovitis/capsulitis) may be a result of tissue injury. A larger volume of synovial fluid is found in injured or diseased joints, making it easier for aspiration and analysis. Considerable reduction in the viscosity of diseased joints has been demonstrated.[23–25] Osteoarthritic and rheumatoid joints cause decreased viscosity of the synovial fluid.[19]

In experimental studies, the viscosity of synovial fluid in slow-moving joints is relatively high as opposed to the low viscosity found during high-velocity movements (i.e., thixotropic behavior). The long and large mucopolysaccharide chains may move parallel along each other during high-velocity movements, whereas these chains may become somewhat "tangled up" during slow movements. Changes in the rate and the amount of loading and temperature of the fluid have been shown to have considerable mechanical effects. The physical and chemical properties of synovial fluid must therefore play an important role in the (patho)mechanics of the joint.

Clinical Relevance of Synovial Fluid

The function of the synovial fluid in the TMJ is basically not different from the function in other synovial joints. An important feature of the TMJ is the presence of two separate joint cavities: the upper and the lower synovial cavities. The articular disc and its attachments are the structures that provide the separation into two independent synovial cavities. Both cavities have their separate flows of synovial fluid. As the condyle–disc complex travels anteriorly during mouth opening, the synovial fluid flows in the opposite direction (i.e., posteriorly, medially, and laterally of the condyle) to form the posterior recess and vice versa. Nourishing and "washing" the articulating surfaces and the synovial lining of the joint are important functions of synovial fluid.

The TMJ can function under extreme loading conditions. For instance, it may function at great speeds and low forces (e.g., speech) or at low speeds and high forces (e.g., clenching/grinding). Particularly, the high and repetitive loads during one-sided bruxing (i.e., tooth grinding) may be considered harmful to the synovia–cartilage function. However, the physical properties of synovia–cartilage complex (i.e., the viscosity) have been found to decrease in cases of osteoarthritis and rheumatoid arthritis (RA).[19]

Jaw immobilization after surgery or a chronic disc displacement without reduction may (temporarily) impede these important functions of the TMJ. Restoring particularly the translatory movements by means of jaw mobilization techniques and exercises is an important goal in the rehabilitation of these patients. However, joint mobilization techniques are generally contraindicated as long as an inflammatory joint condition exists, for it could stimulate the exudation process. Proper (anti-inflammatory) medication should be administered as long as the signs and symptoms of inflammation are dominantly present. Parallel to this therapy, this condition may be treated by a stabilizing occlusal appliance to alter and somewhat diminish the loading of the joint. Yet, in addition to these therapeutic measures, rest seems to be beneficial.

ASPECTS OF JOINT FRICTION AND STIFFNESS

Joint Friction

Particularly for bioengineers and clinicians, the low friction found in synovial joints during function is one of their most outstanding features. Friction can be described as the counteraction to the motion of one object sliding along the surface of another object.[26] Full friction occurs as the object is set in motion and somewhat decreases as the motion continues (i.e., friction of motion). Friction is proportional to the normal force N, which is the force component perpendicular to the surface against which the surface slides (Fig. 2-4).

$F = u \cdot N$, where F is the friction force, u is the coefficient of friction, and N is the normal force. In an animal ankle joint, the coefficient was found to be 0.005.

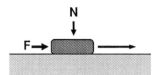

Fig. 2-4. Schematic presentation of a body subjected to friction as this body is being pushed across another surface.

The degeneration or wear of joints is undoubtedly linked to the mechanical properties of cartilage–synovial fluid mechanism. The joint might fail because of mechanical damage to the cartilage. Fibrillation (i.e., vertical lesions) through the full depth of the cartilage layer or a destructive thinning (i.e., erosion) of the cartilage layer may be the result of adverse loading. However, inflammatory processes affecting the synovial membrane may be involved as well, causing a loss of quality of the synovial fluid. It has been hypothesized that in a diseased joint the lubricant may lose its quality even before the surfaces are impaired by the wear that occurs in badly lubricated joints. Analysis of the synovial fluid of the TMJ and other joints can be performed and may give important diagnostic information and perhaps a greater insight into the pathogenesis of TMJ disease.[19]

Joint Stiffness

Similar to joint friction is the coefficient of stiffness for a given joint, which may be used as an index for its mobility. Joint mobility in terms of joint stiffness has been described by Wright[5] as the passive resistance to movement, exhibited by a total joint subjected to a passive displacement. An index for joint stiffness, in terms of the coefficient of resistance to movement, has been described by Barnett[27] as the sideways force needed to move one articular surface on the other divided by the force compressing the two surfaces together (Fig. 2-5).

The active and passive influence of muscles on the stiffness and mobility of joints is another factor to consider.[20] Reflex activity of a muscle will occur when a joint is rapidly moved toward its extreme border position.[27] This mechanism protects the joint from becoming overstretched or displaced. Even fully relaxed muscles will exhibit some passive resistance to movement (i.e., the passive elastic tension) exerted by muscles and tendons. Stiffness of the knee joint was found to be increased in healthy subjects, as the circumference of the thigh muscle increased.[28] Joint size and tendon and ligament thickness demonstrated the same correlation in knee and finger joints of healthy subjects.[29] The total passive resistance depends on the mechanical characteristics of all structures that cross a joint, as well as on the friction between the articular surfaces.

The load-dependent deformation of cartilage and the cohesive, adhesive, and thixotropic behavior of synovial fluid promote excellent coherent function with a minimum of shear rate and wear. It allows sliding surfaces to move at extremely low friction, even during high loading forces.

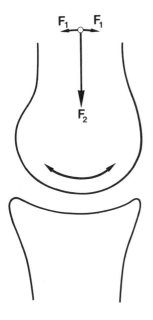

Fig. 2-5. An index for joint mobility as the coefficient of resistance to movement *(Cr)* from Barnett.[27] F_1 = sideways force and F_2 = compressing force. $Cr = F_2/F_2$. When F_2 is 1 kilogramforce (kgf), then only 0.007 kgf on average is needed to move the joint; Cr is then 0.007. (From Hesse and Hansson,[17] with permission.)

Clinical Relevance of Joint Friction and Joint Stiffness

It may be assumed that a healthy TMJ is a joint with a low degree of friction and stiffness. Joint friction and joint stiffness are manifestations of joint functions that are often difficult to detect clinically. Joint friction may become clinically detectable at advanced stages of osteoarthrosis and internal derangements.

Joint stiffness may be found in patients after jaw immobilization, postinflammatory joint conditions, and TMJ surgery. TMJ patients may express a sensation of TMJ stiffness at the onset of movements or intensifying during jaw functions such as chewing and speech. Hereto, jaw stiffness has only been studied in a clinical and experimental investigation by Hesse and colleagues.[30] In a healthy population, a significant higher jaw stiffness during passive mouth opening to the border position was found in the male group. Although the stiffness of the different tissues (i.e., joint capsule/ligaments, muscles, etc.) cannot directly be separately distinguished by the method described by Hesse,[30] different patient subgroups are now being studied for jaw stiffness.

MANDIBULAR MOVEMENTS AND THEIR BASIC BIOMECHANICAL CONSTRAINTS

For many years, mandibular kinematics (i.e., mandibular movements and positions) have been the focus of interest of the dental and physical therapy professions. An understanding of the patterns of mandibular motion under various conditions of guidance and restraint are considered to be of great clinical importance.

In daily practice, an experienced clinician dealing with TMJ disorders on a regular basis is often able to obtain a fair impression of an impeded TMJ function just by listening to the patient's history and by observing the main movements of the mandible. Even small asymmetric jaw movements, occurring during repeated opening and closing movements, with or without audible clicking, can be observed from different views. The teeth usually serve as good landmarks for observation of asymmetric jaw movements.

Different methods of study have been used to observe mandibular motion. The study on the movement of whole bones or any point on the bone is named *osteokinematics*, whereas arthrokinematics focuses on the movements taking place between the articulating surfaces. These particular methods of study are addressed later in this chapter.

Early Observations of Jaw Movement

Many of the modern concepts of mandibular movements arose from the classic work of Posselt.[31] Observation and registration of movements of a fixed point on the mandible, such as near the medial incisor point, were his specific contribution. The projections of condylar movements on the incisor point is a functional approach, because both TMJs function as a single unit. A stylus, attached to the lower incisors, was used to inscribe movement patterns on waxed plates during mandibular movements in the horizontal and sagittal planes. The three-dimensional "banana figure," which can be composed from the two recordings, displays the active border positions of the mandible (Fig. 2-6). The retruded contact position (RCP) is the starting point of the incisor point and is the maximum achieved retruded active jaw position with the condyles located maximally posteriorly and superiorly in the articular fossae. From this position, the jaw can be moved maximally to the left (i.e., the maximum left laterotrusion [MLLT]) under tooth contact guidance. In reverse, the maximum right laterotrusion (MRLT) is found by moving the jaw maximally to the right. Maximum protrusion (MPP) is found by actively moving the mandible forward. The "dip" in the curve displays the temporary lowering of the incisor point below the anterior incisors as the mandible comes forward.

The mobility of the mandible may be expressed by the volume of this figure. Mouth opening starts from the RCP. In this contact position, the condyle is seated as far posteriorly as clinically can be achieved. As the mouth is being opened, the lesser volume remains. Thus, the mobility of the mandible decreases rapidly. It may therefore be assumed that the mobility of the mandible is at its maximum just after the dental arches leave contact. At the most inferior point of the figure, both joints have become completely immobilized toward further opening and will allow only a jaw closing movement.

Since Posselt's work,[31] many other technologically advanced jaw tracking devices have been designed and tested.[32-35] Recording both condylar pathways simultaneously at the site of the joint enables visualization of condylar move-

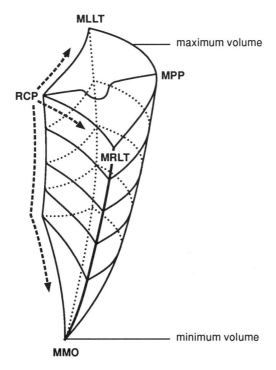

Fig. 2-6. Three-dimensional presentation of the border positions of the mandible, known as Posselt's figures.[31] MMLT, maximum left latcrotrusion; MMO, maximum mouth opening; MRLT, maximum right laterotrusion; MPP, maximum protrusion; RCP, retruded contact position.

ments in three planes. This has become known as gnathography. Asymmetric joint function can be demonstrated with the use of such devices. The asymmetry of jaw functions may be an expression of muscle incoordination and/or mechanical impediments found in the TMJ (i.e., capsule, disc, abnormal viscosity of the synovial fluid, structural defects of the cartilage, etc.) or in the direct vicinity of the TMJ. However, the interpretation of the recordings in patients, and even in healthy subjects, may sometimes lead to erroneous conclusions. A low coordination of jaw muscles in combination with hypermobile TMJs usually display low values of reproducibility. However, marked mechanical impediments, such as found in patients with an acute disc displacement without reduction, usually display highly reproducible figures. Further research is needed to study the clinical and experimental values of gnathography.

Osteokinematics of the Jaw

The science concerned with the interplay of two bones is called osteokinematics. Using this particular kinematic method, researchers have been able to study the motion of healthy and diseased joints. Joint surgery and/or the development of prosthetic devices can help restore natural function based on the knowledge and experience gained with kinematic studies.

Basically, the mandible, considering the constraints, can rotate about and/ or translate along any axis.[36] The complex dynamic functions within the masticatory system have proved difficult to analyze. This prevented most researchers from analyzing the forces and/or movements in different planes. Although predictions made from single-plane models are incomplete, they do serve a purpose in clinical practice. Particularly, observation of the movement of the mandible in the sagittal plane is part of a routine inspection and examination in TMJ patients.

Grant[37] described an instant center technique for the opening movement of the mandible. This technique was earlier described by Reuleaux[38] and allows a description of the relative uniplanar motion of two adjacent segments of a body and the direction of displacement of the contact points between these segments. As one segment rotates about the other, there exists at an instant in time a point that does not move (i.e., a point that has zero velocity).[13] This point is called the *instantaneous center of rotation* (CRo). CRo is found by identifying the displacement of two clear landmarks on the mandible as the mandible moves from one position to the other. The CRo pathway is a collection of CRo points connected by a line and demonstrates the entire range of a bone motion relative to another bone.

Osteokinematic analysis of the mandible can be started by taking successive lateral radiographs of the head. The displacement of two clearly identified landmarks an be observed with such a technique (Fig. 2-7). The displacements of a point A to A'; A' to A''; . . . and B to B'; B' to B''; . . .; etc., may each be connected by a straight line. The perpendicular bisectors of these two lines are then drawn. CRo(S) is found at the start of mouth opening and CRo(E) is found at the end of mouth opening. The figure is a schematic presentation of CRo points that are found during mouth opening.[37,39]

A different CRo pathway will be found during closure of the mouth, because different muscles will come into play at different times. This will lead to a different sequence of roll and slide movements of the condyle on the articular eminence. Further studies are needed to determine the clinical importance of the mouth closure pathway in contrast to the mouth opening pathway.

Although it is generally thought that during the initial mouth opening the mandible rotates about an axis through the long axes of both condyles, the initial CRo is found approximately 1 cm posteriorly and inferiorly of the condyle and not at the center of the condyle.[39]

Although mandibular osteokinematic evaluation involves mainly the observation of mandibular bone movement, some arthrokinematic aspects of this evaluation method are directly addressed here. If the different CRos are known, the specific motion of each of their contact points at the joint surface can be derived. This motion may be characterized as pivoting, sliding, or a combination of both. To determine these particular types of motion at the joint surface, a line is drawn connecting CRo with the surface contact point. A second

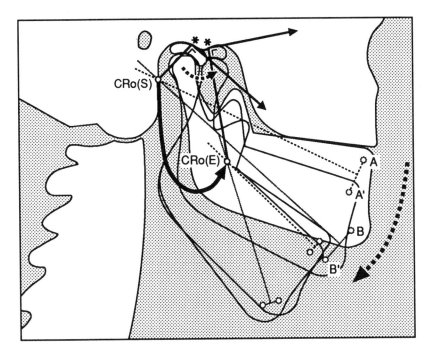

Fig. 2-7. Schematic presentation of a mouth-opening movement in a lateral view and the instantaneous centers of rotation (CRo) pathway. *CRo(S)*, instantaneous center of rotation at the start of mouth opening; *CRo(E)*, instantaneous center of rotation at the end of mouth opening; *, joint surface contact point.

line is then drawn perpendicular to the first line at the surface contact point. A sliding movement will occur at the contact point if the direction of this line is tangential to the surface. This may lead to friction and wear of the articulating surfaces. If, as a result of internal joint derangement, CRo has become displaced, then either compression will occur at the contact point or separation of the articulating surfaces will take place. If CRo lies on the articulating surface, a rolling movement and thus no friction or wear, will occur.[13]

Knowledge and understanding of CRo pathways of joints in healthy subjects may be helpful in those cases in which orthopaedic reconstructive surgery (i.e., internal joint surgery, joint replacement, soft tissue reconstructions near the joint, etc.) is needed.[40] The rehabilitation of patients who have undergone corrective orthopedic surgery may then also be directed more specifically.

Several investigators have reported on the inaccuracies in finding CRo with the Reuleaux method.[40] The inherent error in this method increases when the rotation angle between the bisectors decreases. Ideally, they would have to meet perpendicular. Spiegelman and Woo[40] also reported on the difficulties in locating small line segments during the process of digitizing landmarks, which led to much greater error in locating the intersection of the bisectors. A "rigid-body" method (i.e., an algorithmic calculation method) was designed for the calculation of CRo and angular displacement and was derived from a series of coordinate rotations and translations. Fixed landmarks on the body were the only restriction. When the two landmarks can be well identified before and after the rotation, the angular displacement and CRo can be determined independent of the coordinate system.

Although the rigid-body method is found to be more accurate and will be favored in future studies, the explanation of the Reuleaux method was chosen here for practical understanding. It remains clear that any predictions made from such models only are incomplete because of their uniplanar (and thus simplified) observation and explanation.

Arthrokinematics of the Jaw

To recognize and interpret abnormal jaw mechanics, it is necessary to understand how different biomechanical constraints will influence the different mandibular movements toward their border positions. For instance, a joint partner subjected to constraints does not necessarily move in the direction of an applied force.[41] Muscle actions and gravity will start a joint motion, but throughout the joint surface motion, a changing combination of different constraining factors will come into play. During jaw opening, the articular surface of the temporal bone, as well as the different jaw ligaments, is generally considered a potential constraint. The passive resistance (i.e., the structure's viscoelastic nature) of jaw closure muscles, which are being stretched during mouth opening, must also be considered a constraining factor.

During the past decades, many authors have studied the different biomechanical constraints of the TMJ, particularly during symmetric mouth opening. Various designs of study on the movement of the mandible have been reported in the literature using tracings on radiographs to measure the change in position of different anatomic landmarks on the skull and the mandible.[41] Others have used human cadaver skulls for measurement and calculating purposes for the prediction of the behavior of several (mostly ligamentous) constraining factors. The investigations are based on the premise that ligaments are virtually inextensible and, when pulled taut, act as tension members that tightly constrain movements.[41,42] Elastic (physiologic) deformation of ligaments may range from a 5 to 8 percent lengthening. Beyond 10 percent lengthening irreversible damage (i.e., plastic deformation) of the ligament occurs.[43] However, during this capsule and ligament stretching, mechanoreceptor and nociceptor endings in the joint capsule will reflexly activate muscles. Particularly in manipulative medicine, this protective mechanism should be well understood.

The TMJ capsule is (e.g., particularly anteriorly to the joint) composed of a loose connective tissue enforced laterally by the temporomandibular (TM) ligament and is considered an important constraining factor during most motions of the condyle–disc complex. The posterior fibers of the TMJ capsule particularly will have allowed approximately 10-mm slide before constraining further anterior movement of the condyle.[43]

The lateral enforcement of the TMJ capsule (i.e., the TM ligament) is generally assumed to provide the joint with more passive stability. The passive stability of the TMJ during loading conditions (i.e., during chewing, hard biting, etc.) is assumed to be derived mainly from synergistic muscle actions and to a much lesser degree from the congruency of the articulating TMJ partners.

Most authors agree on the (mainly static) function of the TM ligament; it prevents a combination of posterior and inferior movement of the condyle.[44,45] However, Boucher[46] found no difference toward the most retruded condylar position after sectioning this ligament. A mathematical model of the TMJ acting in three dimensions,[36] as well as a two-dimensional mathematical model,[43] has greatly improved the understanding of the various constraints of the TM articulation.

In most studies, agreement exists on the slackening of the stylomandibular ligament during mouth opening. Full protrusion and overclosure of the mandible (i.e., extreme loss of vertical relation), as well as extreme lateral excursions of the mandible, will make this ligament somewhat taut.[44]

An interesting biomechanical model to the problem of the interplay of the constraining factors during symmetric mouth opening was offered by Osborn.[41] The main constraining factors considered in this study are the TM and sphenomandibular ligaments and the articular eminence. Osborn explained the function of the TM ligament by the mechanism of a swing movement occurring at its upper attachment *U*, while a rotary movement would occur at its lower attachment *L* (Fig. 2-8A and B). During the initial phase of mouth opening, the jaw closure muscles relax and the condyle drops down slightly (i.e., the "swing" motion) following the constraint of the TM ligament. Immediately after this movement, lateral pterygoid activity (e.g., the inferior belly) will move the condyle forward under passive guidance of the TM ligament, causing both a combination of angular motion and translation of the mandible.

The early rotation of the condyle at the lowest attachment of the TM ligament would drive the condyle against the posterior slope of the eminence, after which the condyle would swing downward about the most posterior attachment of the ligament to the articular tubercle (Fig. 2-8C). To achieve full mouth opening, angular rotation must be greater than angular swing. If the swing motion would be greater than the rotation motion, the mouth would be (over)closed and not opened.

Barager and Osborn[36] calculated the slackness of the TM and sphenomandibular ligaments at rest to be, respectively, 0.5 mm and 6 mm. Earlier, Hjortsjö and associates[42] showed that the condyle generally moves forward at the early start of mouth opening, which supports the idea that the TM ligament is particularly taut during the initial phases of mouth opening. Osborn[41] also concluded that the articular disc is well stabilized between the condyle and articular eminence by this ligament action during the full range of mouth opening. However, tightness of the capsule/ligament may displace a disc throughout the early phase of mouth opening and increase the amount of surface loading,

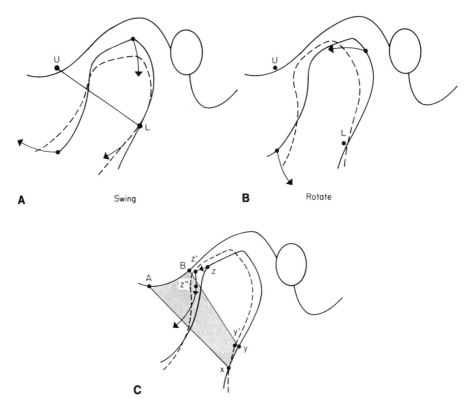

Fig. 2-8. (**A**) During forward "swing" all points of the mandible circle about the upper attachment of the TM ligament, *U*. The jaws are therefore closed, and the condyles drop down. (**B**) During an opening "rotation," the condyle moves toward the articular eminence. Rotation of the condyle takes place around the lower attachment of the TM ligament, *L*. (**C**) With a broad ligament, the centers for "swing" and "rotation" change according to the position of the condyle. *Z* is a point on the condyle moving to *Z'* and *Z''*; *A* and *B* are the upper attachments of the TM ligament; *x* and *y* are the lower attachments of the TM ligament. (From Osborn,[41] with permission.)

possibly initiating surface wear and disc perforation. If this condition is diagnosed, specific TMJ mobilization techniques may be indicated to help relieve the tension on the disc and the attaching structures.

The sphenomandibular ligament is slack at rest and, because of its course, prevents distraction of the condyle (i.e., joint separation) and limits normal mouth opening, as well as protrusion of the mandible.[47] The sphenomandibular ligament becomes taut during the last stage of mouth opening (i.e., particularly when the condyle crosses the articular eminence). Concomitantly, a steep articular eminence may further increase the tension between the articulating surfaces, and audible clicking may be a result as the condyle–disc complex accelerates across the articular eminence.[48]

Finally, a matter that has received little attention yet, although often clinically accepted, is the ill-understood concept of "close- and loose-packed" positions of the TMJ. Rocabado[49] described the close-packed position of the TMJ at the RCP. This jaw position would combine optimum congruency of the joint partners and a maximum tightening of surrounding ligaments. However, the close-packing of the articulating partners may be optimum, but it is not considered the maximum loaded area of the TMJ. This area lies farther down the posterior slope of the articular eminence, where the muscles guide and balance the condyle–disc complex during mastication.[14] Unlike other joints, both TMJs become nearly close-packed when the jaws reach full occlusion of the dental arches. Also, frequently observed in edentulous patients is the further closure of the mouth beyond the "normal" vertical relation. This means that the TMJs are not fully constrained yet at the latter jaw relation.[17] At full mouth opening, the ligamentous and capsular constraints may be at maximum, but the congruency between the joint partners is minimal. The definition of close-packing at this extreme of movement, as described by Rocabado,[49] is not applicable according to the correct definition. It is likely that the maximum loose-packed position of the TMJ is to be found in the direct vicinity of the occlusion of the dental arches (see Fig. 2-6).

The clinical relevance of knowing the maximum loose-packed position of a joint is that it usually serves as the optimum starting point for joint-play examination (i.e., the passive examination of a joint partner relative to its adjacent partner in all possible directions) as well as the starting position for specific mobilization techniques. The maximum close-packed position is a physiologic border position, which may serve as a "locked" joint position when other adjacent joints, for instance, in the spinal column, are the object of specific mobilization or manipulation.

The clinical relevance of these extreme positions of the TMJ needs to be further studied and defined before they are adapted in clinical practice.

Observing and testing joint functions are two of the most important tools in the diagnosis of TMDs. Mechanical impediments of the TMJ, such as caused by a disc displacement without reduction, often demonstrate clear asymmetric movement patterns. It would be an interesting challenge to describe the change in jaw movement patterns for the different disorders affecting the masticatory system. The ligamentous actions controlling jaw movement, as described by Osborn[41] and jaw stiffness in TMJ patient subgroups, as currently studied by Hesse and colleagues,[30] are interesting from a diagnostic as well as a therapy standpoint and could be further studied.

Mobilization techniques applied to the capsule and TM ligament may be useful in the situation of early disc displacement and/or increased loading of the articular surfaces. In physical therapy and dental practices, dislocation of the condyle–disc complex is still treated mostly by stabilizing exercises. However, dislocation of the condyle–disc complex, when caused by sphenomandibular ligament tightness, may request mobilization of this structure at full mouth opening instead of stabilizing techniques. Further development of joint-play and mobilizing techniques will be an important objective in physiodiagnostics and physiotherapy.

The interpretation of diagnostic findings in TMDs and their treatment may improve considerably as we learn more about the biomechanics of the masticatory system.

BIOMECHANICAL ANALYSIS OF THE FORCES IN THE MASTICATORY SYSTEM

During biting on a hard object, there are three contact points between the mandible and the skull (i.e., both TMJs and the point where the object makes contact with the teeth [bite point]). The total force exerted by the jaw muscles is distributed among these three points (the two joint reaction forces and the bite force). The distribution of the total muscle force among these points depends on the magnitude and the orientation of the muscle force and on the position of the bite point along the dental arches. It has been a matter of debate in the literature whether the TMJs are really loaded during biting or chewing.[50] The main argument against the loading hypothesis was that the roof of the fossa of the tuberculum articulare is very thin, too thin to withstand any substantial vertical reaction force. However, the contact point between mandible and skull in the TMJ does not lie in the top of the roof of the fossa but lies more anteriorly. The anterior part of the fossa is much thicker and is more suited to withstand reaction forces than the roof of the fossa. Moreover, no load in the TMJs would imply that only two forces are acting on the mandible (the resultant muscle force and the bite force). Then, for static equilibrium, the resultant muscle force should always pass through the bite point during biting or chewing. Otherwise, a net momentum is acting on the mandible, and the mandible would have the tendency to rotate. This would make very high demands on the control of the muscle forces.

Biomechanical analysis of the masticatory system gives a better understanding of the influence of muscle activity on the masticatory system. A condition for static equilibrium of a body is that the vectorial sum of forces is zero. If this condition is not met, then the body will, because of the resultant force, undergo an acceleration. If more than one force is acting on the body, the points of application of these forces will in general not coincide; think of the muscle forces and the joint reaction forces acting on the mandible. This poses a second condition for static equilibrium on the forces: The vectorial sum of the moments of the forces about any arbitrary axis has to be zero as well. Otherwise, the net momentum of forces will force the body to rotate about that axis.

For a biomechanical analysis of the masticatory system, we often look at the resultant of two forces acting on a body. The resultant of two forces is that force that may replace the two forces without changing the net amount of force and momentum acting on the body. Figure 2-9 shows the resultant F_{res} of two parallel forces F_1 and F_2. The magnitude of the F_{res} is equal to the sum of the two forces; the point of application depends on the magnitude and orientation

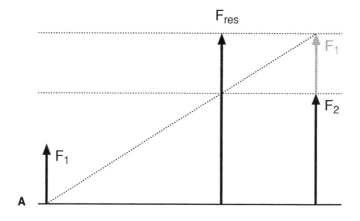

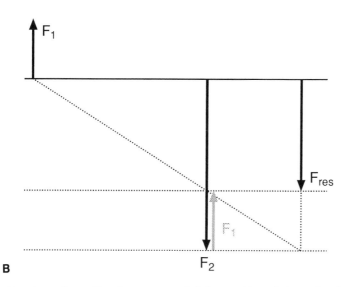

Fig. 2-9. Resultant force F_{res} for two parallel forces F_1 and F_2 acting in the same direction (**A**) or in opposite directions (**B**).

of the forces F_1 and F_2. If F_1 and F_2 have the same orientation, then the point of application of the resultant will lie between F_1 and F_2. If F_1 directs in the opposite orientation of F_2, then F_{res} will lie outside the range of F_1 to F_2 on the side of the greater force, and it will point in the orientation of that force. Thus, the resultant will always lie closest to the greater force.

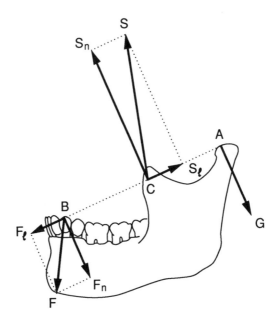

Fig. 2-10. Static symmetric bite. *A, B,* and *C* are the points of application of the joint reaction force *G,* the bite force *F,* and the resultant muscle force *S.*

Static Symmetric Bite

If on equivalent places on the right and the left side of the dental arches the bite forces are the same and the muscle and joint reaction forces are also symmetric with respect to the medial plane, we talk about a static symmetric bite. The resultant forces of the muscle forces, of the joint reaction forces, and of the bite forces then also lie in the medial plane, and a two-dimensional analysis of the biomechanics of the masticatory system in the medial plane is possible (Fig. 2-10). *A, B,* and *C* are the points of application of the resultant muscle force and the resultant of both joint reaction forces and of the bite force. The orientation of the joint reaction force is unknown. However, as the friction in the TMJ is low, the joint reaction force has to pass through the contact point of fossa with condyle and will direct perpendicular to the tangent in that point. In this two-dimensional biomechanical analysis, the joint reaction force is taken to be perpendicular to the line *AB.* The muscle resultant force *S* and the bite force *F* have components S_1 and F_1 parallel to the line *AB* and components S_n and F_n perpendicular to this line. The conditions for static equilibrium are, as a consequence, that the sum of the two parallel components should be zero. Furthermore, the muscle force S_n will be distributed among the joint reaction force *G* and the bite force F_n according to

$$G = \frac{BC}{AB} * S_n; \qquad F_n = \frac{AC}{AB} * S_n$$

This simple two-dimensional model demonstrates that the greater bite forces and the smaller joint reaction forces are found if the bite point *C* lies in the molar region. Then *BC* is short and *AC* is long. If the point of application of the bite force shifts from the molar region to the premolar and incisal region, then the situation becomes biomechanically more unfavorable. A greater percentage of the total muscle force will then be found in the TMJ and a smaller percentage in the bite point. Thus, from a biomechanical point of view, it is more efficient to exert bite forces in the molar region and thus conserve the posterior dental support in patients. If the molars are lacking, patients will perform chewing functions more anteriorly. The maximum attainable bite force will then be smaller, and a greater percentage of the muscle force will be "wasted" in the TMJs.

Experimentally, the heavier bite forces are indeed measured in the molar region.[51] The recorded decrease in maximum bite force for more anteriorly positioned bite forces is even greater than predicted by this simple two-dimensional biomechanical model. The amount of masticatory muscle activation also depends on the position of the bite point. Individuals cannot fully activate the temporal muscles if the bite point is situated more anteriorly. This causes a further decrease in maximum bite force. This decrease in the maximum activation of the temporal muscles also results in a "trade off" effect as far as the loading of the TMJs is concerned: During anterior biting, a higher percentage of the resultant muscle force will be distributed in the TMJ, but the maximum muscle force itself will be smaller than for a more posterior bite. It depends on the individual's anatomy and masticatory muscle activation patterns what the net outcome will be for the loading of the TMJs.

Static Asymmetric Bite

In general, the bite force will not be evenly distributed over the occlusal surfaces. Chewing usually occurs with the food bolus on one side at the time. This makes a three-dimensional analysis of the masticatory system more adequate to describe the mechanics of the masticatory system. However, a full analysis with the magnitude and direction of muscles involved is not possible as the muscle activity patterns of the different parts of the masticatory muscles are not known in detail yet. However, a simplified three-dimensional model of the masticatory system is possible, and this model will deepen our insight into some of the interrelationships between muscle activities, joint reaction forces, and bite force. Figure 2-11 shows the mandible with its three contact point with the skull, the bite point *B* and both condyles *Q* and *R*. In this simplified analysis, only those force components perpendicular to the plane *BQR* will be taken into account. All force components parallel to this plane will be neglected. Also, in this three-dimensional analysis, three forces are acting on the mandible: the resultant muscle force S_n, the resultant joint reaction force *G*, and the bite force F_n. For a situation of static equilibrium, these three forces must lie on a straight line. If this condition is not met, then there would be a net momentum

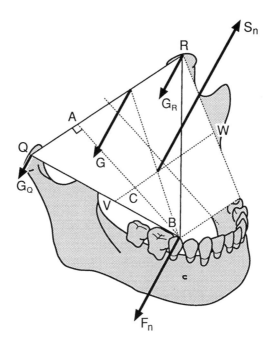

Fig. 2-11. Static asymmetric bite. *B* is the point of application of the bite force *F; Q* and *R* are the points of application of the TMJ reaction forces. The points of application of the resultant muscle force S_n and the resultant joint reaction force *G* lie on the line *VW* and *QR*, respectively, dependent on the relative ipsi- and contralateral masticatory muscle activity.

acting on the mandible with respect to an axis through two of the three forces and the mandible would rotate around this axis. The rule that the three forces acting on the mandible must lie on a straight line makes it clear that for a given bite force point, the loading of both TMJs is strongly determined by the point of application of the resultant muscle force, thus by the left–right masticatory muscle activities.

The point of application of the resultant muscle force will lie on the line *VW*, which is located closely behind the third molars. The exact position of the point of application depends on the relation between the activity of the ipsi- and contralateral masticatory muscles. With symmetric muscle activity, the point of application of the resultant muscle force will lie exactly between *VW*, thus in the medial plane (Fig. 2-12). The point of application of the resultant joint reaction force, which lies on the line *QR*, will lie closer to the contralateral joint, indicating that this joint is heavier than the ipsilateral joint in case of symmetric muscle activity.

If the two TMJs are evenly loaded, then the point of application of the resultant condylar reaction forces will lie in the medial plane. Figure 2-13 shows that for an asymmetric bite point, symmetric joint loads are only possible when the ipsilateral masticatory muscles are more active. Indeed, during chewing,

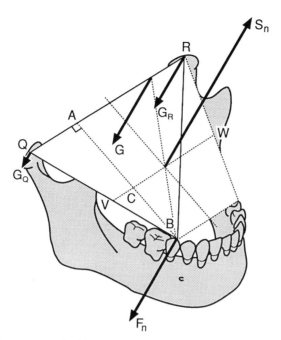

Fig. 2-12. Static asymmetric bite with symmetric masticatory muscle activity. See Figure 2-11 legend for definitions.

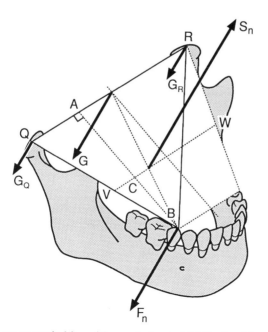

Fig. 2-13. Static asymmetric bite with evenly loaded TMJ. See Figure 2-11 legend for definitions.

the ipsilateral muscles are usually found to be more active than the contralateral muscles, making it likely that both joints are more or less evenly loaded.

Figure 2-11 shows the general situation in which both the masticatory muscle forces and the joint reaction forces are asymmetric. When the bite point shifts along the dental arch to a more posterior position, closer to the line *VW*, then the resultant joint reaction force will shift away from the ipsilateral joint and closer to the contralateral joint. Thus, the more posterior the bite point is, the heavier the contralateral joint is loaded and less compression in the ipsilateral joint occurs. For rather posterior bite points, such as in the third molar region, the resultant joint reaction force may even be lateral to the contralateral joint, indicating heavy compression in the contralateral joint and tension (a tendency to be lifted off the tuberculum articulare) in the ipsilateral joint. Experimentally, it has been verified[52] that under very limited and restricted conditions (e.g., powerful isometric biting along the M_3), the ipsilateral TMJ is either unloaded or loaded in tension. Thus, this simplified three-dimensional model also provides a biomechanical explanation for the clinical observation that patients with a fracture in the ramus ascendens mandibulae can chew at the fracture side provided the activation of the masticatory muscles is such that mainly the contralateral joint is loaded.

Generally speaking, the following applies for the asymmetric static bite:

The relationship between the bite force, the resultant muscle force, and the resultant joint reaction force is the same as the one for the symmetric static bite.

The magnitude of the bite force is independent of the relationship between the ipsi- and contralateral muscle force.

It is more favorable to activate the jaw muscles bilaterally, because then twice as many muscles contribute to the same bite force.

The load of the ipsilateral joint will decrease and that of the contralateral joint will increase when the contralateral muscles are more activated. This may even lead to a reversal of the load in the ipsilateral joint, tension instead of compression and a tendency of the condyle to drop and put tension on the joint capsule.

A simple two-dimensional biomechanical analysis of the masticatory system already shows that biting in a more posterior position is biomechanically more efficient: a higher percentage of the exerted masticatory muscle force is found as bite force in the bite point and a smaller percentage is wasted as joint reaction force in the TMJs. Fortunately, the effect of the relatively high percentage of muscle force distributed to the TMJs at more anterior bite points is counteracted by the observation that the maximum muscle force itself is lower at more anterior bite points. This is due to the fact that it is impossible to fully activate the temporal muscle when the bite point is in a more anterior position.

A three-dimensional analysis demonstrates that the TMJ reaction forces are very sensitive to the left–right masticatory muscle activities. If the muscle activity at the ipsilateral side, where the bite point is, is much higher than at the contralateral side, then the ipsilateral joint will be heavily loaded. However, the more the contralateral muscles are activated, the more the joint load will shift to the contralateral TMJ. With the proper contralateral muscle activity, the ipsilateral joint may even get a distraction (unloading) of the condyle from the fossa. This may explain the observation that patients with a fracture in the ramus ascendens mandibulae are still able to chew with the food bolus on the fractured side. With the proper left–right masticatory muscle activity, their fractured joint may be unloaded during chewing.

REFERENCES

1. Hsieh HH, Walker PS: Stabilizing mechanisms of the loaded and unloaded knee. J Bone Surg 58a:87, 1976
2. Mennell JM: Joint Pain: Diagnosis and Treatment Using Manipulative Techniques. Little, Brown, Boston, 1978
3. Mankin HJ, Radin E: Structure and function of joints. p. 179. In McCarty DJ (ed): Arthritis and Allied Conditions: A Textbook of Rheumatology. 10th Ed. Lea & Febiger, Philadelphia, 1985
4. De Bont LGM: Temporomandibular joint articular cartilage structure and function. Thesis, University of Groningen, 1985
5. Wright V: Lubrication and Wear in Joints. Sector Publishing Limited, London, 1969
6. Yamada H: Strength of Biological Materials. Williams & Wilkins, Baltimore, 1970
7. Gay S, Millr EJ: Collagen in the Physiology and Pathology of Connective Tissue. Gustav Fisher Verlag, Stuttgart, 1978
8. Solberg WK, Hansson TL, Nordstrom B: The temporomandibular joint in young adults at autopsy: a morphologic classification and evaluation. J Oral Rehabil 12: 303, 1985
9. Woelfel JB: Dental Anatomy: Its Relevance to Denistry. 4th Ed. Lea & Febiger, Philadelphia, London, 1990
10. Sprintz R: Temporomandibular menisectomy in rabbits. J Anat 88:514, 1954
11. McDonald F: The condylar disc as a controlling factor in the form of the condylar head. J Craniomandib Disord Facial Oral Pain 3:83, 1989
12. Hjortsjö CH: The significance of the articular disc and the accentuated grinding joint. Odontologisk Revy 4:203, 1953
13. Frankel VH, Nordin M: Basic Biomechanics of the Skeletal System. Lea & Febiger, Philadelphia, 1980
14. Osborn JW: The disc of the human TMJ: design, function and failure. J Oral Rehabil 12:279, 1985
15. Costen JB: Syndrome of ear and sinus symptoms dependent upon disturbed function of the temporomandibular joint. Ann Otol Rhinol Laryngol 3:1, 1934
16. Hansson TL, Nilner M: A study of the occurrence of symptoms of diseases of the temporomandibular joint, masticatory muscles and related structures. J Oral Rehabil 2:313, 1975
17. Hesse JR, Hansson TL: Factors influencing joint mobility in general and particular respect of the craniomandibular articulation: a literature review. J Craniomandib Disord Facial Oral Pain 2:19, 1988
18. Seligman DA, Pullinger AG: TMJ derangement and osteoarthrosis subgroups dif-

ferentiated according to active range of mandibular opening. J Craniomandib Disord Facial Oral Pain 2:35, 1988

19. Israel HA: Synovial fluid analysis. p. 85. In Merrill RG (ed): Disorders of the TMJ 1: Diagnosis and Arthroscopy. WB Saunders, Philadelphia, 1989
20. Roxendal RH: Inleiding tot de kinesiologie van de mens. Stam technische boeken. Culemborg, Porz, Birmingham, 1974
21. Buchbinder D, Kaplan AS: Biology. p. 11. In Kaplan AS, Assael LA (eds): Temporomandibular Disorders: Diagnosis and Treatment. WB Saunders, Philadelphia, 1991
22. Toller PA: The synovial apparatus and the temporomandibular joint function. Br Dent J 50:4, 1968
23. Schmid FR, Ogata RL: The composition and examination of synovial fluid. J Prosthet Dent 18:449, 1967
24. Cohen AS, Brand KD, Krey PR: Synovial fluid. p. 1. In Cohen AS (ed): Laboratory Diagnostic Procedures in Rheumatic Diseases. 2nd Ed. Little, Brown, and Co., Boston, 1975
25. Larkin JG, Lowe GDO, Sturrock RD: The correlation of clinical assessment of synovial fluid with its measured viscosity. Br J Rheumatol 23:195, 1984
26. Von Heyne Witkorin C, Nordin M: Introduction to Problem Solving in Biomechanics. Lea & Febiger, Philadelphia, 1986
27. Barnett CH: The mobility of synovial joints. Rheum Phys Med 11:20, 1971
28. Such CH, Unsworth A, Wright V: Quantitative study of stiffness in the knee. Ann Rheum Dis 34:286, 1975
29. Howe A, Thompson D, Wright V: Reference values for metacarpophalangeal joint stiffness in normals. Ann Rheum Dis 44:469, 1985
30. Hesse JR, Naeije M, Hansson TL: Craniomandibular stiffness toward maximum mouth opening in healthy subjects: a clinical and experimental investigation. J Craniomandib Disord Facial Oral Pain 4:257, 1990
31. Posselt U: Studies in the mobility of the human mandible. Acta Odont Scand 10: 19, 1952
32. Jankelson B, Swain C, Crane P: Kinesiometric instrumentation: a new technology. J Am Dent Assoc 90:834, 1975
33. Hannam AC, De Cou R, Scott J: Kinesiographic measurement of jaw displacement. J Prosthet Dent 44:88, 1980
34. Lewin A: Electrognathographics: Atlas of Diagnostic Procedures and Interpretation. Quintessence Publishing Co., Chicago, 1985
35. Bessette RW: Role of mandibular tracking in temporomandibular joint surgery. p. 205. In Merrill RG (ed): Disorders of the TMJ II: Arthrotomy. WB Saunders, Philadelphia, 1989
36. Barager FA, Osborn JW: A model relating patterns of human jaw movement to biomechanical constraints. J Biomech 17:757, 1984
37. Grant PG: Biomechanical significance of the instantaneous center of rotation: the human temporomandibular joint. J Biomech 6:109, 1973
38. Reuleaux F: Theoretische kinematic: Grundzuge einer Theorie des Maschinenwesens. Vieweg Verlag, Braunschweig, 1875
39. Falkenström CH, Boering G, Cool JC: The temporomandibular joint: an in vivo experiment for locating the instantaneous center of rotation. 7th Meeting of the European Soceity of Biomechanics, July 8–11, Aarhus, Denmark, 1990
40. Spiegelman JJ, Woo SLY: A rigid-body method for finding centers of rotation and angular displacements of planar joint motion. J Biomech 20:715, 1987

41. Osborn JW: The temporomandibular ligament and the articular eminence as constraints during jaw opening. J Oral Rehabil 16:323, 1989
42. Hjortsjö CH, Persson PI, Sonesson A, Sonesson B: A tomographic study of the rotation movements in the temporomandibular joint during lowering and forward movement of the mandible. Odontologisk Revy 8:1, 1954
43. Freesmeyer WB, Stehle CM: Zur Biomechanik der Kiefergelenk-bewegung. Dtsch Zahnarttl Z 43:194, 1988
44. Burch JG: Activity of the accessory ligaments of the temporomandibular joint. J Prosthet Dent 24:621, 1970
45. Saizar P: Centric relation and condylar movement: anatomic mechanisms. J Prosthet Dent 26:581, 1971
46. Boucher L: Limiting factors in posterior movements of mandibular condyles. J Prosthet Dent 11:23, 1961
47. Dubrul EL: Sichers' Oral Anatomy. CV Mosby, St. Louis, 1980
48. Kerstens HCJ: The influence of surgical and anatomical factors on the function of the temporomandibular joint. Thesis, Free University, Amsterdam, 1989
49. Rocabado M: Arthrokinematics of the TMJ. In Gelb H (ed): Clinical Management of the Head, Neck and TMJ Pain and Dysfunction. WB Saunders, Philadelphia, 1985
50. Hylander WL: The human mandible: lever or link? Am J Phys Anthropol 43:227, 1975
51. Pruim GJ, de Jongh HJ, ten Bosch JJ: Forces acting on the mandible during bilateral static bite at different bite force levels. J Biomech 13:755, 1980
52. Hylander WL: An experimental analysis of temporomandibular joint reaction force in macaques. Am J Phys Anthropol 51:443, 1979

3 | History and Physical Examination for TMD

Peter W. Benoit

NATURE AND SCOPE OF TMD

In 1934, Costen,[1] an otolaryngologist, described a complex of symptoms presumed caused by disorder of the TMJ. After Zimmerman's exhaustive critique of the proposed mechanisms for the symptoms in 1951,[2] the term *Costen's syndrome* gradually fell from favor. However, until recently, the concept of a rather consistent symptom complex caused by a variety of TMJ and/or masticatory muscle disorders has persisted, and many syndrome names and features have appeared in the literature. This has resulted in considerable diagnostic confusion. During the past 20 years, significant progress has been made in our understanding of TMJ and masticatory muscle disorders, particularly intracapsular joint disorders and interpretation of joint sounds. This has resulted in the current emphasis on diagnosis of specific muscle and joint conditions rather than a single syndrome.

Although universal agreement has not been reached, the emerging consensus defines TMD as various musculoskeletal disorders of the masticatory system usually manifested by one or more of the following: joint sounds, limitation of jaw movement, muscle tenderness, joint tenderness, and pain, particularly in the preauricular area.[3-6] The specific TMD can be limited to the joint, or the masticatory musculature, or can involve both.[7] This definition of TMD usually includes arthritides but excludes diseases of the teeth, mouth, and sinuses, as well as many pathologies of local tissues, such as infection.

At this time, reliable epidemiologic data on the incidence and prevalence of specific TMD are lacking. However, cross-sectional studies of nonpatient populations indicate that approximately 75 percent of persons have at least one sign of joint dysfunction, and 33 percent have at least one symptom.[8,9]

71

For purposes of uniformity, the following diagnostic classification for TMD from the International Headache Society,[10] which also represents the consensus of the American Academy of Craniomandibular Disorders[11] (now the American Academy of Orofacial Pain), is used throughout this text. The latter organization is composed of persons with academic credentials, advanced education and training, and/or extensive clinical experience, particularly regarding TMD, and therefore arguably represents the most authoritative group in this field.

Deviation in Form
Articular Disc Displacement
   Disc Displacement With Reduction
   Disc Displacement Without Reduction
      Acute
      Chronic
TMJ Hypermobility
Dislocation
Inflammatory Conditions
   Synovitis
   Capsulitis
Arthritides
   Osteoarthritis
   Osteoarthrosis
   Polyarthritides
Ankylosis
   Fibrous Ankylosis
   Bony Ankylosis
Masticatory Muscle Disorders
   Myofascial Pain
   Myositis
   Spasm
   Reflex Splinting
   Muscle Contracture
   Hypertrophy
   Neoplasm
      Malignant
      Benign

OTHER HEAD AND NECK PAIN

When a patient presents with one or more complaints of joint sounds, jaw movement limitation, pain in or near the jaws, headache, or neck pain, the clinician cannot initially be certain that the complaints are caused by a TMD or some other condition completely unrelated to the jaw joints or muscles. This is particularly true when pain is the primary, or only, presenting complaint, as is often the case. Therefore, diagnosis and treatment of TMD requires thorough familiarity with the many head and neck pain entities. It can be fairly stated that the head and neck comprise the most neurologically and anatomically complex region of the body. Moreover, the variety of underlying conditions that can give rise to head and neck pain is far greater than are variations in the clinical presentation of pain. Recently, a major effort to classify and present clear diagnostic criteria for the entire spectrum of headaches and facial pain disorders was published.[10] This compendium, which includes the major categories listed below, serves as a useful guide to practitioners dealing with head and neck pain and provides a stimulus for further cooperation and standardization in a complex, evolving field.

Headache Types
  Migraine
  Tension
  Cluster and Chronic Paroxysmal Hemicrania
  Miscellaneous, Not Associated With Structural Lesions
Headaches Associated With
  Head Trauma
  Vascular Disorders
  Nonvascular Intracranial Disorder
  Substances or Their Withdrawal
  Noncephalic Infection
  Metabolic Disorder
Headache or Facial Pain Associated With Disorder of the Cranium, Neck, Eyes, Ears, Nose, Sinuses, Teeth, Mouth, or Other Facial or Cranial Structures (TMD is included in this major category)
Cranial Neuralgias, Nerve Trunk Pain, and Deafferentation Pain
Headache Not Classifiable

Because there is considerable overlap in the clinical presentation of diverse and unrelated pain disorders and because many patients present with more than one condition contributing to their complaints, the challenge to the diagnostician is considerable. These considerations demand a thorough, systematic approach to every patient. In many short continuing education courses dealing with TMD, the diagnosis is often taken for granted, and attention is focused on treatment of various joint and muscle conditions. This is most unfortunate because diagnostic decisions are often more difficult than treatment decisions. Moreover, the success of treatment largely depends on accurate diagnosis. When the diagnosis is erroneous or incomplete, patients with TMD are likely to receive ineffective, or even counterproductive, treatment. Worse, patients without TMD will not only receive inappropriate treatment, but referral to other specialists for needed evaluation will at least be delayed.

HISTORY

"The diagnosis is in the history if we but choose to listen. Unfortunately, we are deaf."

Sir William Osler, MD

The preeminence of historical information in reaching an accurate diagnosis of the presenting condition is particularly evident in cases in which pain is the primary, or only, complaint. For the sake of simplicity, *pain* will be used in this chapter to include other terms that the patient might use (such as *tightness, stiffness,* or *tension*) to describe discomfort. As is seen later, in these cases the physical examination often provides relatively little additional diagnostic information. In the absence of laboratory tests or other objective procedures to quantify or otherwise characterize pain, reliance must be placed on the patient's account. Even when the patient can thoroughly describe the pain, more information is needed because, as noted above, the variants of pain expression are considerably less than the variety of possible causative conditions. Beyond information needed for categorizing the pain, the history is important in revealing important causative and exacerbating factors, which, in turn, will influence treatment decisions. This is a particularly important consideration in painful musculoskeletal conditions in which the causes of similar pain can vary considerably. Relevant to this point, it is now widely recognized that multiple etiologic factors are usually involved in TMD.[12] Although discussion of the causes of TMD is beyond the scope of this chapter, it is generally recognized that gender, macrotrauma, microtrauma, anatomic, pathophysiologic, and psychosocial factors can all be implicated in the etiology of TMD.

General Medical History

Given the broad scope of the general medical history, it is efficient common practice for the patient to fill out a standard medical history form (Fig. 3-1) before seeing the physician. After the form has been filled out, further details can generally be elicited in a brief review with the patient. The medical history provides an essential overview of the patient's general health. Although past or present conditions identified may not significantly relate to the presenting complaint, it is important to be aware of them and to question the patient further when relevance is obvious or suspected. In cases in which the medical history is extensive, review should not be rushed. When the patient has a lengthy history, complicating psychological factors might be present. The importance of psychological factors in TMD is discussed further below, along with selected areas particularly relevant to head and neck pain disorders.

MEDICAL HISTORY

Dentist: _____ Phone: _____

    Address: _____

Physician: _____ Phone: _____

    Address: _____

Height: _____ Weight: _____ Age: _____

1) Date and reason for last medical examination: _____

2) Current medical problems: _____

3) Current medications: _____

4) Dates of previous surgeries and/or hospitalizations: _____
_____

5) Problems associated with general anesthesia: _____

6) Are you allergic to:

Local anesthetics	YES	NO	Penicillin	YES	NO
Sulfa Drugs	YES	NO	Other antibiotics	YES	NO
Aspirin	YES	NO	Codeine	YES	NO
Other: _____					

7) Do you have or have you had any of the following diseases or problems?

Congestive Heart Disease	YES	NO	Diabetes	YES	NO
High Blood Pressure	YES	NO	Thyroid Disease	YES	NO
Heart Birth Defect	YES	NO	Hepatitis or Liver Disease	YES	NO
Heart Attack	YES	NO	Stomach Ulcers	YES	NO
Angina Pectoris	YES	NO	Venereal Disease	YES	NO
Rheumatic Fever	YES	NO	Immune Deficiency	YES	NO
Heart Murmur	YES	NO	AIDS / HIV Positive	YES	NO
Collagen or Vascular Disease	YES	NO	Arthritis	YES	NO
Anemia	YES	NO	Hay Fever	YES	NO
Bleeding Problem	YES	NO	Respiratory Disease	YES	NO
Other Blood Disorder	YES	NO	Sinusitis	YES	NO
Stroke	YES	NO	Asthma	YES	NO
Convulsions or Seizures	YES	NO	Tuberculosis	YES	NO
Neurologic Disorder	YES	NO	Emphysema	YES	NO
Nervous or Psychiatric Condition	YES	NO	Bronchitis	YES	NO
Fainting Spells	YES	NO	Glaucoma	YES	NO
Kidney Disease	YES	NO	Cancer	YES	NO

    Please specify any medical conditions you have that are not listed: _____

8) Have you ever had a neck injury? .... YES   NO

9) Have you had radiation treatment or chemotherapy for any tumor or growth? .... YES   NO

10) Do you smoke or have you ever smoked? .... YES   NO

11) Do you have or have you had an alcohol or drug abuse problem? .... YES   NO

12) Are you pregnant? .... YES   NO

Signature: _____ Date: _____

Reviewed By: _____ Date: _____

Fig. 3-1. Medical history form.

Chief Complaint

After the general medical history has been reviewed, a detailed history of the presenting condition must be elicited. The chief complaint is a brief statement of the presenting condition in the patient's own words. When pain is the primary manifestation, the chief complaint statement is often of limited diagnostic value and is generally embellished by other complaints that emerge on further questioning.

The method of eliciting a detailed history relevant to the chief complaint is largely a matter of personal preference. The goal is to gather information accurately and efficiently in a manner comfortable for both physician and patient. The major choice is whether to have the patient fill out an additional questionnaire, focused on the presenting condition, before interview. A recent study comparing the use of patient-completed questionnaires to interview in the evaluation of headache concluded that interview provides more reliable information.[13] If patient-completed questionnaires are used, interview will still be needed to clarify and embellish the patient's responses. When patient-completed questionnaires and are not used, a pre-printed form with categories and space for taking notes during the interview can become part of the permanent record. Using this method during interview helps to provide flexibility and to avoid omissions. Interviewing effectively is a skill that cannot easily be taught and requires considerable experience to develop. It is most important to guide the patient, being sure that all information is efficiently obtained, without suggesting answers. The interviewer should also be reasonably flexible regarding the order in which information is elicited because some patients are not easily lead through a predetermined sequence.

It is not possible to mention every category or item of information that might be encountered in a thorough history of the presenting condition, nor is it intended to present a rigid format or sequence for taking the history. Personal style and preference are extremely variable when it comes to communicating with patients. The information discussed in sections below is of value in the history pertinent to TMD and can be organized in a variety of ways to produce questionnaires or forms for interview notes as determined by individual preference.

Head and Neck Pain Description

Obtaining an accurate description of the patient's pain is the most difficult, and most important, part of the history. Reliance is on the patient's ability to characterize pain. Unfortunately, the emotional aspects of pain can cause the patient's description to be erratic or incoherent. With this in mind, and because pain can be inherently difficult to describe, there is probably more temptation to put words into the patient's mouth while taking this portion of the history than with other areas. This tendency should be resisted, because the patient's phrasing and word selection can provide important diagnostic clues that would otherwise be missed. For example, pain described as "burning" or "like an electric jolt" might indicate a classic neuralgia or other neuropathic (nerve dysfunction) pain. If a patient describes pain as "punishing" or "vengeful," a significant psychological influence in pain generation or perpetuation might be suspected. Occasionally, when a patient is incapable of describing the pain, prompting or suggestions of common pain patterns by the clinician may be necessary.

A complete description of pain should include the location as precisely as possible, quality, intensity, duration, and timing patterns. It is convenient to record relative pain intensity by asking the patient to place a mark on an un-graduated horizontal line (with highest intensity at the right end); use of the visual analog scale is superior to verbal descriptors, whose meanings vary considerably among patients. It is critical to include all current head and neck pains. Some patients might state that they have pain in many areas and attempt to describe them as a single entity. This is generally uninformative as well as confusing, and every attempt should be made to distinguish separate pain entities. When more than one pain pattern appears to be present, as is often the case, care must be devoted to characterizing each according to the descriptors enumerated above. It is also important to obtain a history of prior head and neck pains, but the degree of detail needed is often less. This will depend largely on how remote the history is and judgment of apparent relevance to current pain. Family history, particularly regarding various forms of headache, may also be helpful.

Other Symptoms

In addition to pain description, other symptoms associated with the pain often provide important diagnostic and/or etiologic clues. The patient should be questioned regarding the occurrence of nausea, vomiting, numbness, paresthesia, and disturbances of motor function, vision, hearing, taste, or smell. Local autonomic phenomena, such as sweating, flushing, lacrimation, or nasal discharge, should also be noted. The presence of any of these and their timing relative to pain episodes are particularly helpful in determining the classification of headache and may provide insight into causation.

A history of allergies or upper respiratory congestion correlating with pain can help distinguish sinus headache from TMD and other facial pains.

Symptoms such as tinnitus and sensations of blockage, fullness, pressure, or fluid accumulation in the ears can be suggestive of primary otologic disturbances. True vertigo, which is dizziness with a distinct sensation of movement of self or surroundings, is usually indicative of an inner ear problem.[14] Other forms of dizziness, such as light-headedness or disequilibrium, can be due to a wider range of problems.[14] However, any of these symptoms can also be caused by TMD. Although the mechanisms for the association of ear symptoms with TMD are uncertain, many plausible theories have been proposed.

Finally, sleep disturbances, such as difficulty falling asleep, frequent waking, or nonrestorative sleep, can provide diagnostic clues. Any of these symptoms, particularly combined with unexplained aching in other parts of the body and tenderness at certain specific sites, can be suggestive of fibromyalgia.[15] When fibromyalgia is suspected, referral for rheumatologic evaluation should be considered.

Associated Factors

Although recognizing patterns of pain and other symptoms generally leads to diagnosis, factors associated with the initiation and perpetuation of symptoms often provide critical etiologic information that can influence treatment decisions. For example, many factors can be responsible for persistent muscle pain, and the most effective management strategies will be directed at elimination of those most important; in one case, permanent occlusal change may be required, whereas in another, stress management might be needed most. Detection of important causative factors can be accomplished only by carefully questioning the patient. The histories of physical factors, including overt trauma, oral and other habits, perception of bite discomfort, recent dental treatment, working conditions, and exercise activities, are important areas to be explored.

In most patients, many potential contributing factors are likely to be encountered, and the challenge to the clinician is to identify the important ones. This can be completed only by searching for convincing correlations between potential factors and the patient's symptoms. A patient with a history of repeated episodes of limited opening that resolve when the joint clicks, suggesting disc displacement, can serve to illustrate application of these principles. For example, if limitation is present only on waking, then nocturnal jaw habits can be presumed to be important in causing episodic disc displacement, and use of an occlusal appliance at night is likely to prevent the disc displacement. If, however, the patient has episodes only while eating, an appliance worn at night is not likely to be effective.

In addition to physical factors, emotional issues can be significant contributors to head and neck pain disorders. Psychological factors may be secondary to long-term physical suffering and limitations. Conversely, emotional problems may be primarily responsible for the development of painful somatic conditions. Whether psychological factors are primary or secondary, these patients are likely to exhibit signs of anxiety and/or depression and are likely to present special management problems, particularly if pain is an important feature of their presenting complaints. Questioning patients about their own insights into stress factors often can help detect the presence of strong primary psychological factors. The patient with the primary emotional factors is generally more difficult to manage successfully, and referral to specialists for further evaluation and stress management may be necessary, either before somatic treatment is begun or at some point during treatment.

Joint Sounds

A full history of joint sounds audible to the patient, although not necessarily to others, should be obtained up to the present. The patient should be asked to distinguish between clicking, grating, or dull, thudding sounds in their description, and asked if there is pain or other sensations within the joint coincident with the sound. The frequency and quality of sounds, as well as their association with specific functional movements and pain, might provide important clues regarding the condition of bony and soft tissues within the joint. For example, a definite click or pop sound on opening and/or closing, often accompanied by a coincident palpable jarring of joint movement, probably indicates a disc displacement with reduction. A grating sound often indicates a perforation of the disc and/or posterior attachment tissue, possibly with associated arthrotic changes of the functional bony surfaces.

Mandibular Movement Abnormalities

Any history of difficulty with opening, closing, lateral, or protrusive movements should be thoroughly described. An understanding of normal joint and masticatory muscle mechanics and function is necessary before attempting to interpret movement abnormalities. The occurrence or disappearance of joint sounds with the onset or resolution of movement limitations or irregularity of joint movement can help to differentiate arthrogenous from muscular causes. For example, limited opening that suddenly resolves after a click occurs in the joint indicates that the limitation was caused by anterior disc displacement rather than by muscle dysfunction.

Prior Evaluations and Treatment

The patient's prior evaluation and treatment experience relevant to the presenting complaints should be explored before further diagnostic decisions and management strategies are reached. It is important to identify medications and other treatments that have been beneficial as well as those that have not. Results of previous tests and imaging studies must also be recorded.

After the history has been obtained, the clinician should have a generally coherent sense of the patient, and a fairly clear impression of the diagnostic possibilities. If this is not the case, requestioning the patient in areas that are unclear or seem incomplete should be performed before proceeding with the examination. This will most often prove fruitful, although some patients are unable to provide a comprehensive history regardless of how skillfully they are questioned.

PHYSICAL EXAMINATION

Although the history generally provides a feeling for what the examination findings are likely to be, the examination must always be performed thoroughly and objectively. It is not unusual to encounter unanticipated findings, and the examination should never be approached with a perfunctory attitude. When unexpected discoveries are made, it may be necessary to requestion the patient for additional historical information relevant to the finding. The examination procedures described below are generally performed by a dentist, who is most often the primary care manager in TMD cases.

Asymptomatic variations from ideals or norms of jaw configuration, mandibular movement, joint anatomy, or occlusion have not generally been shown to lead predictably to significant symptoms or deteriorations.[7,16–18] In view of this, the major justification for treatment is the fact that the patient has presented with a complaint that is sufficiently bothersome to motivate seeking care. Accordingly, the primary aim of the physical examination is to determine the locations of tissue damage, pain, and tenderness; it is not to document every measurable deviation from the ''ideal'' temporomandibular (TM) apparatus.

These goals should be attained by the simplest, most practical means available. As is discussed in Chapter 4, there is no justification for using sophisticated (often expensive) techniques in routine clinical practice when simpler means to gather needed information are available. There is also no point to gathering data that may not materially influence diagnostic or treatment decisions. A clinical examination for TMD usually can be accomplished with the items shown in Figure 3-2. Routine examination should include assessment not only of the TMJs, but also of the jaw and neck muscles and the occlusion. It is convenient to record data on a standard form with space provided for special tests and comments. A concise example is shown in Figure 3-3. On this form, the 0 to 3 scale is used to rate joint and muscle tenderness to palpation. The severe rating (3) is used only when the patient exhibits pain behavior, such as flinching or crying out, in addition to their verbal rating.

TMJs

The full range of vertical and horizontal mandibular movements should be measured (Fig. 3-4). This provides information relevant to both joint and muscle function. It is important to ask if the patient is aware of changes from their customary range, because individual limits vary, and reliance on average figures can be misleading. The smoothness and overall coordination of active movements should be observed, as well as deviations from symmetric trajectories. The patient should report frank pain or notable sensations of tension, pressure, or other discomfort during the movements. When there is limited or uncomfortable active movement, the mandible should be manipulated passively to determine true limits and to assess the degree of rigidity or resistance at end points, which can provide diagnostic clues. For example, in cases of muscle trismus, there is usually a very rigid resistance felt at the end point of opening, whereas when opening is limited by disc displacement without reduction, the end point usually is not this firm.

Joint palpation technique is shown in Figure 3-5. Lateral palpation should be performed with the jaw closed and also as the mandible moves through its range. This is best accomplished with the finger tip over the lateral aspect of

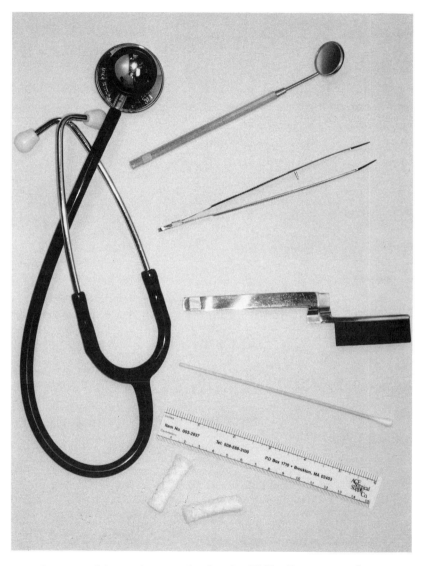

Fig. 3-2. Items used in routine examination for TMD. From top to bottom: mouth mirror, cotton forceps, forceps with articulating paper, cotton swab, rule (mm), cotton rolls. Stethoscope (left).

EXAMINATION

Nodes: _____ Lips: _____ Comments & Special Tests:

Oral Mucosa: _____ _____

Dental Tx Summary: _____ _____

Teeth Missing: _____ Crssbt: _____ _____

Angle: _____ H-Obt: _____mm. V-Obt _____mm. _____

Mobil: _____ Perc: _____ Facets: _____ _____

Slide CR-IP: None _____ Ant _____ Vert _____ Lat _____ _____

Excursions: work _____ balance _____ work Protr. _____

R	TMJ	L		R	Muscles	L
____	pain, lat.	____	0 = none / 1 = mild / 2 = moderate / 3 = severe	____	masseter, super.	____
____	pain, post.	____		____	masseter, deep	____
____	pain, vert.	____		____	temporalis, ant.	____
____	click, open	____		____	temporalis, post.	____
____	click, close	____		____	splenius capitis	____
____	click, ipsilat.	____		____	trapezius, insert.	____
____	click, contra.	____		____	trapezius, lateral	____
____	crep., vert.	____		____	posterior triangle	____
____	crep., ipsilat.	____		____	SCM, upper	____
____	crep., contra.	____		____	SCM, lower	____

ROM: max. open _____mm., pain: _____   ____ digastric, post. ____

lat. R _____, L _____mm., pain: _____   ____ digastric, ant. ____

protrusive _____mm., pain: _____   ____ medial pterygoid ____

R	Arteries	L	Comments: _____
____	carotid	____	_____
____	facial	____	_____
____	temporal	____	_____

Radiology/Imaging: _____

Fig. 3-3. Physical examination form including sections for entries concerned with dental occlusion, TMJ, and masticatory and cervical musculature.

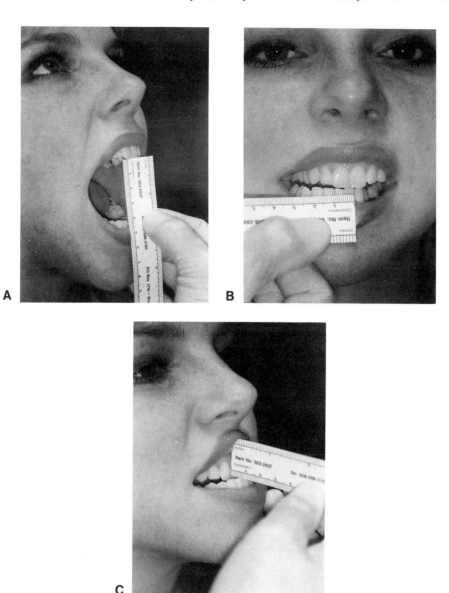

Fig. 3-4. The maximum range of mandibular movement from IP is measured (**A**) vertically, and horizontally in (**B**) right and left lateral, and (**C**) anterior directions. It is preferable to record the vertical measurement as the distance between the biting edges of the maxillary and mandibular central incisors at maximum opening plus the vertical overbite (see Fig. 3-10). Thus, if the maximum interincisal opening is 42 mm and the vertical overbite is 3 mm, then the actual mandibular movement to maximum opening, measured at the incisors, is 45 mm. Similarly, the horizontal overbite measurement (Fig. 3-10) should be added to the anterior movement (protrusive) measurement to obtain the actual maximum anterior mandibular movement.

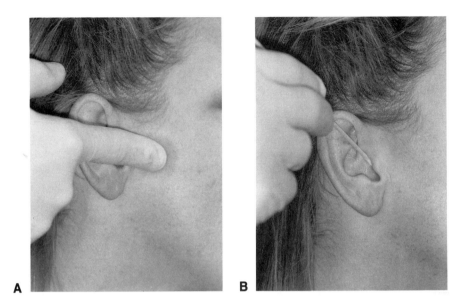

Fig. 3-5. Palpation of the (**A**) lateral and (**B**) posterior aspects of the TMJ. A cotton swab placed in the auditory canal and directed forward, inward, and downward will apply pressure to the lateral aspect of posterior joint soft tissues and is usually more effective than attempting digital palpation in the small canal. Pressure against posterior joint tissues can be confirmed by feeling for condylar movement when the patient opens and closes slightly during palpation.

the condyle. A cotton swab placed in the auditory meatus can be used to palpate the posterolateral aspect of the joint. Joint palpation provides information regarding the source of jaw pain and also helps to detect internal joint derangements by feeling for abnormal condyle or disc movement during lateral palpation. Abnormal disc movement during intrameatal palpation must be interpreted with caution. This is because the pressure of the palpating swab or finger against the posterior joint soft tissues during mouth closure can cause a temporary anterior disc displacement in a normal joint. For this reason, joint movements during posterior palpation should be minimal. Unfortunately, the anterior, medial, and posteromedial aspects of the joint cannot be palpated. This limitation, coupled with the possibility of pain referred from muscles being perceived at or near the joint, can make determination of joint damage difficult.

Applying a vertical load to the joint can help detect pain emanating from the joint. This can be performed either by pushing the mandible superiorly while the teeth are kept apart or by having the patient bite forcefully on a cotton roll between posterior teeth on each side separately. During the latter test, joint pain is often greatest when the cotton roll is between the teeth of the opposite side. This might be because greater joint loading occurs on the side in which the posterior teeth are not separated by the cotton. Joint loading must be performed and interpreted carefully, because a report of pain does not necessarily mean that the joint is the source. When the load is applied manually, the patient might mistake local hand pressure against the mandible for joint pain. When the patient loads the joint by biting a cotton roll, muscle pain might be misinterpreted as joint pain. Careful communication with the patient helps to identify the source of pain.

In addition to movement irregularities, joint palpation, and loading, stethoscopic auscultation of the joint is performed to detect sounds that might indicate joint abnormalities. Joint sounds should be characterized according to quality, frequency, repeatability, palpability, timing relative to mandibular movements, correlation with movement irregularities, and association with pain. Definite clicking sounds generally indicate abnormal disc movement relative to the condyle, but they might also be caused by surface irregularities of soft and/or hard tissues or might possibly even indicate joint fluid disturbances. Crepitant sounds very often indicate soft tissue perforation and/or bony abnormalities.[19] Special maneuvers sometimes provide further diagnostic information or can help determine the type of appliance needed to control disc derangement. Having the patient close normally on cotton rolls between the molars (or to a protruded mandibular position) after an opening click has occurred can often prevent further clicking on subsequent opening from the altered mandibular position. When this occurs, the opening click is likely caused by reduction of an anteriorly displaced disc. If the click is not thus eliminated, it might be caused by posterior disc displacement on opening. The latter condition has recently been documented with arthrotomograms in some patients with hypermobile joints when condyles translate anterior to the temporal eminences during opening.[20]

In some instances, treatment strategies will be affected significantly depending on whether pain is largely originating from the joints or from muscles. When the primary pain source remains unclear after examination, local anesthetic block of the auriculotemporal nerve posteromedial to the neck of the condylar process can help resolve the question. If the joint is the primary pain source, both joint discomfort and regional muscle tenderness will often disappear or be sharply reduced during the period of anesthesia. The effect of auriculotemporal nerve block on headache and neck pain, in addition to jaw pain, can also help to predict results in cases in which joint surgery is being considered to control pain.

By the above methods, condylar hypertranslation, abnormalities of disc position, perforations, and other soft tissue irregularities often can be detected. However, joint diagnoses frequently must be tentative because many recent studies have clearly shown that clinical findings are not entirely reliable predictors of internal derangements or other joint abnormalities.[19,21–25] Both false-positive and false-negative conclusions can be reached. For example, it is particularly noteworthy that chronic anterior disc displacement without reduction has been documented by disc-imaging studies in completely asymptomatic persons with no clinical signs of joint abnormality.[25] Frequently, imaging studies of joint hard or soft tissues are required for complete diagnosis and treatment planning. Joint radiology is discussed in Chapter 5.

Masticatory Muscles

The major muscles of mastication are the masseter, temporalis, medial pterygoid, and lateral pterygoid. The digastric is an accessory masticatory muscle that assists the lateral pterygoid in depression of the mandible. Because of their large size and external location, the masseter and temporalis can be inspected for evidence of enlargement or atrophy. All the muscles, except the lateral pterygoid, can be palpated to assess texture and tenderness. To elicit tenderness, digital pressures of approximately 4 kg/cm^2 should be applied over muscles. This method has been shown to be more discriminatory for eliciting pain than use of dolorimetry devices.[15] Although it is assumed that the reader is generally familiar with locations of the masticatory muscles and nearby structures that could influence patient response to palpation, Figures 3-6 and 3-7 illustrate palpation sites. Most portions of the masseter, temporalis, and digastric can be palpated, whereas only a limited portion of the medial pterygoid is accessible; because this area is near the tonsil, the muscle is difficult or impossible to evaluate in patients with prominent gagging. A very small portion of the lateral pterygoid might be accessible from the maxillary buccal vestibule. However, because both the buccinator and anterior head of the medial pterygoid are interposed (Fig. 3-8), the muscle cannot be convincingly evaluated by palpation. Because oral tissues are generally more sensitive to deep pressure

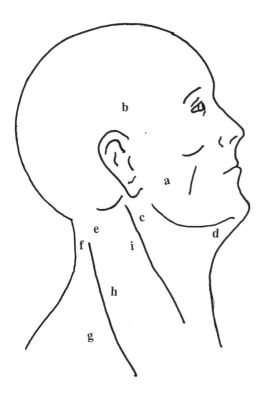

Fig. 3-6. Approximate sites for extraoral palpation of muscles: masseter *(a)*, temporalis *(b)*, posterior *(c)* and anterior *(d)* bellies of digastric, splenius capitis insertion *(e)*, trapezius insertion *(f)*, upper lateral portion of trapezius *(g)*, floor muscles of the lower posterior triangle *(h)*, and sternocleidomastoid *(i)*.

Fig. 3-7. Semischematic view of the right side of the oral cavity showing the internal surface of the cheek and approximate sites for intraoral palpation of masticatory muscles: anterior portion of masseter *(a)*, lower portions of temporalis insertions *(b)*, and midanterior portion of medial pterygoid *(c)*. The *dotted line* represents the position of the anterior edge of the mandibular ramus, which is easily palpable through the mucosa of the posterior cheek. Pterygomandibular fold or raphe *(d)*; position of palatine tonsil *(e)*.

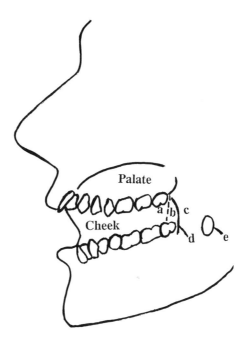

Fig. 3-8. Cut-away view of the right infratemporal fossa showing that the bulk of the lateral pterygoid *(a)* is located well superior and posterior to the oral cavity. Medial pterygoid *(b)*, showing the superficial anterior head overlying the most anteroinferior portion of the lateral pterygoid. Buccinator *(c)*.

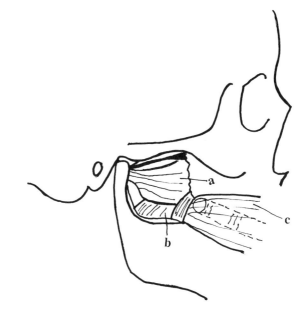

than cutaneous sites, response to intraoral muscle palpation should be interpreted with caution, particularly when positive responses are equal bilaterally. It sometimes is helpful to palpate a muscle during contraction, as well as when at rest or stretched, particularly when there is doubt regarding the source of tenderness. Palpation should cover as much of the muscle as possible, because tenderness is often focal, particularly when trigger points are present. To assess for active trigger points, sustained pressure over the tender area is often necessary to provoke pain in the reference zone. When the patient's responses to palpation are suspect, observing the response to palpation of bony areas not covered by muscle (e.g., the supraorbital ridges, crown, or malar and chin prominences) might help to detect malingering or hyperreactiveness. However, this test is not infallible, because pain from muscle can be referred to non-muscular areas.

In addition to inspection and palpation, intramuscular injection of local anesthetic is sometimes of diagnostic value. Effects of the muscle anesthesia can help to identify sources of pain. Also, resultant muscle relaxation can help to differentiate muscular from joint causes of abnormal mandibular movement or changes in dental occlusion. It has been found that skeletal muscle undergoes rapid necrosis when directly exposed to common local anesthetics, followed by complete regeneration within a few weeks.[26] Muscle tenderness for a few days after injection might be at least partially due to this response. To minimize the possibility of permanent muscle damage, it is recommended that use of vasoconstrictors in the anesthetic solution,[27] as well as frequently repeated injections,[28] be avoided. In some instances, application of the vapocoolant stretch and spray technique[29] can be used in lieu of injection for evoking muscle relaxation.

Although the specific muscle diagnostic entities listed at the beginning of this chapter serve as a guide for differentiating various conditions, there is no universal agreement on the meaning of the terms, and some are often used interchangeably. Although the confusion is partially caused by carelessness or ignorance, it also reflects the genuine complexity and overlap of muscle disorders, as well as our incomplete understanding of them. The differentiations suggested by the terms are frequently not clearly distinguishable on examination. Because of this, treatment strategies will largely depend on the apparent causes of muscle pain, revealed to a large extent by the history. Except for some cases of contracture, or rare instances of neoplasia, in which pain may not be present, myalgia is generally a major complaint and is usually confirmed by tenderness at examination.

Pain originating from muscles is present in the great majority of TMD patients. Despite the preeminent position of myalgia in TMD and many other conditions, the precise mechanisms of muscle pain remain partially obscure, although many theories exist.[30] However, it is known that there is more than one type of muscle pain,[31,32] and mechanisms probably vary with the type of pain. Clinicians have long known that muscle pain is poorly localized and that dysfunctional muscles can refer pain to remote sites. Recent studies involving experimental stimulation of small-diameter neurons in the masseter have documented, for the first time, resultant sensitivity changes in brain stem nociceptive neurons that may help explain both the diffuse localization and referral of muscle pain to other tissues, such as skin.[33] It is not surprising that skeletal muscle is prominently subject to pain, because it is the most exquisitely neuroregulated basic tissue, with complex motor and sensory innervations. Fully two-thirds of the sensory innervation is composed of small-diameter fibers.[34] Many of the small-diameter neurons appear specialized to respond to either pressure, contraction, or temperature at physiologic levels, but all will also respond to painful stimulation.[35] These neurons end almost exclusively in the muscle connective tissues, closer to blood vessels than to muscle fibers.[34,36] Interestingly, there is evidence that the small-diameter neurons are far more concentrated in muscle areas rich in slow, oxidative, fatigue-resistant muscle fibers than in areas composed largely of fast, glycolytic, easily fatigued fibers.[36] Masticatory muscles are particularly rich in the former type of myofiber.[37] Beyond the number and complexity of motor and sensory endings within skeletal muscles, in the mesencephalic nucleus, the cell bodies of primary afferents from the masticatory muscles are directly innervated by hypothalamic neurons.[38,39] The functional implications of this unique innervation are not yet understood. However, it appears to provide a neuroanatomic basis for possible direct modulation of masticatory muscle function by neural activity in emotional centers, which, in turn, might further our understanding of stress-related bruxing and masticatory muscle pain.

Cervical Examination

It is now generally recognized that TMD patients often complain of neck pain. In trauma cases, such as hyperextension injury from motor vehicle accidents, often there is damage to both the neck and jaw. In these situations, identification of pain sources can present a considerable diagnostic challenge. This is because of overlapping areas of pain referred from neck and jaw structures, which, in turn, are at least partially based on overlap of upper cervical spinal segments and the trigeminal system in the brain stem. Because of the neuroanatomic conjunction of the two areas, it is also theoretically possible for a primary jaw condition to cause secondary neck symptoms, and the converse might also occur. Clinical experience with TMD patients generally supports the reality of both situations.

In light of the above considerations, neck symptoms certainly should be included in the history. It also follows that there should be an examination of the neck, which is a highly complex structure with many pain-sensitive structures, including intervertebral discs and annuli, dura, nerve roots, zygapophyseal joints, vertebral arteries, and a multitude of muscles and ligaments.[40] In addition to pain within the neck itself, the concept of cervicogenic headache[41] has been studied rather extensively in recent years and is becoming generally recognized. The extent of neck examination will depend on expertise and training; when the examiner is a dentist, there may be significant constraints imposed by state practice acts. For dentists who are comfortable with their knowledge of at least superficial cervical anatomy, it is reasonable to conduct a gentle palpation examination of major surface muscles and muscle groups as indicated in Figure 3-6. More vigorous examination, involving forced movements or deeper manipulations, are potentially dangerous when the examiner is not specifically trained. When to refer a patient for further cervical evaluation is a matter of clinical judgment and experience. Prominent symptoms such as nausea or dizziness with certain neck movements or positioning, significant movement limitations, or sharp, reproducible pain with movement will usually warrant referral to a medical or physical therapy specialist.

Occlusion

Beyond noting obvious jaw size discrepancies, tooth misalignment, and crowded, missing, or worn teeth, the physical therapist should not be concerned with the details of dental examination. This is partially because of training limitations and also because the role of objective occlusal findings in the genesis or perpetuation of TMD is problematic, as discussed further below. General occlusal examination by a dentist should note the Angle bite classification and any jaw or dental arch asymmetries, as well as incompatibilities of maxillary and mandibular arch size or shape. Missing teeth should be noted, with particular attention to lost molars. Excessive tooth mobility or sensitivity can provide clues to functional discrepancies. In the absence of periodontal disease, these findings can be suggestive of significant tooth malalignment and/or parafunctional habits that place excessive stress on teeth and their supporting tissues. Presence of attrition also provides clues to possibly important dysfunctional relations or noxious habits such as bruxism. In assessing wear, the patient should be questioned about the location and extent of previous occlusal adjustments to identify tooth morphology changes intentionally made by dentists. The surface appearance of wear facets can help determine if bruxing is occurring currently; a shiny facet suggests that enamel has been abraded recently. In patients with essentially normal occlusal configurations, wear from bruxing is most likely to be seen on the cuspids and incisors, because these teeth most often guide mandibular movements discussed below.

Closer inspection of the occlusion should include evaluation of both static and functional dental relationships. The relaxed mandible should be manually guided to closure in the "centric relation" (CR) position and initial tooth contacts noted (Fig. 3-9). The direction and magnitude of subsequent mandibular slide required to reach the maximum intercuspation position (IP) should then be recorded. The same can be performed on voluntary closure of the mandible into the position dictated by the neuromuscular system, noting any discrepancy between this and the IP position. In the IP position, horizontal and vertical overbites should be measured (Fig. 3-10). Existence of nonideal dental relationships in IP should be noted. This will include crossbites, anterior or posterior open bites, and any other irregularities. Finally, the patient should be

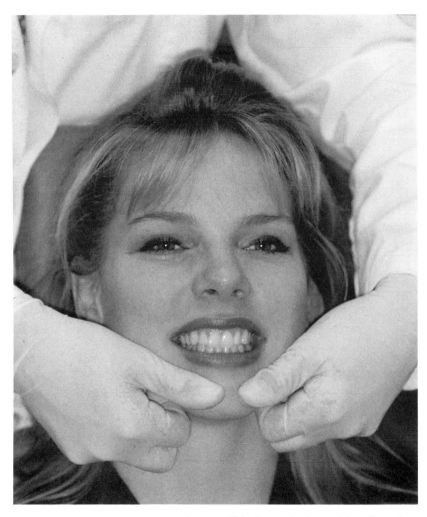

Fig. 3-9. With the patient relaxed, the mandible is passively positioned to place the condyles in their fully seated superior position. The arc of closure from this position (CR) is determined by joint anatomy rather than by the neuromuscular system. The significance of occlusal discrepancies between the CR and intercuspation positions (IP) in the genesis or perpetuation of TMD remains unknown and probably varies considerably among individuals.

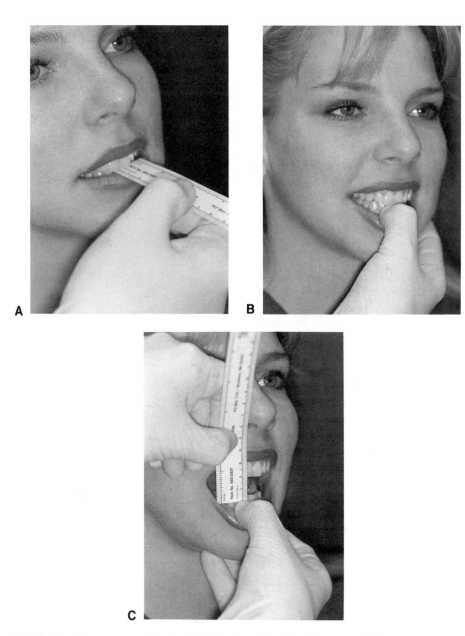

Fig. 3-10.   Measurement (mm) of (**A**) horizontal and (**B & C**) vertical overbites of the maxillary incisors. In rare instances when the mandibular incisors are anterior to the maxillary incisors in intercuspation (IP), similar measurements are made of the degree of underbite.

instructed to slide the mandible to each side and forward, keeping the guiding teeth touching during movements, to detect functional contacts (Fig. 3-11). In addition to visualizing the contacts, questioning the patient and checking with articulating paper may be necessary for complete assessment. Casts of the dentition are not routinely needed, but they may be necessary when occlusion is believed to be a significant etiologic factor, and permanent occlusal changes are anticipated in treatment.

Considerable controversy surrounds the question of the importance of occlusal factors in the etiology or perpetuation of TMD. In recent years, critical reviews generally have not shown strong epidemiologic correlations between occurrence of various nonideal occlusal features and incidence of TMD.[42,43] This certainly does not mean that occlusal factors may not be of primary importance in an individual case; however, it does indicate that objective occlusal findings must be interpreted carefully. Clues to the importance of occlusal factors in the individual case are likely to be found in the history and the patient's perceptions of occlusal discomfort. For example, if a previously asymptomatic patient develops persistent muscle aching and tenderness very shortly after a new crown is placed and also states that the bite feels uncomfortable, occlusal adjustment is likely to eliminate the problem. In most cases, however, the history is not this compelling, and despite careful assessment efforts, the importance of occlusal factors often remains in doubt. Therefore,

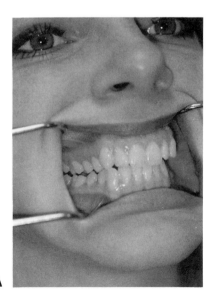 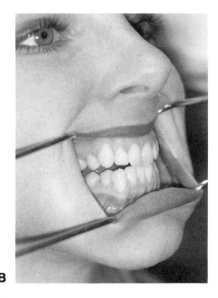

A   **B**

Fig. 3-11. Observation of anterior dental guidance in mandibular (**A**) lateral and (**B**) protrusive movements. In this patient, right lateral movement is cuspid-guided, and protrusion is incisor-guided.

caution is generally warranted before recommendations for permanent occlusal change are made.

DIAGNOSIS AND TREATMENT

After the history has been elicited and the examination completed, the clinician's total knowledge and experience are applied in reaching diagnoses and planning effective management. Although detailed discussion of specific diagnoses and treatment strategies is beyond the scope of this chapter, some general comments regarding these matters are appropriate.

It is sometimes evident, or suspected, that at least some symptoms are caused by conditions other than TMD. In such instances, referral to other specialists may be warranted. These usually will involve evaluation for cervical orthopedic, ear, nose, throat, or neurologic disorders.

Even when a case does not appear complicated by the existence of conditions other than TMD, the complete TM diagnosis may not always be clear at the initial visit. In this situation, the first decision centers on whether further diagnostic procedures are needed immediately. If the initial treatment plan will be influenced by the issues in doubt, then further investigations (such as disc-imaging studies) should be accomplished forthwith. However, when the initial treatment plan will not be altered by the availability of further diagnostic information, observation of the patient's response to early conservative treatment often will clarify the diagnosis. Whether the initial treatment plan will be affected in cases in which there is diagnostic doubt will depend largely on the individual clinicians' overall treatment philosophy.

Regarding TMD, differences in fundamental philosophy will have profound impact on whether, when, and how patients will be treated. This is most evident in the management of joint disorders. Recent literature indicates that most TMDs, including internal joint derangements, are usually benign and self-limiting.[44] With this in mind, many clinicians have adopted a conservative approach to treatment, with the goal of restoring comfortable jaw function by the simplest and preferably most reversible means possible. Others are more strongly oriented toward correcting anatomic or pathologic abnormalities presumably associated with symptoms. In other words, the former group is primarily concerned with treating subjective symptoms, whereas the latter is primarily concerned with treating objective findings. The latter philosophy assumes that the patient cannot function comfortably indefinitely if anatomic abnormalities, or deviations from the ideal, are not corrected. This notion is intuitively appealing but is not well supported by the TMD literature. As mentioned above, it appears that objective joint findings are rather poor predictors of pain or functional impairment. Although there is no doubt that derangements can be extremely painful and cause unacceptable functional limitations, such conditions do not occur in all patients; they appear to be an individual-specific, rather than a condition-specific, phenomenon. A parallel exists in medicine where it has been found that the epidemiologic correlations between detectable abnormalities or pathologies of the spine and incidence of back pain are weak.[45]

REFERENCES

1. Costen JB: Syndrome of ear and sinus symptoms dependent upon disturbed function of the temporomandibular joint. Ann Otol Rhinol Laryngol 43:1, 1934
2. Zimmerman AA: An evaluation of Costen's syndrome from an anatomic point of view. p. 82. In Sarnat BG (ed): The Temporomandibular Joint. Charles C. Thomas, Springfield, Illinois, 1951
3. Clark GT, Seligman DA, Solberg WK et al: Guidelines for the examination and diagnosis of temporomandibular disorders. J Craniomandib Disord Facial Oral Pain 3:7, 1989
4. Dworkin SF, LeResche L, DeRouen T et al: Assessing clinical signs of temporomandibular disorders: reliability of clinical examiners. J Prosthet Dent 63:574, 1990
5. Mohl ND, McCall WD, Lund JP, Plesh O: Devices for the diagnosis and treatment of temporomandibular disorders. Part I: introduction, scientific evidence, and jaw tracking. J Prosthet Dent 63:198, 1990
6. Pertes RA, Cohen HV: Guidelines for clinical management of temporomandibular disorders: part 1. Compend Contin Educ Dent 13:268, 1992
7. American Academy of Orofacial Pain, McNeill CE (ed): Temporomandibular Disorders, Guidelines for Classification, Assessment and Management. Quintessence, Chicago, 1993
8. Rugh JD, Solberg WK: Oral health status in the United States. Temporomandibular disorders. J Dent Educ 49:398, 1985
9. Schiffman E, Fricton JR: Epidemiology of TMJ and craniofacial pain. p. 1. In Fricton JR, Kroening RJ, Hathaway KM (eds): TMJ and Craniofacial Pain: Diagnosis and Management. IEA Publ, St. Louis, 1988
10. Headache Classification Committee of the International Headache Society: Classification and diagnostic criteria for headache disorders, cranial neuralgias and facial pain. Cephalalgia 8:1, 1988
11. American Academy of Craniomandibular Disorders: Craniomandibular Disorders, Guidelines for Evaluation, Diagnosis and Management. Quintessence, Chicago, 1990
12. American Academy of Pediatric Dentistry, University of Texas Health Science Center at San Antonio Dental School: Treatment of temporomandibular disorders in children: summary statements and recommendations. J Am Dent Assoc 120:265, 1990
13. Rasmussen BK, Jensen R, Olesen J: Questionnaire versus clinical interview in the diagnosis of headache. Headache 31:290, 1991
14. DeWeese DD: Differential diagnosis of dizziness and vertigo. p. 1871. In Paparella MM, Shumrick DA (eds): Otolaryngology. The Ear. Vol. II. 2nd Ed. WB Saunders, Philadelphia, 1980
15. Wolfe F, Smythe HA, Yunus MB et al: The American College of Rheumatology 1990 criteria for the classification of fibromyalgia: report of the multicenter criteria committee. Arthritis Rheum 33:160, 1990
16. Mohl ND, Lund JP, Widmer CG, McCall WD: Devices for the diagnosis and treatment of temporomandibular disorders. Part II: electromyography and sonography. J Prosthet Dent 63:332, 1990
17. Mohl ND, Orbach RK, Crow HC, Gross AJ: Devices for the diagnosis and treatment of temporomandibular disorders. Part III: thermography, ultrasound, electrical stimulation, and electromyographic biofeedback. J Prosthet Dent 63:472, 1990
18. Mohl ND, Orbach R: The dilemma of scientific knowledge versus clinical management of temporomandibular disorders. J Prosthet Dent 67:113, 1992

19. Takahashi A, Murakami S, Nishiyama H et al: The clinicoradiologic predictability of perforations of the soft tissue of the temporomandibular joint. Oral Surg Oral Med Oral Pathol 74:243, 1992

20. Sadako K, Hiroyuki K, Nakayama E et al: Clinical symptoms of open lock position of the condyle. Oral Surg Oral Med Oral Pathol 74:143, 1992

21. Paesani D, Westesson P-L, Hatala MP et al: Accuracy of clinical diagnosis for TMJ internal derangement and arthrosis. Oral Surg Oral Med Oral Pathol 73:360, 1992

22. Roberts C, Katzberg RW, Tallents RH et al: The clinical predictability of internal derangements of the temporomandibular joint. Oral Surg Oral Med Oral Pathol 71: 412, 1991

23. Roberts CA, Tallents RH, Espeland MA et al: Mandibular range of motion versus arthrographic diagnosis of the temporomandibular joint. Oral Surg Oral Med Oral Pathol 60:244, 1985

24. Roberts CA, Tallents RH, Katzberg RW et al: Clinical and arthrographic evaluation of the location of temporomandibular joint pain. Oral Surg Oral Med Oral Pathol 64:6, 1987

25. Westesson P-L, Eriksson L, Kurita K: Reliability of a negative clinical temporomandibular joint examination: prevalence of disk displacement in asymptomatic temporomandibular joints. Oral Surg Oral Med Oral Pathol 68:551, 1989

26. Benoit PW, Belt WD: Some effects of local anesthetic agents on skeletal muscle. Exp Neurol 34:264, 1972

27. Benoit PW: Reversible skeletal muscle damage after administration of local anesthetics with and without epinephrine. J Oral Surg 36:198, 1978

28. Benoit PW: Microscarring in skeletal muscle after repeated exposures to lidocaine with epinephrine. J Oral Surg 36:530, 1978

29. Travell JG, Simons DG: Apropos of all muscles. p. 45. In: Myofascial Pain and Dysfunction: The Trigger Point Manual. Williams & Wilkins, Baltimore, 1983

30. Miller CS, Thrash WJ, Glass BJ et al: Progressive deep muscle relaxation for the treatment of myofascial pain dysfunction. J Oral Med 42:216, 1987

31. Jones DA, Newham DJ, Obletter G, Giamberardino MA: Nature of exercise-induced muscle pain. p. 207. In Tiengo M, Eccles J, Cuello AC, Ottoson D (eds): Advances in Pain Research and Therapy. Pain and Mobility. Vol. 10. Raven Press, New York, 1987

32. Vecchiet L, Giamberardino MA, Marini I: Immediate muscular pain from physical activity. p. 193. In Tiengo M, Eccles J, Cuello AC, Ottoson D (eds): Advances in Pain Research and Therapy. Pain and Mobility. Vol. 10. Raven Press, New York, 1987

33. Hu JW, Sessle BJ, Raboisson P et al: Stimulation of craniofacial muscle afferents induces prolonged facilitory effects in trigeminal nociceptive brain-stem neurons. Pain 48:53, 1992

34. Stacey MJ: Free nerve endings in skeletal muscle of the cat. J Anat 105:231, 1969

35. Mense S, Meyer H: Different types of slowly conducting afferent units in cat skeletal muscle and tendon. J Physiol 363:403, 1985

36. Zenker W, Sandoz PA, Neuhuber W: The distribution of anterogradely labeled I–IV primary afferents in histochemically defined compartments of the rat's sternomastoid muscle. Anat Embryol 177:235, 1988

37. Eriksson P-O: Muscle-fibre composition of the human mandibular locomotor system. Enzyme-histochemical and morphological characteristics of functionally different parts. Swed Dent J (Suppl) 12:1, 1982

38. Nagy JI, Buss M, Daddona PE: On the innervation of trigeminal mesencephalic

primary afferent neurons by adenosine deaminase-containing projections from the hypothalamus in the rat. Neuroscience 17:141, 1986

39. Yamamoto T, Shiosaka S, Daddona PE, Nagy JI: Further observations on the relationship between adenosine deaminase-containing axons and trigeminal mesencephalic neurons: an electron microscopic, immunohistochemical and anterograde tracing study. Neuroscience 26:669, 1988
40. Wilson PR: Chronic neck pain and cervicogenic headache. Clin J Pain 7:5, 1991
41. Sjaastad O, Saunte C, Hovdal H et al: "Cervicogenic" headache: an hypothesis. Cephalalgia 3:249, 1983
42. Seligman DA, Pullinger AG: The role of intercuspal occlusal relationships in temporomandibular disorders: a review. J Craniomandib Disord Facial Oral Pain 5:96, 1991
43. Seligman DA, Pullinger AG: The role of functional occlusal relationships in temporomandibular disorders: a review. J Craniomandib Disord Facial Oral Pain 5: 265, 1991
44. Dworkin SF, Huggins KH, LeResche L et al: Epidemiology of signs and symptoms in temporomandibular disorders: clinical signs in cases and controls. J Am Dent Assoc 120:273, 1990
45. Haldeman S: Presidential address, North American Spine Society: failure of the pathology model to predict back pain. Spine 15:718, 1990

4 | Evaluation of Diagnostic Tests for TMD

Charles G. Widmer

As new developments are made toward understanding the pathology of TMDs, it becomes necessary to re-evaluate diagnostic techniques to verify their validity (accurately diagnose patients from nonpatients). This process occurs by various methods: one is an informal, less rigorous, nonscientific process that can only provide empirical conclusions regarding the diagnostic capability, and the other is a scientifically based process that uses well-defined patient samples, matched control groups, and standardized assessment protocols so that calculated values of measurement reliability and validity and diagnostic validity (i.e., sensitivity, specificity, and predictive values) can be used to compare the diagnostic abilities of various tests. More recently, it has become apparent that the scientifically based process is required to evaluate conditions such as chronic pain because there are no definitive assays that are available and it is easy to be misled by presumed etiologic factors when, in fact, no evidence exists for their role as a causative factor. Occlusion is a good example of this presumed etiologic factor in TMD, although there is no evidence to establish occlusal factors such as interferences or Angle classification as a primary cause for TMD.[1]

As an example of an informal, less rigorous process, Zeman[2] described four phases of evolution of diagnostic techniques. At first, the test evolves from anecdotal findings and descriptive research. As the test becomes popular, the second phase begins, during which it is touted as being superior to all conventional tests. In the third phase, a backlash occurs as the shortcomings of the new technique and its inferiority to prior tests are stressed. In the fourth and final phase, the true cost-effectiveness and impact on patient care are established. The test then either achieves general acceptance or is abandoned. Recognizing that this system of evaluation for diagnostic tests is commonly used, it is important to note that this process is not preferable to a well-structured method that is free of bias.

A more scientific approach to this problem of evaluation is to critically assess the diagnostic test to understand the true potential before its introduction as a clinical tool. This information should be provided by the manufacturers and should be based on data from well-controlled, blinded clinical trials. The specific information needed to assess the ability of the technique should include parameters of measurement reliability and validity as well as diagnostic reliability and validity. These topics are addressed in detail later in this chapter.

In discussing additional diagnostic tests for TMD, we must consider whether the test will provide new information to establish the diagnosis rather than duplicate existing information. All the tests that are discussed have been advocated for screening patients to separate TMD patients from asymptomatic subjects and are the focus of this discussion. When considering screening tests, it is imperative that the benefit of the test outweighs any potential risk for the patient under study. This includes physical risks, psychological risks or financial risks. As an example of physical risks, if the diagnostic test involves ionizing radiation, is the benefit of screening for the disease far better than the actual disease? If one is considering a life-threatening disease such as cancer in a population known to be at high risk, then the answer would be positive. However, for chronic musculoskeletal conditions such as TMD, which are not life-threatening and are cyclic and self-limiting, unnecessary screening tests that involve radiation are inappropriate.

Another issue to consider is the psychological aspects of screening tests. If the diagnostic test has a high degree of false-positive diagnoses (i.e., incorrectly identifying a normal as diseased), then the use of such a test can sensitize normal individuals to constantly seek treatment for a condition that either does not exist or has no association with their pain complaint. For many patients with pain, reinforcement of a physical explanation for their pain problem is commonplace among health care practitioners and, for some patients, may cause the patient to become psychosocially dysfunctional.[3] For example, many patients who were told that their pain problem was caused by a particular aspect of their occlusion were treated by occlusal rehabilitation and later became "occlusophobics," who continuously demanded occlusal treatment for their minor masticatory musculoskeletal pain conditions. Therefore, it is imperative that the assessment techniques are based on current knowledge regarding the etiology and pathophysiology of TMD to minimize the *creation* of chronic pain patients. Our current knowledge does not support an identified etiologic factor for chronic musculoskeletal pain conditions, and our treatment strategies are directed toward management of symptomatology. So it becomes increasingly difficult to accept a new screening diagnostic test when there are no identified etiologic factors to be targeted.

The cost of diagnostic tests must also be a primary consideration when evaluating patients. As previously stated, it is important that diagnostic tests provide new, supplementary information necessary for diagnosis of a condition, not just confirm or repeat the results of the primary evaluation. Using electronic instruments to amplify and record TMJ sounds would be an example of a test that is more expensive than using direct palpation or a stethoscope, but the results and how they are used for diagnosis are no different. Therefore, risk issues are important to consider when screening tests are to applied to the general population for discovery of disease.

RELIABILITY AND VALIDITY OF DIAGNOSTIC TESTS

Evaluation of diagnostic tests have been described in detail,[4-6] and there are standard measures that can be calculated to determine the efficacy of the test. Unfortunately, there are few studies in the literature of TMD that fulfill the requirement of a well-conducted clinical trial or epidemiologic study so that these values can be calculated. For conditions of chronic pain, it is essential to account for potential sources of bias when evaluating TMD diagnostic tests, and this can only be accomplished with well-designed studies.

The theoretical basis of a diagnostic test should also be examined when considering the applicability of the test. Tests that measure factors directly related to the etiology of the condition (not the result of the condition) are the ones that will have the greatest application. Unfortunately, these tests do not exist for TMDs because an etiologic factor (or factors) has not been identified.

Various measures of reliability and validity can provide some indication of the ability of the diagnostic test. The measurement process of the instrument must have the ability to be repeated over time *(measurement reliability)* and must provide an accurate measure of the phenomenon *(measurement validity)*. For example, measuring the distance between two bony landmarks on a cephalometric radiograph of a patient using calipers will provide a measure that can be repeated over time and will be very reliable and, therefore, has high measurement reliability. This is because there is no variation of the bony landmarks in the radiograph. However, the validity of the actual measure is not good because of the 12 percent magnification of the skull in the film, and all radiograph measures would have to be corrected by this factor to approach the *true* distance between the landmarks, assuming that they are in the same two-dimensional plane as the cephalometric radiograph. So, in this example, one can repeatedly obtain measurements that are nearly the same, but they do not accurately represent the true phenomenon that is desired to be measured. This example emphasizes that measurement reliability and measurement validity are two very important parameters that need to be examined and verified before using the measurement as a basis for diagnosis.

Once a reliable and valid measure can be obtained, assessment of diagnostic validity can be performed. Diagnostic validity is determined by measuring a characteristic or parameter in a group having the disease under study and comparing these measurements to an appropriately selected control group that does not have signs and symptoms of the disorder. Appropriate selection means that individuals in the control group should have as much similarity to the patient group as possible (e.g., same proportion of males and females, similar age range).

Determining that there are statistically significant differences between two groups, such as a patient and control group, does *not* establish that the test has diagnostic validity. The value of a diagnostic test depends on its ability to identify those who are really suffering from the disease *(sensitivity)* and also be able to identify successfully members of the general population who do not have the disease *(specificity)*. A perfect test has a sensitivity of 1.0 (it correctly found 100 percent of the patients) *and* a specificity of 1.0. However, when the measurements from the two groups overlap, sensitivity and specificity cannot both be 1.0. The actual sensitivity and specificity of each test are determined by where one draws the line (cutoff) that separates the two populations. The cutoff criteria are adjusted according to the nature of the test. For instance, if the diagnostic test is for a potentially fatal disease, sensitivity should be set very high to maximize the number of correct diagnoses of the patients, even if the number of false-positive diagnoses is very high because of low specificity. However, TMDs are conditions of low morbidity. It is therefore important not to subject normal individuals to unnecessary treatment by misdiagnosing them as diseased. Specificity, therefore, needs to be very high.

Finally, the performance of any screening test depends on the prevalence

Population of 100 people
Prevalence of TMD = 12%, therefore 12 diseased and 88 non-diseased people
Sensitivity of Dx test = 0.50
Specificity of Dx test = 0.50

	Diseased	Non-Diseased
Positive Dx	6	44
Negative Dx	6	44
Total	12	88

$$\text{Sensitivity} = \frac{\text{true positives}}{\text{total diseased}} = \frac{6}{12} = 50\% \text{ or } 0.50$$

$$\text{Specificity} = \frac{\text{true negatives}}{\text{total non-diseased}} = \frac{44}{88} = 50\% \text{ or } 0.50$$

$$\text{Positive Predictive Value (PPV)} = \frac{\text{true positives}}{\text{total positives}} = \frac{6}{6 + 44} = 12\% \text{ or } 0.12$$

Fig. 4-1.   An example of calculating sensitivity, specificity and positive predictive value using an assumed prevalence rate and sensitivity and specificity of the diagnostic test.

of the disease being studied. The most important measure of this performance is the *positive predictive value* (PPV) of the test. To calculate this value, the proportion of true-positive and false-positive diagnoses are adjusted for the prevalence of the disease. The prevalence of TMD is approximately 12 percent or less of the general population.[7] Therefore, if the ability to diagnose patients from nonpatients was essentially random (or the flip of a coin = 0.50), then the PPV would only be 0.12 (or the prevalence of the disease in the population). An example of the calculations for sensitivity, specificity, and PPV is shown in Figure 4-1. Most of the techniques other than those used in the "gold standard" (history, clinical examination such as palpable joint and muscle tenderness) do not have a PPV much greater than 0.12 (random selection) and, therefore, do not provide additional diagnostic information to distinguish patient from nonpatient.

ASSESSMENT OF VARIOUS DIAGNOSTIC TECHNIQUES FOR TMD

The following sections examine the measurement and diagnostic capabilities of various techniques that have been suggested to screen for TMD. Whenever possible, theoretical validity is assessed to determine if a scientific basis is supported for use of the technique.

Mandibular Kinesiology

Reduced mandibular movement has been classically used as a diagnostic criterion for TMD.[8] A restriction of the range of motion (ROM) caused by an arthrogenous condition such as a disc displacement without reduction or muscular co-contraction in the presence of pain[9] supports the theoretical validity of measuring mandibular movement. Manual measurements using a millimeter ruler have been reported for large population studies of TMD patients and asymptomatic individuals[7] and have also been assessed for measurement reliability and validity. Electronic instruments have also been marketed to assess mandibular ROM as well as other parameters including speed of movement, anterior/vertical ratio, regularity of movement, vertical freeway space, closure trajectory, and chewing movements. However, there is very little information on the measurement reliability and validity of these electronic instruments, and the information that is available documents significant error in the measurement validity. For example, one instrument has a vertical error range of 3 to 31 percent and an oblique error range of 1 to 66 percent,[10] whereas another instrument has a vertical error range of 9.4 to 30 percent and a z-axis error up to 15 percent.[11] However, millimeter rulers have high measurement reliability and validity.[12–14]

With the exception of opening amplitude, all other movement parameters have low sensitivity or specificity levels and PPVs that range from 0.11 to 0.15.

Table 4-1. Jaw Movement

Diagnostic Test	Cutoff Value	Sensitivity	Specificity	PPV
Opening amplitude[7]				
Male	35 mm	0.216	0.978	0.58
Female	30 mm	0.218	0.975	0.59
Speed of movement[52,53]	300 mm/sec	—	0.24	—
	250 mm/sec	1.0	0.20	0.15
Anterior/vertical ratio[53]	1:2	0.86	0.30	0.14
Chewing movements[53]	Descriptive	0.26	0.70	0.11
Dyskinesia	No data	No data	No data	No data

These are unacceptable levels and document the inability to distinguish asymptomatic individuals (low specificity) and cannot predict a patient status with a positive test (low PPV) any better than random selection. Reviews of sensitivity and specificity have been reported elsewhere,[15,16] and a summary of these values is shown in Table 4-1. Therefore, use of jaw tracking instrumentation does not improve the accuracy of measurement and, in fact, consistently underestimates the mandibular movement. Consequently, if a clinician compares these values with normative values, the patient will be classified as limited mandibular movement when it may be normal. This can lead to overdiagnosis of TMD conditions. The low specificity values of other parameters calculated from electronic mandibular movement recordings will also incorrectly identify normal patients as abnormal and can also lead to an overdiagnosis of TMD. These limitations of the technique do not support their use in clinical practice.

Surface Electromyography

Electromyography (EMG) has been suggested as a clinical tool to assess the status of the jaw musculature by classifying electrical activity recorded by surface electrodes as normal or abnormal. Muscle hyperactivity, spasm, and imbalance have been suggested in the dental literature for many years as a major feature of TMD patients, but evidence to support such concepts is lacking.[15,17,18] Moreover, other chronic muscle pain conditions such as fibromyalgia, myofascial pain, chronic lower back pain, and tension headache also lack evidence of muscle hyperactivity and spasm and have been reviewed in detail.[9] In fact, the lack of evidence was so compelling for tension headache that the International Headache Classification Committee of the International Headache Society renamed the category of "tension headache" to "tension-type headache" because no association was found from multiple studies of muscle contraction levels and headaches.[19] This gradual realization of the lack of muscle hyperactivity in chronic muscle pain conditions has overcome a long history of assumptions, proclamations, and conjectures since Travell introduced the pain–spasm cycle theory in the 1940s.[20]

The problems in the methodology of recording surface EMG in masticatory muscle disorders has been described previously.[17] Briefly, the need to control for such parameters as age, sex, facial form, and history of bruxism is essential to allow for comparison of absolute EMG levels. Bruxism is very important because these patients have a higher level of resting EMG activity.[21] Normalizing levels to the maximum voluntary contraction (MVC) is inappropriate for patients with facial pain because their MVC decreases during the pain episode and does not provide a common denominator for normalizing muscle activity.[17] Newer evidence has also documented the need to consider facial expression (recruiting facial muscles) as a source of additional EMG levels recorded by surface electrodes.[22,23] Facial muscle activity increases during emotional conditions of sadness and anger as well as pain in chronic pain patients.[24–26]

In dentistry, as in other allied health professions, the need to document the status of the patient as accurately and objectively as possible is the goal of every practitioner. However, measuring the EMG activity of a patient with palpable muscle tenderness does not provide the "objective" assessment of muscle function that has been promoted by many advocates and does not discriminate those patients from the ones without muscle pain. The ability of EMG to discriminate patients from nonpatients is shown in Table 4-2 and illustrates the lack of discrimination of the nonpatient group using the criteria suggested by the instrument manufacturers. In the only study where PPV could be calculated, it is no better than the prevalence in the population. Therefore, the use of EMG as a diagnostic indicator of muscle status is contraindicated based on the evidence of well-controlled clinical studies.

Electrical Stimulation Devices

Devices have been advocated to stimulate the jaw muscles and move the mandible into a more "physiologic" position to establish the "correct neuromuscular position" of the condyle in the fossa and the appropriate interdigitation of the teeth. This concept has been challenged many times in the literature because there has been no evidence to support direct neural stimulation of the motor root of the fifth cranial nerve by their technique.[27–30] Recent evidence has demonstrated that the stimulation paradigm only recruits the ef-

Table 4-2. Electromyography

Diagnostic Test	Cutoff Value	Sensitivity	Specificity	PPV
Resting EMG[52,54]	EM1 = 10 μV EM2 = 2.5 μV	0.89	0.19	0.13
Resting EMG[55]	EM2 = 2.5 μV	No data	0.0	No data
"Balanced" muscle function[52]	Not defined	No data	0.19	No data
Maximum clench levels	160 μV	No data	No data	No data

Table 4-3. Electrical Stimulation Devices

Diagnostic Test	Cutoff Value	Sensitivity	Specificity	PPV
Freeway space before stimulation[52,54]	<0.75 mm or >2.0 mm	0.42	0.62	0.17
Freeway space after stimulation[52,54]	<0.75 mm or >2.0 mm	0.76	0.19	0.11
Stimulated versus habitual trajectory[52,54]	Not defined	0.75	0.27	0.12

ferents (motor axons) of the masseteric nerve or, at higher levels of stimulation, directly stimulates the muscle fibers.[29] No other muscles of mastication were found to be directly or indirectly recruited, and therefore, the mandibular position achieved by this technique is completely dependent on the orientation of the superficial muscle fibers of the masseter muscle. This would account for the more anterior position of the mandible because of the anterior inclination of the superficial masseter muscle fibers. Facial muscles underlying the stimulating electrodes are also recruited during stimulation and, to a lesser degree, will affect mandibular position. Recruitment of the masseter muscles and various nearby facial muscles does *not* establish a "physiologic" jaw position and should not be used as an indicator of mandibular misalignment and does *not* document the need for occlusal or mandibular repositioning. Nor do these instruments indicate variation of mandibular rest position. The diagnostic ability of electrical stimulating devices is shown in Table 4-3 and have low sensitivity, specificity, and PPV levels. Therefore, there is no indication for their use in diagnosis of muscle-related conditions.

Sonography and Doppler Ultrasound

TMJ sounds have been included in the definition of TMD for many years. However, recent information from cross-sectional and longitudinal studies of patient populations with TMJ sounds[7,31,32] have led some authors to question the diagnostic validity of joint sounds and their relationship to painful TMJ or masticatory muscle conditions.[15,18,32–34] Evidence of joint sounds as a part of the pathophysiology of TMD still remains unresolved. If the estimate that 33 to 65 percent of the asymptomatic population has some form of TMJ sounds is accurate and that patients with clicks followed longitudinally become click-free rather than locked (disc displacement without reduction) on a 2:1 ratio,[31] then there is lack of support for clicking joints as a vital part of the pathophysiology of TMDs. Also, painful clicking joints can be treated to a nonpain condition yet the clicking pattern persists, suggesting that a cause-and-effect relationship between the chronic clicking joint and pain does not exist.

The consistency of joint sounds from one measurement to the next in the same individual has been found to be highly variable.[35] The instability of this measure combined with the lack of agreement among examiners to common sounds heard on a tape recording suggest that this measure may have too much variability to be of diagnostic value.[35,36] Other sources of sounds that are unrelated to the joint may also contribute to the perception or recording detected by various techniques (palpation, auscultation, sonography, electrovibratography). Examples include skin and hair sounds, blood flow, respiration, and room sounds. In fact, in one study, Gallo et al[37] detected sounds by a microphone over the TMJ even without moving the mandible. These contaminating sources must be identified, particularly in techniques that do not use the human perception of an examiner to identify the background sounds.

Another aspect to joint sounds that has been used diagnostically is the timing of the occurrence of the sound (such as a click) during the opening and closing movement of the mandible. This method has been described as a means for discriminating the reciprocal click associated with a disc displacement with reduction from other joint conditions. The reciprocal click is identified as a pair of clicks; the first is detected during mandibular opening and the second is detected at a smaller vertical dimension than the opening click during the closing movement. Many times the closing click is difficult to detect unless the joint is loaded to accentuate sound or vibration from the articular tissues. Crepitus can also be detected during the full range of mandibular movement and has been positively correlated with osteoarthritic or osteoarthritic changes in the TMJ.[38] Unfortunately, the presence of crepitus remains even after the arthritic processes have subsided within the joint. Thus, distinct crepitus is only indicative of bony remodeling of the joint and cannot be used to stage the disease process. Also, extensive bony remodeling in the TMJ can even be present without joint sounds, further complicating the diagnostic process.[38,39]

Identification of specific types of clicks or other joint sounds such as crepitus may aid in subdividing the TMD patient population, but it still remains unclear whether the basic issue of TMJ sounds can be used as diagnostic criteria for TMD, particularly when the patient is pain-free. Given the high prevalence of TMJ sounds in the asymptomatic population and the observations that most sounds (clicks or crepitus) do not progress to a painful involvement of the TMJ, using sonography as a predictive test for TMD, is unfounded. It has long been assumed that joint sounds, clicks in particular, must be treated before they progress to degenerative joint disease (DJD). However, without the longitudinal data to support this hypothesis, TMJ sounds should be regarded as variation of normal. Further, these sounds have not been shown to affect the prognosis and have not reliably improved with treatment interventions.[40] Altogether, it would seem that TMJ sounds, by themselves, have no predictive, screening, or differential diagnostic capability and may mislead a clinician to a diagnosis of TMD rather than aid in establishing the presence of active disease or dysfunction. The summary of different joint sounds and their diagnostic significance is shown in Table 4-4.

In summary, existing evidence does not support the use of sonography for diagnosis of TMD pathophysiology and, in fact, can distract the clinician by emphasizing structural incongruities that may occur as a part of normal variation. Because joint sounds may be present in patients without pain or dys-

Table 4-4. TMJ Sounds

Diagnostic Test	Cutoff Value	Sensitivity	Specificity	PPV
Digital palpation	Presence of click	0.43	0.75	0.19
Digital palpation	Presence of crepitus	0.08	0.92	0.12
Digital palpation	Presence of grating	0.06	0.99	0.45
Digital palpation	Presence of any sound	0.57	0.66	0.19

(Data from Dworkin et al.[7])

function in at least one-third of the normal population, diagnosis of intracapsular conditions should be based on clinical presentation (e.g., history of pain, masticatory functional pain) and clinical examination (e.g., palpable joint or muscle tenderness).

Thermography

Thermography is the measurement of the temperature of a body and is expressed as hot or cold relative to a standard. Heat, as a form of temperature, can be transferred by conduction or radiation, and devices measure heat by one of these processes. For example, heat conduction is measured by thermometers, thermocouples, and contact liquid crystal thermographic units, whereas radiation of heat is measured by infrared detectors or electromagnetic detection. The use of thermography for detection of surface facial temperature abnormalities has been based on the premise that altered blood flow occurs in cutaneous, subcutaneous, or underlying structures that directly affect the temperature measured on the skin surface. Usually, side-to-side comparisons are made to determine asymmetric temperature distributions and differences of 0.5 to 1.0°C are considered to be asymmetric. The protocol requires that the patient be equilibrated to a room temperature of 22 to 25°C, and then three thermograms separated by 10- to 15-minute intervals are usually recorded to determine the consistency of the surface temperature.[41] Various external factors have been identified that can affect the measurement, such as sunburn, smoking, and skin lotions.

As with any diagnostic technique, the theoretical basis for using thermography to diagnose painful muscle and TMJ conditions must be established. The presumed basis for detecting hot areas on the surface of the skin overlying the masseter and TMJs is that inflammation is present in these structures and, by thermal conduction or radiation, it can be accurately detected by the thermographic technique[42,43] or the condition causes cutaneous vasomotor activity reflected as localized changes in cutaneous blood flow.[43,44] Some authors have equated the presence of increased skin temperature as a diagnostic sign for muscular pain conditions due to involvement of the autonomic system.[44] However, there are no data to support this assertion, and a recent study demonstrated the lack of correlation of active myofascial trigger points and hot spots observed on the upper back.[45]

Most of the studies evaluating thermograms of the face used either liquid crystal thermography or infrared thermography. Both of these techniques are routinely used with a resolution of 0.5 to 1.0°C because a greater sensitivity would produce thermograms that showed asymmetry in both patients and normals.[46] Unfortunately, most of the asymmetries that have been reported for various TMD conditions are less than 0.5°C.[47]

Given the small temperature differential (0.1 to 1.0°C) and the large amount of overlap of the facial surface temperatures of patients and controls, thermography cannot adequately distinguish between these groups as shown by the low PPVs. Also, facial temperatures do not necessarily rise in the presence of a TMD condition. For example, three studies reported a *decrease* of surface temperature for the skin overlying painful jaw muscles rather than an increase.[42,43,48] This variability of presentation further confounds the diagnosis of TMD conditions.

The vast majority of the studies evaluating facial thermography have not been properly conducted. For example, most studies fail to describe the diagnostic criteria for TMD patients, fail to describe how the thermograms are quantitatively compared, fail to provide detailed results of their study, fail to have a control group, or were biased in their assessment of the thermograms by previously reviewing the patient's symptomatology.[41-44,49] One study, which deserves more attention, has evaluated both asymptomatic subjects and defined TMD patients in a blinded manner so that the evaluator of the liquid crystal thermograms had no information regarding the clinical history of the patients.[47] This study evaluated asymptomatic controls, asymptomatic sides of patients, painless clicks, painful TMJs, myofascial pain, or patients with a combination of myofascial pain and painful TMJs. Statistically significant differences of mean surface temperatures of the masseter, TMJ, and temporalis were found for the patients with myofascial pain, painful TMJs, or a combination of the two when compared with controls. These differences ranged from 0.10 to 0.97°C, and standard deviations ranged from 0.61 to 0.95. The mean surface temperature differences found between patients and controls in this study, although statistically difficult, cannot be used diagnostically because there is substantial overlap of the measures from the control group and the various patient groups. Unfortunately, no data are available to calculate sensitivity, specificity, and PPV. Therefore, at the current time there is no support for the use of thermography to diagnose various conditions affecting the TMJ or masticatory muscles.

Although various proponents of thermography claim that this technique can distinguish muscle conditions, TMJ conditions such as internal derangement, specific headache patterns, reflex sympathetic dystrophy, or atypical odontalgia, the data are either lacking or have not been evaluated in a population of pain patients with different conditions.[50,51] Discriminating normal subjects from these different pain conditions have shown unacceptable sensitivity and specificity levels.

Some preliminary studies have described surface temperatures to change to more symmetric patterns after resolution of the TMD condition for 80 percent of the patients that were evaluated and treated.[42,43] However, none of these studies have described the basis on which they quantitate the symmetry or asymmetry. Also, it is unclear that the temperature variations actually reflect the underlying disease process. Instead, it may be an indirect response to the patient's pain or other conditions such as stress. Better studies are required to establish any relationship of the changes in the thermogram and the painful TMD condition.

In summary, studies evaluating surface temperature as a method to diagnose various TMD conditions have reported small (0.1 to 1.0°C) differences between patient and nonpatient samples. However, because of the substantial overlap of thermal measurements from masseter, TMJ, or temporalis of both patient and nonpatient groups, resulting in low PPVs, use of thermography as a diagnostic technique is not supported. Side-to-side comparisons to evaluate asymmetry have an even lower thermal difference (0.1 to 0.5°C), and this thermal difference is lower than the sensitivity of the thermographic techniques that are advocated. Finally, many studies have demonstrated that facial temperatures of TMD patients can decrease rather than increase at specific sites such as the masseter and further confounds the use of surface temperature as a diagnostic test for TMD.

Algometer or Pain Threshold Meter

Algometers have been used to measure the pressure exerted by the examiner for assessing reliability and validity of joint and muscle palpation assessment techniques for TMD.[14] For examination of large populations, such as during an epidemiologic study, algometers provide the necessary standardization required to compare findings of different examiners. For routine clinical examination, however, the use of these instruments may not provide any additional diagnostic information to the clinician over traditional manual techniques. The assessment of palpable muscle or joint tenderness will depend on the amount of pressure used, the site and direction of palpation, the area of surface contact, and the anatomic knowledge of the practitioner. Although algometers can help to establish a uniform surface area and palpation pressure, the site and direction and anatomic correlation remain the judgment of the clinician. Therefore, the use of algometers (or some means of calibrating examiners) is a requirement to standardize examiners in research studies, but no advantages have been documented for routine clinical use in diagnosis.

FALLACIES OF TREATMENT SUCCESS AS DIAGNOSTIC INDICATORS

In chronic pain conditions, it is imperative to conduct well-controlled studies to investigate the etiology of the condition because of multiple factors that can also affect the effectiveness and intensity of the pain. For example, increasing the patient's ability for pain control (through some form of treatment) or coping skills (through education) can affect a patient's pain report. Similarly, the time of day or the amount of sleep can also affect pain perception. This makes the interpretation of clinical reports of treatment success and, by inference an association of cause and effect, to be misleading and uninformative. In dentistry during the past 30 to 40 years, such reports have been the mainstay for suggesting that occlusion is the primary etiology for TMD. Proof for such a concept has been suggested from the success of occlusal equilibration and intraoral appliance therapy. However, treatment success cannot be the standard for assessing etiologies of chronic pain conditions. This naive approach has led to many clinical concepts that are now considered unsupported in medical and dental literature and should no longer be accepted as proof of cause and effect for pain conditions.

THE "GOLD STANDARD"

So what is the "gold standard" to use as a base for comparison of newer diagnostic screening assessment techniques? Essentially, diagnosis of a masticatory musculoskeletal condition requires a thorough history to determine a recent experience of pain and/or sudden mandibular restriction and a clinical examination that involves palpation of joint and muscle to duplicate the patient's pain report and isolate it to the masticatory musculoskeletal system. Because joint sounds can occur in asymptomatic patients who do not progress to a pain condition and because mandibular ROM of symptomatic and asymptomatic patients also has a high degree of overlap, consideration of these signs as independent diagnostic indicators for TMD should be viewed with caution.

The documentation of a thorough history and clinical examination (which may include TMJ imaging as necessary) provides the clinician with the necessary information to make an assessment for TMD and provides a baseline for subsequent re-evaluations of the patient. This documentation also supports the clinician during any cases of litigation because it accurately reflects the clinician's historical perspective based on the patient interview and the patient's clinical presentation based on the clinical examination to establish the diagnosis.

CONCLUSION

Diagnosis of TMD and facial pain conditions should be based on a comprehensive history of the patient's disorder combined with a thorough clinical examination. The examination should include examination of the masticatory musculoskeletal system and other systems such as adjacent musculoskeletal systems (e.g., cervical spine) and neurologic, vascular, or otolaryngologic systems to determine the source(s) of the patient's complaint. Imaging of the masticatory skeletal system may also be obtained as necessary to establish the diagnosis. At the present time, adjunctive tests such as electronic mandibular kinesiology, EMG, electrical stimulation devices, sonography, or thermography do not provide additional diagnostic information over that gained during a comprehensive clinical examination. In fact, use of these instruments may allow overdiagnosis of TMDs and subsequent overtreatment of asymptomatic patients.

There is a need to continually refine the definition of TMDs to more accurately reflect the characteristics of the condition, and this may be achieved by examining asymptomatic patient populations and establishing subcategories of the musculoskeletal condition. We may find that the relative importance of signs and symptoms included in traditional definitions of TMD (TMJ sounds, restriction of mandibular motion, palpable joint or masticatory muscle tenderness) need to be modified to simply history of pain in the masticatory system and palpable joint or muscle tenderness to exclude asymptomatic individuals from unnecessary treatment. However, we must use caution in developing new diagnostic strategies and maintain the overview that the need for diagnosis implies that specific treatment strategies exist for specific diagnostic classifications.

REFERENCES

1. Magnusson T, Enbom L: Signs and symptoms of mandibular dysfunction after introduction of experimental balancing-side interferences. Acta Odontol Scand 42: 129, 1984
2. Zeman RK: Foreword. Radiol Clin North Am 23:379, 1985
3. Dworkin SF: Illness behavior and dysfunction: review of concepts and application to chronic pain. Can J Physiol Pharmacol 69:662, 1991
4. Swets JA: Measuring the accuracy of diagnostic systems. Science 240:1285, 1988
5. Begg CB: Statistical methods in medical diagnosis. Crit Rev Med Inform 1:1, 1986
6. McNeil BJ, Keller E, Adelstein SJ: Primer on certain elements of medical decision making. N Engl J Med 293:211, 1975
7. Dworkin SF, Huggins KH, Le Resche L et al: Epidemiology of signs and symptoms in temporomandibular disorders: clinical signs in cases and controls. J Am Dent Assoc 120:273, 1990
8. Griffiths RH: Report of the president's conference on the examination, diagnosis, and management of temporomandibular disorders. J Am Dent Assoc 106:75, 1983
9. Lund JP, Donga R, Widmer CG, Stohler CS: The pain-adaptation model: a discussion of the relationship between chronic musculoskeletal pain and motor activity. Can J Physiol Pharmacol 69:683, 1991
10. Throckmorton GS, Teenier TJ, Ellis E: Reproducibility of mandibular motion and muscle activity levels using a commercial computer recording system. J Prosthet Dent 68:348, 1992
11. Tsolka P, Woelfel JB, Man WK, Preiskel HW: A laboratory assessment of recording reliability and analysis of the K6 diagnostic system. J Craniomandib Disord Facial Oral Pain 6:273, 1992
12. Dworkin SF, Le Resche L, Derouen T: Reliability of clinical measurement in temporomandibular disorders. Clin J Pain 4:88, 1988
13. Dworkin SF, LeResche L, Derouen T, Von Korff MR: Assessing clinical signs of temporomandibular disorders: reliability of clinical examiners. J Prosthet Dent 63: 574, 1990

14. Goulet J, Clark GT: Clinical TMJ examination methods. J Calif Dent Assoc 18:25, 1990
15. Widmer CG, Lund JP, Feine JS: Evaluation of diagnostic tests for TMD. J Calif Dent Assoc 18:53, 1990
16. Mohl ND, McCall WD Jr, Lund JP, Plesh O: Devices for the diagnosis and treatment of temporomandibular disorders. Part I: introduction, scientific evidence, and jaw tracking. J Prosthet Dent 63:198, 1990
17. Lund JP, Widmer CG: An evaluation of the use of surface electromyography in the diagnosis, documentation and treatment of dental patients. J Craniomandib Disord Facial Oral Pain 3:125, 1989
18. Mohl ND, Lund JP, Widmer CG, McCall WD Jr: Devices for the diagnosis and treatment of temporomandibular disorders. Part II: electromyography and sonography. J Prosthet Dent 63:332, 1990
19. Headache Classification Committee of the International Headache Society: Classification and diagnostic criteria for headache disorders, cranial neuralgias and facial pain. Cephalgia 8 (Suppl. 7):1, 1988
20. Travell J, Rinzler S, Herman M: Pain and disability of the shoulder and arm. Treatment by intramuscular infiltration with procaine hydrochloride. JAMA 120:417, 1942
21. Sherman RA: Relationships between jaw pain and jaw muscle contraction level: underlying factors and treatment effectiveness. J Prosthet Dent 54:114, 1985
22. Lund JP, Stohler CS, Widmer CG: The relationship between pain and muscle activity in fibromyalgia and similar conditions. p. 307. In Vaeroy H, Merskey H (eds): Progress in Fibromyalgia and Myofascial Pain. Elsevier Science Publishers B. V., Amsterdam, 1993
23. Large RG, Lamb AM: Electromyographic (EMG) feedback in chronic musculoskeletal pain: a controlled trial. Pain 17:167, 1983
24. Schwartz GE, Fair PL, Salt P et al: Facial expression and imagery in depression: an electromyographic study. Psychosom Med 38:337, 1976
25. Schwartz GE, Fair PL, Salt P et al: Facial muscle patterning to affective imagery in depressed and nondepressed subjects. Science 192:489, 1976
26. Tassinary LG, Cacioppo JT, Geen TR: A psychometric study of surface electrode placements for facial electromyographic recording: I. The brow and cheek muscle regions. Psychophysiology 26:1, 1989
27. Bessette RW, Quinlivan JT: Electromyographic evaluation for the Myo-monitor. J Prosthet Dent 30:19, 1973
28. De Boever JA, McCall WD Jr: Physiological aspects of masticatory muscle stimulation: the Myo-monitor. Quintessence Int 3:57, 1972
29. Dao TTT, Feine JS, Lund JP: Can electrical stimulation be used to establish a physiologic occlusal position. J Prosthet Dent 60:509, 1988
30. Mohl ND, Ohrbach RK, Crow HC, Gross AJ: Devices for the diagnosis and treatment of temporomandibular disorders. Part III: thermography, ultrasound, electrical stimulation, and EMG biofeedback. J Prosthet Dent 63:472, 1990
31. Lundh H, Westesson P-L, Kopp S: A three year follow-up of patients with reciprocal temporomandibular joint clicking. Oral Surg Oral Med Oral Pathol 63:530, 1987
32. Greene CS, Laskin DM: Long-term status of TMJ clicking in patients with myofascial pain and dysfunction. J Am Dent Assoc 117:461, 1988
33. Widmer CG: Temporomandibular joint sounds: a critique of techniques for recording and analysis. J Craniomandib Disord Facial Oral Pain 3:213, 1989

34. Widmer CG: Reliability and validation of examination methods. J Craniomandib Disord Facial Oral Pain 6:318, 1992
35. Truelove E, LeResche L, Sommers E et al: Reliability of TMJ sounds in patients and controls. J Dent Res 66:336, 1987 (Abstract)
36. Eriksson L, Westesson P-L, Sjoberg H: Observer performance in describing temporomandibular joint sounds. J Craniomandib Pract 5:32, 1987
37. Gallo LM, Airoldi R, Ernst B, Palla S: TMJ sounds: quantitative spectral analysis of asymptomatic subjects. J Dent Res 70:371, 1991 (Abstract)
38. Rohlin M, Westesson P-L, Eriksson L: The correlation of temporomandibular joint sounds with joint morphology in fifty-five autopsy specimens. J Oral Maxillofac Surg 43:194, 1985.
39. Eriksson L, Westesson P-L, Rohlin M: Temporomandibular joint sounds in patients with disc displacement. Int J Oral Surg 14:428, 1985
40. Clark GT: A critical evaluation of orthopedic interocclusal appliance therapy: effectiveness for specific symptoms. J Am Dent Assoc 108:364, 1984
41. Weinstein SA, Weinstein G: The validation of TMJ dysfunction with standardized computerized electronic thermography. Mod Med 55 (Special Ed): 35, 1987
42. Berry DC, Yemm R: A further study of facial temperature in patients with mandibular dysfunctions. J Oral Rehabil 1:255, 1974
43. Steed PA: The utilization of contact liquid crystal thermography in the evaluation of temporomandibular dysfunction. J Craniomandib Pract 9:120, 1991
44. Weinstein SA, Weinstein G, Weinstein EL, Gelb M: Facial thermography, basis, protocol, and clinical value. J Craniomandib Pract 9:201, 1991
45. Swerdlow B, Dieter JNI: An evaluation of the sensitivity and specificity of medical thermography for the documentation of myofascial trigger points. Pain 48:205, 1992
46. Gratt BM, Pullinger AG, Sickles EA, Lee JJ: Electronic thermography of normal facial structures: a pilot study. Oral Surg Oral Med Oral Pathol 68:346, 1989
47. Pogrel MA, Erbez G, Taylor RC, Dodson TB: Liquid crystal thermography as a diagnostic aid and objective monitor for TMJ dysfunction and myogenic facial pain. J Craniomandib Disord Facial Oral Pain 3:65, 1989
48. Finney JW, Holt CR, Pearce KB: Thermographic diagnosis of temporomandibular joint disease and associated neuromuscular disorders. Postgrad Med 79 (Special Ed): 93, 1986
49. Berry DC, Yemm R: Variations in skin temperature of the face in normal subjects and in patients with mandibular dysfunction. Br J Oral Surg 8:242, 1971
50. Farman AG: Electronic thermography in the diagnosis of atypical odontalgia: a pilot study. Oral Surg Oral Med Oral Pathol 68:472, 1989
51. Gratt BM, Sickles EA, Ross JB: Electronic thermography in the assessment of internal derangement of the temporomandibular joint. Oral Surg Oral Med Oral Pathol 71:364, 1991
52. Cooper BC, Rabuzzi DD: Myofacial pain dysfunction syndrome: a clinical study of asymptomatic subjects. Laryngoscope 94:68, 1984
53. Feine JS, Hutchins MO, Lund JP: An evaluation of the criteria used to diagnose mandibular dysfunction with the mandibular kinesiograph. J Prosthet Dent 60:374, 1988
54. Cooper BC, Alleva M, Cooper DL, Lucente FE: Myofacial pain dysfunction: an analysis of 476 patients. Laryngoscope 96:1099, 1986
55. Manns A, Zuazola RV, Sirhan R et al: Relationship between the tonic elevator mandibular activity and the vertical dimension during the states of vigilance and hypnosis. J Craniomandibular Pract 8:163, 1990

5 | TMJ Imaging

Peter W. Benoit
Samuel J. Razook

In the century since Roentgen produced the first x-ray image in 1895, advances in radiation physics and the development of computers have enabled production of spectacular detailed images of both hard and soft internal body tissues. Today, many imaging methods, some using regions of the electromagnetic spectrum other than x rays, are used in ever-increasing medical applications. Fundamental techniques include plain radiography, conventional tomography, computed tomography (CT), magnetic resonance imaging (MRI), thermography, and nuclear imaging generated by radioactive isotopes within body tissues. Xeroradiography and arthrography represent variations of fundamental techniques. In the former, the x-ray image is formed on a charged plate by a dry process rather than on conventional film; in the latter, a radiopaque contrast medium is injected, usually into a joint space, before conventional radiographs, ordinary noncomputerized tomograms, or CT images are made.

The usefulness of thermography and nuclear imaging relative to TMD has not yet been established, although both are being studied in this context. Plain radiography, conventional tomography, arthrography, CT, and MRI are all commonly used for TMJ studies. During the past decade, the virtues and limitations for each have become clearer, as interest in TMD has intensified. The practical applications of each technique for TMD, as reflected in the current literature, are discussed briefly below. For detailed technical information, or images of TMJ pathologies, the reader is referred to the list of suggested reading at the end of the chapter.

PLAIN RADIOGRAPHY

Conventional radiographs of the TMJ can be readily produced in most dental or medical offices, and a variety of equipment variations is available for this purpose. Projections include lateral transcranial, transpharyngeal, and

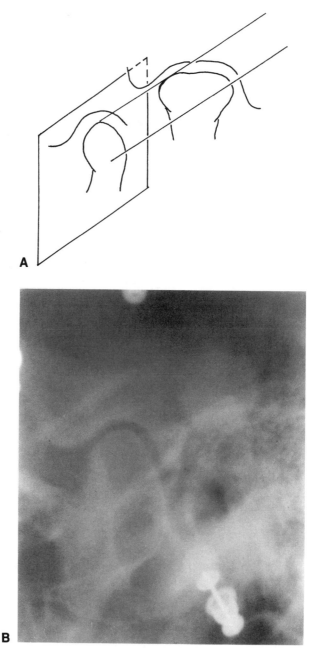

Fig. 5-1.   Lateral transcranial projection. (**A**) Angulation of x-ray beam through the condyle to the laterally positioned film. (**B**) Lateral transcranial view of a normal adult right TMJ with the condyle seated in the mandibular fossa in the closed-mouth position.

transorbital. Each provides relatively limited information regarding a different aspect of joint bony anatomy. None of the projections provides direct information regarding the condition of joint soft tissues; moreover, research has indicated that soft tissue conditions cannot be reliably determined indirectly by inference from bony findings. Therefore, plain radiography is limited to screening assessment of relatively gross bony abnormalities, most commonly developmental anomalies or damage secondary to trauma or arthritides.

Lateral Transcranial Projection

An often-used projection in plain radiography of the TMJ is the lateral transcranial, in which the x-ray beam is directed downward from the opposite side of the head through the joint to be imaged. This is performed to avoid superimposition of the dense petrous portion of the temporal bone on the joint image. The lateral transcranial image does not include the condylar neck, and only the lateral one-third to one-half of the condyle and fossa articulating surfaces are well visualized (Fig. 5-1). The lateral portion of the joint is the region where functional hard tissue changes are likely to be most pronounced.

A refinement of the basic technique involves taking an initial submental-vertex view of the skull to determine the angulation of the long axis of each condyle to the frontal plane (Fig. 5-2). This information is then used to orient the beam parallel to this (horizontal) aspect of the condylar long axis to produce a "corrected" lateral transcranial projection. It is also possible to similarly use an anteroposterior (AP) view of the skull beforehand to measure the vertical angulation of the condylar long axis to the horizontal plane and to use this information to reorient the beam further to produce a fully corrected lateral transcranial view. In routine practice, however, it is most common to use average settings for both the horizontal and vertical angulations of the x-ray beam; for corrected views, generally only the horizontal angle is individualized.

Some have contended that disc position and normality of mandibular position can be assessed or confirmed by evaluating the centricity of the condyle–fossa relationship seen in lateral transcranial projections. Recent literature has not supported these contentions, even when corrected views are used.

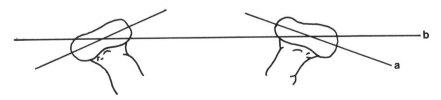

Fig. 5-2. Superior-inferior view of condyles as in a submental-vertex radiograph, showing angulation of condylar mediolateral axes (*a*) to the frontal plane (*b*).

Transpharyngeal and Transorbital Projections

In some instances, it is desirable to screen bone condition in parts of the joint not well visualized on lateral transcranial projections. The transpharyngeal projection provides a lateral view, appearing similar to the lateral transcranial but with a clear image of the medial portion of the condyle. Perhaps more useful is the transorbital projection, which provides an AP view of the condyle, often somewhat obscured, depending on variations of individual skull anatomy. In both views, the condylar neck is visualized, which is of particular advantage in trauma cases.

TOMOGRAPHY

Tomograms are views of a preselected plane of joint anatomy, from 0.5- to 10-mm thickness, produced by synchronous movement of the x-ray source and the film during exposure. With this technique, several "slices" can be made through the joint either perpendicular or parallel to the condylar long axis to produce mediolateral (Fig. 5-3) or AP images, respectively. The major advantage over plain films is that clear images of all portions of the bony articulating surfaces are provided, so that abnormalities not shown in conventional films are revealed. Major disadvantages include inconvenience, considerably higher radiation exposure, and cost.

As with the lateral transcranial projection, lateral tomograms can be corrected for individual inclinations of the condylar long axis in an attempt to

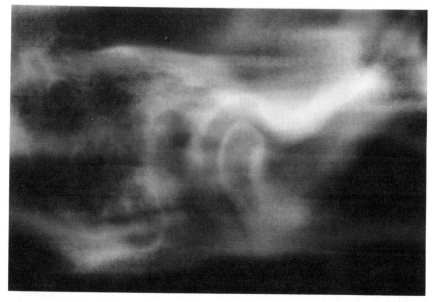

Fig. 5-3. Lateral tomogram of a normal adult TMJ in the closed-mouth position.

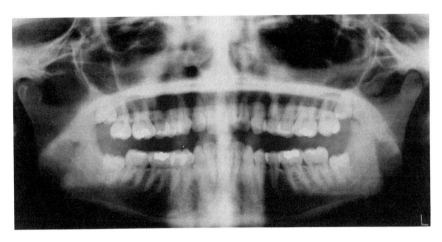

Fig. 5-4. Panoramic radiograph showing normal adult TMJs. In this instance, the fossae and eminences are more clearly shown than in most panoramic films.

produce more accurate estimation of joint space and the condyle–fossa relationship. Although fully corrected tomograms produce accurate estimations of true condyle position, the questions of "correct" condyle position and the relevance of variations of condyle position to the incidence of TMD are not resolved. This is not surprising, considering the well-documented considerable variations in normal condyle and fossa anatomy, even between sides in the same individual. The soft tissue coverings of the condyle and fossa have been shown to vary in thickness and not to faithfully reflect the bony contours; this introduces another source of error in the assessment of joint "space" seen in tomograms or plain films.

Panoramic Radiography

The panoramic radiograph, commonly used in dental offices, is a modified tomogram that provides a rather comprehensive image of the maxilla and mandible on a single film (Fig. 5-4). It is an excellent, convenient, relatively low-radiation technique for screening the jaws for a wide variety of bony and dental abnormalities. The view of the joint is inferior to finer tomographic studies in that only a single plane is imaged, and the mandibular fossa and articular eminence are generally not well visualized.

ARTHROGRAPHY

Arthrography is used for the diagnosis of joint soft tissue abnormalities. The introduction of a radiopaque contrast medium into the TMJ for the purpose of assessing disc position or to detect perforation of the disc or posterior attachment tissues can be combined with any of the above imaging techniques, usually lateral transcranial or lateral tomographic views. The joint is anesthetized with local anesthetic before the contrast medium is injected under fluoroscopic visualization. The lower joint space is generally used, particularly when a nontomographic technique is used; this minimizes obscuring of the image that occurs when the contrast medium fills the relatively large superior joint space. The size and shape of the image formed by the contrast medium in the anterior recess is evaluated to indirectly determine disc position. When a perforation is present in the disc or posterior attachment, the medium will flow from the injected inferior joint space into the uninjected superior space. A typical arthrogram, confirming disc displacement, is shown in Figure 5-5.

One advantage of arthrography over other techniques to determine disc position is that a dynamic study can be performed under fluoroscopic observation while the patient is instructed to perform mandibular movements. Another advantage is that movement of the joint during intracapsular infusion with a fluid medium is sometimes of therapeutic value, resulting in a lasting improvement of joint range of motion (ROM), possibly with pain reduction. This might occur, for instance, in joints with nonreducing anteriorly displaced discs and/or fibrous adhesions, presumably as a result of mechanical joint inflation by the introduced fluid. Finally, arthrography is the most sensitive technique for detecting soft tissue perforation, even surpassing direct arthroscopic visualization.

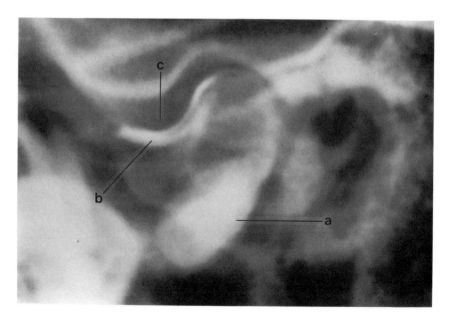

Fig. 5-5.   TMJ arthrogram in the closed-mouth position showing radiopaque contrast medium in the lower joint space posterior (*a*) and anterior (*b*) to the condyle. Note the abnormal position of the anteriorly displaced disc (*c*).

However, disadvantages are considerable and must be weighed when contemplating use of arthrography. Radiation exposure is relatively high, and the technique is often painful. Arthrography is also time-consuming and requires high technical skill as well as considerable experience in interpretation, because the disc is not visualized directly and perforations can be produced inadvertently by mistakes in needle placement. Because the joint is disturbed by introduction of the contrast medium, joint dynamics during the procedure may not accurately reflect the prearthrographic condition. Allergic reactions to contrast media can also occur. Finally, because arthrography is an invasive technique, it is contraindicated when local superficial or periarticular infections are present.

COMPUTED TOMOGRAPHY

In CT, selected planes (usually axial) of the body are exposed to x-ray beams from many angles. Beam attenuation, after passing through the subject, is computer analyzed to construct images whose contrast is a sensitive representation of differing tissue densities. Images of both hard and soft tissue are thus produced. Information from 1- to 13-mm-thick axial CT sections can be computer-reconstructed to create sagittal, frontal, or even three-dimensional images of the TMJ, although at some reduction in resolution. It is also possible to make direct images in the more conventional planes, but necessary patient positioning is sometimes difficult or impossible. Because the TMJ soft tissues are relatively scant and closely surrounded by bone, their resolution is generally poor. Therefore, the major application of CT in TMD is for analysis of bone structure and density, particularly applicable to cases involving trauma or degeneration of the hard tissues. CT involves less radiation exposure than tomography, and it is a more sensitive detector of density changes.

MAGNETIC RESONANCE IMAGING

Contrasts in MRI are dependent on the concentration of hydrogen ions in the tissues. The orientations of hydrogen nuclei are affected by exposure to a strong magnetic field and to radio waves. When exposed differentially to both, the nuclei transmit radio signals that are computer analyzed to form images in which the highest intensity signals are from hydrogen-rich sources, particularly water and fat. Because bone tissue contains relatively little water, MRI is inferior to CT for bone studies. However, it is superior for imaging TMJ soft tissues and is particularly applicable for assessing disc position and, to a limited extent, disc condition. Large perforations can be detected with MRI, but arthrography remains superior for that purpose. The major advantages of MRI over arthrography are noninvasiveness and no exposure to ionizing radiation. Also most patients are more comfortable with MRI unless they are claustrophobic and cannot tolerate relatively long periods holding still in a small, noisy

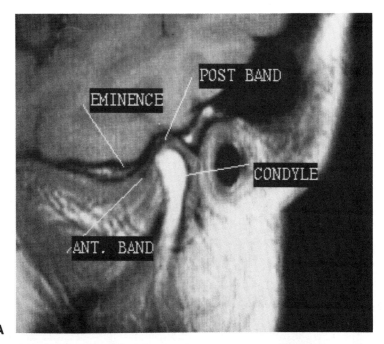

A

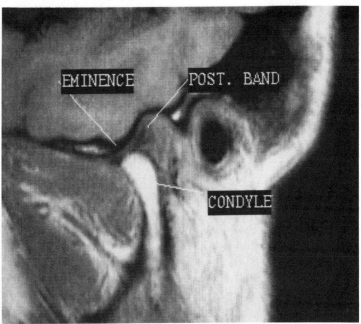

B

Fig. 5-6.   MRI images of a normal adult TMJ **(A)** Mouth closed; **(B)** mouth open.

chamber. It is to be recalled, however, that MRI studies are not dynamic; full assessment of disc position generally requires joint views in the closed and fully opened positions, in each of which the patient must hold still for several minutes (Fig. 5-6).

IMAGING DECISIONS

General applications for the various joint imaging techniques in TMD have been indicated above. However, decisions to use them are dependent on clinical judgment, which, in turn, depends on the practitioner's overall philosophy in managing TMD, as briefly discussed at the end of Chapter 3. Commonly accepted indications for joint imaging in this controversial field will clarify further only as practice standards continue to evolve. This will largely depend on continuing research into the natural course, and response to treatment, of the various TMDs. In the meantime, the most authoritative existing literature on the subject should be used to support imaging decisions. At this point, aside from plain screening films, which can reasonably be routinely justified, it seems prudent that special studies should be ordered only when the diagnosis is in doubt after history review and clinical examination, particularly if initial treatment decisions will be affected by the results.

Beyond the strictly medical concerns, legal questions must be considered in the current practice environment. At this time of increasing national concern over burgeoning health care costs, the practice of defensive medicine can be expected to come under closer scrutiny, and policy decisions can be anticipated. Until outcomes of that debate clarify, decisions regarding TMJ imaging will be guided more by individual practitioner judgment, within reasonable limits, than by clear consensus.

SUGGESTED READINGS

Brand JW: Temporomandibular joint arthrography. p. 635. In DelBalso AM (ed): Maxillofacial Imaging. WB Saunders, Philadelphia, 1990

DelBalso AM: Radiography of the temporomandibular joint. p. 607. In DelBalso AM (ed): Maxillofacial Imaging. WB Saunders, Philadelphia, 1990

Helms CA, Kaplan P: Diagnostic imaging of the temporomandibular joint: recommendations for use of the various techniques. Am J Roentgenol 154:319, 1990

Kaplan PA, Helms CA: Current status of temporomandibular joint imaging for the diagnosis of internal derangements. Am J Roentgenol 152:697, 1989

Kircos LT, Ortendahl DA: Magnetic resonance imaging of the temporomandibular joint. p. 675. In DelBalso AM (ed): Maxillofacial Imaging. WB Saunders, Philadelphia, 1990

Knoernschild KL, Aquilino SA, Ruprecht A: Transcranial radiography and linear tomography: a comparative study. J Prosthet Dent 66:239, 1991

Ludlow JB, Nolan PJ, McNamara JA: Accuracy of measurements of temporomandibular joint space and condylar position with three tomographic techniques. Oral Surg Oral Med Oral Pathol 72:364, 1991

Mahan PE, Alling CC: Imaging. In: Facial Pain, 3rd Ed. Lea & Febiger, Malvern, Pennsylvania, 1991

Raustia AM, Pyhtinen J: Computed tomography of the temporomandibular joint. p. 653. In DelBalso AM (ed): Maxillofacial Imaging. WB Saunders, Philadelphia, 1990

6 | Nonsurgical Management of Mandibular Disorders

Eric S. Lawrence
Samuel J. Razook

The criteria for initiating treatment for disturbances that involve the TMJ and associated structures vary according to the practitioners' ability to diagnose and their ability to predict if the value of the treatment will outweigh the time, expense, and personal demands placed on the patient now and in the future.

Diagnosis entails not only an understanding of mandibular function and dysfunctional structures but also requires a recognition of the many facets of pain and pain behavior that may accompany the dysfunction as a primary, secondary, or independent entity. Realistic treatment goals regarding the elimination of pain and the restoration of normal function are developed with this in mind (Table 6-1).

The diagnosis of facial pain can be complex. Pains of vascular, neurogenic, visceral, and psychogenic origin are often present in the patient with a TMD and can mimic musculoskeletal pain both in quality and distribution. Although it is beyond the scope of this chapter to address, the need for a basic clinical understanding of these various categories of facial pain cannot be overstressed and is a requisite for proper patient care.

Musculoskeletal disorders in the head and neck are multicausal and can be classified according to organic or nonorganic etiology. Although this classification is convenient to use, it is unusual to find these entities isolated in the clinical setting. Aberrant mandibular function of organic origin may be caused by occlusal disharmonies, disturbances within the TMJs, skeletal imbalances involving head posturing, maxillomandibular size discrepancies, or

Table 6-1. Summary of Treatment Decisions and Diagnosis

I.   Masticatory Muscle Involvement (No Disc Displacement)
   A.   Diagnostic Factors
      1.   Patient's history (lack of clicking)
      2.   Muscle palpation
      3.   Range of opening
         a.   Average normal maximum opening is 47 mm—muscle spasm generally results in a decreased opening
         b.   Generally more than 30 mm if less than 30 mm may indicate an intracapsular problem such as an acute disc displacement without reduction or fibrosis
      4.   Absence of joint sounds
      5.   Emotional factors may be involved
   B.   Treatment Procedures
      1.   Treat with intraoral orthotic appliance
      2.   Referral for physical therapy for the treatment of mandibular and or cervical spine muscle involvement
      3.   Referral for psychological situation—possible counseling and/or biofeedback
      4.   When joint is stabilized and muscles are functioning normally, treat the malocclusion least invasively
         a.   Equilibration
         b.   Restoration
         c.   Orthodontics
         d.   Orthodontics with orthognathic surgery
II. Disc Displacement
   A.   Diagnostic factors
      1.   Patient's history and chief complaint (clicking)
      2.   Pain to palpation lateral to joint capsule or by pressure in the external auditory meatus
      3.   Decreased maximum opening—if less than 30 mm, then possible acute disc displacement without reduction
      4.   Clicking
         a.   Painful click may indicate disc displacement with reduction
         b.   Nonpainful click may indicate chronic disc displacement without reduction or congenital malformation
   B.   Treatment procedures
      1.   Mild click without pain
         a.   Diagnose and inform patient of condition
         b.   No treatment necessary unless clicking is progressively increasing
      2.   Clicking without pain—chief complaint is click
         a.   Treat with anterior repositioning splints followed by superior repositioning splints
         b.   Treat malocclusion least invasively
      3.   Clicking with pain—chief complaint is joint pain
         a.   Treat with anterior repositioning splints followed by superior repositioning splints
         b.   Treat malocclusion least invasively
      4.   Acute disc displacement without reduction with pain
         a.   Mandibular manipulation to "stretch out" mandibular opening
         b.   Anterior repositioning splints followed by superior repositioning splints if reduced
         c.   Intracapsular surgery or arthroscopy if conservative disc reduction is unsuccessful
         d.   Treat malocclusion least invasively
      5.   Acute disc displacement without reduction without pain
         a.   Mandibular manipulation to "stretch out" mandibular opening
         c.   Anterior repositioning splints followed by superior repositioning splints if reduced
         d.   Superior repositioning splint alone if mandibular opening is "stretched" (treat off disc)
         e.   Treat malocclusion least invasively

any combination of these factors. It is the action of the muscle and relative forces of muscle that define the interaction between these units, which otherwise would be functioning independently. Pain and stress of nonorganic origin can also affect mandibular function by altering muscle function. In this way, nonorganic problems can lead to physical use and abuse of structures that appear to be either degenerating or dysfunctional when the patient is first seen in the clinical setting. Thus, disorders of nonorganic origin can cause organic problems in much the same way that organic imbalances that cause pain and stress may initiate intolerable conditions for the patient to manage psychologically.

FACTORS INFLUENCING MANDIBULAR POSTURE AT REST

Key to the treatment of mandibular problems is an understanding of the factors that can influence and are influenced by the position of the mandible during function and the posture of the mandible at rest.

Ligaments are structures that limit joint movement. As such, they determine the borders in three dimensions, beyond which the joint cannot move. The temporomandibular (TM) ligament, the TMJ capsule, and to some degree, the stylomandibular and sphenomandibular ligaments determine the borders of movement of the mandible. Movement of the TMJs and thus the mandible along its upper border or seated position in the glenoid fossa is influenced significantly by the dental occlusion. These borders describe an envelope of motion within which the mandible functions and rests. At any particular time, the mandible at rest is in a relatively static position determined by muscle tone of the jaw-opening and jaw-closing muscles and the associated soft tissue factors as they react to gravitational pull (Fig. 6-1).

Dental Occlusion

One of the factors that influences the position of the mandible during function and rest is the dental occlusion. Surrounding the teeth, the periodontal ligaments provide an abundance of sensory input to the central nervous system (CNS) regarding the position and quality of the masticatory load. During chewing, this sensory input makes possible the alteration of masticatory muscle activity to adjust the position of the mandible to minimize or avoid aberrant loading of the teeth and joints at any given time. Therefore, the manner in which the occluding surfaces contact one another significantly influences masticatory muscle function.

When the mouth is empty, sensory input from the periodontal ligaments also influences the position that the mandible assumes at rest. When the masticatory muscle is not actively contracting, muscle activity is still detectable electromyographically. This is said to be muscle tone. The resultant position

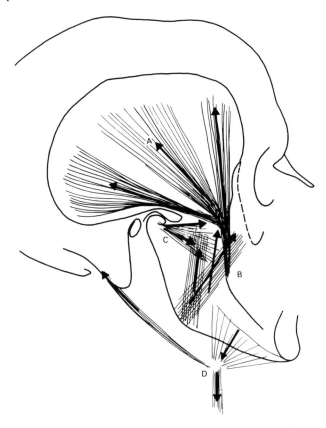

Fig. 6-1. The mechanisms of growth abnormalities in the mandible can be explained by the force couple systems involved in mandibular posture. *(A)* Mean upward and backward direction of the temporalis. *(B)* Mean upward and forward pull of the masseteric complex. *(C)* Downward and forward inclination of the pull of the external pterygoid in reciprocity to the posterior fibers of the temporalis. *(D)* Effects of the drag on the chin by the hyoid musculature. The mandible is often thought to function as a class III lever; however, it is actually a force couple system with a class I lever operating off the coronoid process and perhaps the condylar head, with the external pterygoid acting as a fulcrum. This helps explain the complex physiology of the opening and closing movements of the mandible. (From Ricketts,[8] with permission.)

of the mandible is within the borders of movement and is a position in which the teeth are separated by approximately 2 to 5 mm as measured intraincisally. This has been termed the rest position of the mandible. Voluntary closure of the mouth from this position has been shown to be a series of small arcs that grossly appear as a single smooth arc into maximum intercuspation. This rest position will change when the intercuspal position of the teeth changes to preserve smooth closure into intercuspation of the teeth.

During swallowing, the masticatory muscles contract, bracing the mandible to allow appropriate tongue movement to complete the swallowing act.

This act moves the mandible so that the teeth come into or approach a position of maximum intercuspation. Movement occurs in such a way as to avoid occlusal areas that would prevent simultaneous contact or near contact of the teeth. This movement requires muscle contraction and activity that is altered based on periodontal ligament input. A malocclusion is any imbalance in the intercuspal relationship of the teeth preventing the smooth closure of the mandible from its rest position to maximum intercuspation.

Therefore, if the posture or position of the mandible at rest does not allow for a smooth closure into intercuspation, the muscles will adjust the mandible into another position of rest. This occurs in large part from sensory input from the periodontal ligaments. Thus, an avoidance mechanism is created. This avoidance phenomenon appears to be protective in that it prevents the adverse or uneven loading of teeth, which could result in abnormal wear and/or mobility. Also, because it is through the occlusion that the TMJs are loaded, this mechanism also appears to minimize adverse joint loading.

This phenomenon of avoidance is achieved through the alteration of muscle activity. Muscles do not know innately where to position the mandible at rest to achieve smooth movements into closure. The mandible assumes its mandibular posture at rest by default as a result of avoiding other positions that are less compatible with even tooth contact. Consequently, altering the occluding surfaces of the teeth permanently or through intraoral appliances alters masticatory muscle activity by causing a change in the rest position through a mechanism of avoidance.

TMJ Sensory Input

A second factor that can alter the mandibular positioning is sensory input from the mechanoreceptors of the TMJs. This input allows for joint position sense. In all joints, function on the borders occurs, but only transiently. In the TMJs, this proprioceptive input alters masticatory muscle function to avoid the mandible from functioning on its border positions except transiently during function. In the diseased joint, nociceptive input from degeneration or inflammation acts in a similar manner to alter muscle function in positioning the mandible to minimize stimulation of pain receptors. The position of posture or rest is the result of avoiding other positions that would have resulted in a greater amount of noxious stimuli to the CNS.

Tongue Position and Nasal Airway

A third factor that influences the mandibular posture is tongue position and nasal airway patency. If obstruction of the nasal airway does not allow adequate flow through the nasal cavity, the lips will separate, and if necessary, the tongue position will change, allowing more room for air to flow between it and the palate. The tongue will often come forward, and the mandible will be slightly more depressed. If severe, this can contribute to alterations in growth of the middle and lower face. Also, posturing the head in an extended position on the neck can occur to allow slight alterations of the position of the mandible and tongue to decrease oral obstruction to air flow if nasal obstruction is present. Just as an elevation in the partial pressure of carbon dioxide in the blood can increase the respiratory rate through autonomic mechanisms, changes in tongue position to allow adequate air flow to the lungs is an involuntary adaptive response to maintain adequate ventilation. An alteration in the position of the mandible secondary to alterations in masticatory muscle function allows this to occur.

There is a close association between nasal obstruction, facial maldevelopment, dental malocclusion, and TMJ function. Individuals with nasorespiratory obstruction often exhibit common characteristics, which have been described as the "respiratory obstructive syndrome" (Fig. 6-2). These characteristics are:

1. Primary unilateral or bilateral crossbite (Fig. 6-3)
2. Functional unilateral crossbite with mandibular deflection
3. Presence of enlarged adenoids or tonsils or history of it

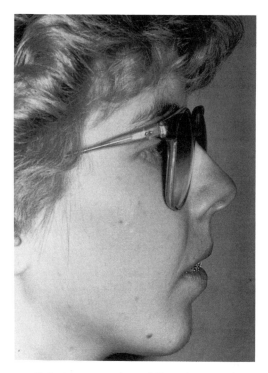

Fig. 6-2. A common clinical presentation of "respiratory obstructive syndrome" is the excessive development of the lower third of the face. This has given rise to the term *long face syndrome*. (From Lawrence and Lawrence,[9] with permission.)

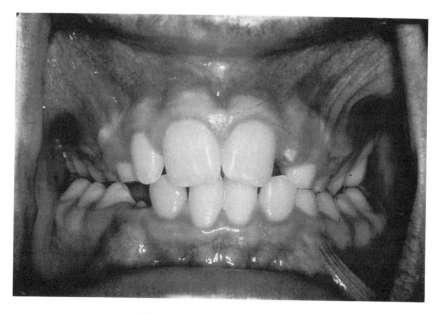

Fig. 6-3. Bilateral crossbite.

4. Open bite (Fig. 6-4)
5. Lowered tongue posture (Fig. 6-5)
6. Tongue thrust
7. Narrow upper arch
8. Chronic mouth-breathing
9. Secondary problems in the TMJ and maxilla
10. Pseudo-class I condition in bilateral crossbite with anterior mandibular deflection
11. Head tipped back on cervical spine
12. Narrow nasal cavity
13. Opening of mandibular angle

It is difficult in humans to establish a direct one-to-one relationship involving factors affecting growth and development. Fortunately, a series of experiments on young, growing rhesus monkeys conducted by Harvold have established this relationship. In one experiment, Harvold and colleagues[1] caused the animals to be obligate mouth-breathers by obstructing the animals' nasal passages with silicone plugs. Harvold et al followed these monkeys for 3 years, collecting a series of photographs, dental casts, radiographs, and electromyographic (EMG) recordings. They observed that the monkeys with nasal blockage kept their mouths open continuously, whereas the control animals kept their mouths closed. Cephalometric analysis showed a significant increase in the distance from nasion to the chin in the mouth-breather. The distance from nasion to the hard palate also increased, but the distance from the hard palate to the chin did not. This demonstrates that the lowering of the mandible to

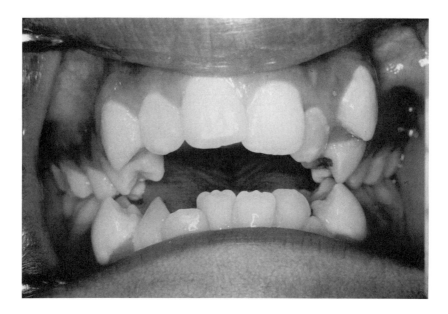

Fig. 6-4.   Open bite.

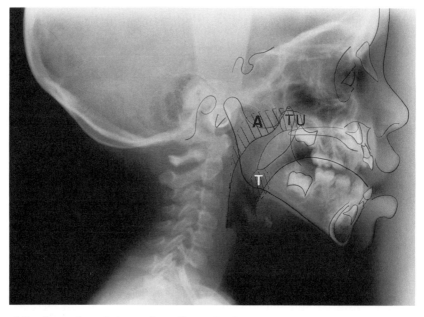

Fig. 6-5.   Lateral cephalometric radiograph. Structural nasorespiratory obstruction may involve any one or a combination of *A*, adenoids; *TU*, inferior turbinate; *T*, tonsils. Also shown is a lowered tongue position and lip separation.

open an oral airway was followed by a downward migration of the entire maxilla. The lower border of the mandible became more steeply inclined in the experimental group as the gonial angle increased. Although these findings were consistent throughout the entire experimental group, the extent and severity of the malformations varied. The differential treatment response appeared to be linked to the manner in which the animal adapted to the nasal obstruction.

Another study conducted by Harvold[2] placed acrylic blocks in the palatal vault of 36 rhesus monkeys to assess the change involved with abnormal tongue position. This condition is not unlike that experienced with enlarged tonsils. The acrylic blocks created a continuous stimulus to the tongue, resulting in an altered tonus of the muscles involved in postural positioning of the mandible. The new stimuli caused the animals to respond initially by lowering the mandible. After only 6 months of this behavior, a statistically significant difference in the ratio between facial height and mandibular length was noted. The mandible in all the experimental animals changed dramatically because of bone resorption at the gonial angle and bone apposition at the chin. After 1 year, the experimental animals showed a greater increase in facial height, an open gonial angle, and prominent bone apposition to the chin, resulting in an increase in the mandibular symphysis. There was a significant morphologic change involving notching at the gonial angle.

Based on a series of experiments on primates, Harvold[3] postulated that oral respiration in monkeys is associated with the recruitment of certain muscles of the orofacial system usually not used for that purpose. The muscle development depends, within certain limits, on the use of the muscle. The change in bone morphology as well as tooth position depends on bone reorganization.

The tongue normally occupies a neutral position in the oral cavity. The tongue is normally in contact with the soft palate in the posterior, with its center located no lower than halfway between the crowns of the upper molars and the palatal vault. In this position, the tongue provides an outward force on the developing dentition to balance the constant inward force placed by the cheek musculature, predominantly the buccinator. Under ideal conditions, an equilibrium exists in which the teeth are positioned in a "neutral space" between these opposing forces. Mouth-breathing results in a displacement of the tongue inferiorly in an effort to open the oral airway. This movement creates an imbalance in muscle forces. There is no longer any opposition to the inward directed force that the buccal musculature is placing on the maxilla, thus a narrow maxilla and dental arch develops, often resulting in a crossbite development and occlusal interferences.

Nasal airway obstruction may be caused by several factors, some of which are transitory and difficult to control, such as allergic rhinitis, and others of a more structural nature that can easily be identified and alleviated, such as enlargement of adenoidal tissue, tonsils, and inferior turbinates (Fig. 6-5). There may also be a narrowing of the external nares or a deviation of the nasal septum, restricting proper nasal respiration.

Nasal-breathing obstruction is only one factor contributing to an altered tongue posture. Lingual tonsils, because of their location and contiguous relationship to the surface of the throat and location at the tongue base when enlarged, displace the tongue forward (Fig. 6-6). This occurs as the enlarged tonsils cause the soft palate to rest on the upper pole rather than the dorsum of the tongue, resulting in a downward and forward displacement of the dorsum. The forward posturing of the tongue may be even more marked when the nasopharynx is filled with adenoids. A short lingual frenum may also "hold" the tongue in an inferior position. Habits may also be involved; a tongue thrust results in a low resting tongue posture, as is also the case with a digital habit that displaces the tongue in a downward direction.

Dentoalveolar changes as a consequence of nasorespiratory obstruction may in itself adversely affect the functioning of the TMJ. A common result of mouth-breathing is a narrow maxillary arch and possible development of a posterior crossbite. To maintain the best possible occlusal contact, the body compensates for this skeletal discrepancy by flaring the upper molars buccally. In this situation, the mandibular arch may be normal or wider than normal because of the new tongue position. The main consequence of this action is that the flaring of the maxillary molars causes their mesiolingual cusps to "hang down" beyond the occlusal plane and to act as an interference in the lateral mandibular movements. This type of interference is very damaging to the integrity of the joint.

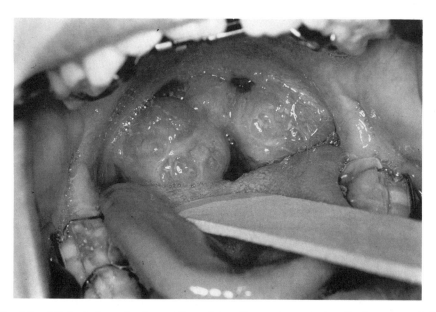

Fig. 6-6. Clinical view of enlarged lingual tonsils causing anterior displacement of the tongue.

Cervical Spine Positioning and Mobility

A fourth factor that influences the rest position of the mandible is cervical spine positioning and mobility (see Ch. 11). The mandible is suspended in a sling of muscles from the cranium. Gravitational forces remain constant and in a direction perpendicular to the ground. Changes in head posture alone can alter the position the mandible assumes relative to the cranium, therefore altering the resting posture of the mandible. Mandibular posture at rest is not static but is within a range. This has been recognized for years and, along with changes in muscle tone caused by normal fatigue during the day, accounts for the variability in the intraincisal distances (2 to 5 mm) during rest. More detail of head–neck positioning influencing the rest position (upright postural position) of the mandible is covered in Chapter 11.

Although the dentist alters tooth structure and uses prosthetic materials of an apparently unyielding nature, the teeth and dental occlusion are not part of a rigid, hard tissue system. Instead, they are truly part of a soft tissue system and dynamic in all respects.

Because alterations in the dental occlusions of the teeth affect muscular performance, the dentist is offered a mechanism to change joint position, joint loading, and muscle activity in an indirect and reasonably predictable fashion. For the masticatory system to remain functional and comfortable, however, the importance of the other factors mentioned above must be appreciated for appropriate diagnosis and treatment of the dysfunctional patient.

Key variables to consider that influence the patient's response to treatment are not only TMJ pathology, masticatory muscle dysfunction, the occlusal relationships of the teeth, and outside stress relationships, but also cervical spine positioning and mobility. Key variables to be considered by the physical therapist in the treatment of cervical spine dysfunction must include dental relationships and TM function. The relationship is direct and predictable because both act and react to mandibular positioning through the interplay of the synergistic and antagonistic activity of the cervical and masticatory musculature.

The relationship between abnormal head posture, enlarged adenoids, blocked nasal airway, and malocclusion was demonstrated in a study conducted by Linder-Aronson and Woodside.[4] They studied lateral and PA cephalometric radiographs of 120 patients in the Burlington growth study. This study consisted on longitudinal records taken every 2 to 3 years between the ages of 6 and 20 years. Linder-Aronson and Woodside found that in patients with an increasing lower anterior facial height, the mean size of the airway through the nose was narrower than in the control subjects. The researchers concluded that the lower anterior facial height is dependent on the growth direction of the mandible and the neuromuscular factors influencing mandibular posture, such as mouth-breathing and head posture. Nasal airway obstruction results in an extended head posture. The process of lowering the mandible to compensate for nasal obstruction actually results in a reduction of size of the oropharynx. To compensate and thus restore the airway volume, the hyoid bone must be elevated and moved anteriorly. This repositioning is accomplished by changing the head posture (tilting backward) or by sustained muscular contraction.

Even though most studies have linked postural changes of the head and neck to airway resistance, head and neck postural changes may be a primary condition, thereby influencing the functional matrix and dentoalveolar-craniofacial morphology. (For further understanding of primary changes in head and neck posture, refer to Chapter 11.) Patients with deep anterior overbites with little overjet commonly have symptoms of joint dysfunction. The most commonly observed symptom is consistent clicking of the TMJ. These patients fall into several categories, with a common denominator being a restriction of freedom of mandibular movement.

NONSURGICAL TREATMENT OF SPECIFIC DISORDERS

Treatment of mandibular dysfunction and head and neck muscle disorders should be reversible and noninvasive whenever possible. Treatment has its goals: (1) relief of pain by resolution of muscle spasm and intra-articular inflammation, and (2) restoration of normal mandibular motion and function in the setting of a stable dental occlusion, acceptable craniocervical relationship, and normal disc–condyle relationship. If the relief of pain, the restoration of acceptable mandibular opening, and the elimination of factors that may herald a relapse are achieved, no further treatment is required regardless of the intracapsular, skeletal, or occlusal abnormalities that exist.

The basic treatment of disorders of both organic and nonorganic origin is not unlike that used for musculoskeletal pain in other joint–muscle systems in the body. Initial symptomatic treatment may include all or some of the following reversible modalities:

1. Establish rapport with the patients, letting them know you understand the problem and are willing to work through this problem with them.
2. Educate the patient as to the etiology, affected anatomy, and the need for treatment over a period of time, emphasizing that there are no "overnight cures."
3. In addition to a gross evaluation of the patient's mental status, the use of a screening evaluation (i.e., stress inventory) or more in-depth testing or psychologic consultation may be indicated.
4. Nonsteroidal anti-inflammatory drugs (NSAIDs) can provide significant analgesia and anti-inflammatory activity directed toward the muscles and the joints. Narcotic analgesics in the patients with chronic pain are indicated only very rarely.
5. The application of heat to painful muscles will increase blood flow and reduce spasm.

6. Application of vapocoolant sprays or the injection of local anesthetics without vasoconstrictor into muscle trigger points assists in reversing the pain–muscle spasm cycle.

7. Muscle relaxants in small doses may provide relief in some patients throughout the day. Sedative doses should be avoided.

8. Resting the jaw and adhering to the use of a soft, nonchewy diet is recommended.

9. Transcutaneous electrical nerve stimulation (TENS), ultrasound, and diathermy are often effective therapeutic modalities.

10. The patient should be made aware of parafunctional habits of clenching and bruxism, if suspect, and should refrain from them if possible. The presence or absence of wear on the occlusal surfaces of the teeth, in and of itself, is not diagnostic of bruxism or clenching.

11. It is important to encourage patients to continue with their normal work and exercise. This helps to keep their mind off pain. Certain postural positions and exercises can aggravate pain, however. Patients are to follow guidelines offered by their dentist or physical therapist as covered in Chapter 11.

This may be all that is necessary to reduce symptoms significantly in many patients while the underlying cause is being determined or other treatment is being planned.

Treatment should entail the use of reversible modalities when possible until symptoms have been relieved and a stable maxillomandibular relationship is maintained. This treatment may include, separately or in combination, any of the following:

1. Use of intraoral orthotic appliances to help alter the masticatory and cervical muscle response to the existing occlusal scheme or to change the mandibular condyle position

2. Physical therapy to modify mandibular and/or cervical posture by normalizing facet joint, soft tissue, and muscular relationships in the cervical and thoracic spine

3. Behavior modification to control muscle tone and tension and stop parafunctional habits through the use of biofeedback, hypnosis, and psychotherapy

Occlusal adjustment by the dentist is irreversible and rarely indicated as an initial treatment except when gross interferences prevent the effective use of intraoral appliances to stabilize the desired maxillomandibular relationship. Further adjustment at a time when muscle spasm and/or intracapsular edema occurs prevents the disc–condyle assemble from assuming its normal concentric position within the glenoid fossa. Also, adjustment at a time when a disc is displaced may worsen the occlusal problems after muscle spasm, edema, or disc displacement is resolved.

Nonarticular Disturbances

Neuromuscular Conditions

Increased muscle tonus progressing to acute or chronic myospasm can occur secondary to imbalances in the occlusion, cervical spine dysfunction, TMJ dysfunction, and changes in the psychological state. Because of the synergistic and antagonistic relationships that exist between the masticatory and cervical musculature, it is not uncommon that both muscle groups are involved. Depending on the degree and the amount of time the hyperactivity remains, the following muscle conditions can result.

Muscle splinting (muscle cramp, acute myospasm) is a protective reflex or guarding mechanism. This generally occurs as a result of acute trauma, causing the skeletal muscles to contract and remain in a hypertonic state, preventing further movement of the part. The trauma can be as gross as a blow to the jaw or head or as innocent as maintaining the head or jaw in one position for prolonged periods. Because this is of an acute nature, metabolic changes that can occur as a result of the vasoconstriction from long-term contraction have not had time to develop. Stretching and spraying the muscle with a vapocoolant spray is often effective in breaking the spasm, restoring normal function, and relieving pain almost immediately. If left untreated, the acute state can progress into a chronic state in which the metabolism of the muscle is altered.

Chronic hyperactivity, contraction, or prolonged muscle splinting can result in metabolic changes leading to chronic myospasm. Often, chronic myospasm does not develop as a result of prolonged acute spasm. Instead, it begins insidiously, developing over long periods of time, and can be secondary to stress, parafunctional habits, the microtrauma of overuse and abuse of the neck and jaws, dental malocclusions, or joint pathology. Chronic hypercontraction of the muscle from whatever source leads to vasoconstriction, resulting in a decrease of the supply of oxygen and nutrients to the muscle. Muscle fatigue occurs as a result of adenosine triphosphate (ATP) depletion, which is critical for both muscle contraction and relaxation. Without sufficient ATP and oxygen, hypertonicity and further vasoconstriction persist. The muscle lacks the ability to thoroughly eliminate waste products such as lactic acid because of the decreased blood flow. This can result in focal areas of inflammation. Pain produced by inflammation causes further muscle contraction and can initiate a self-perpetuating pain–spasm–pain cycle. Predisposing, precipitating, and/or perpetuating factors involving the TMJs, dental occlusion, head posture, or the psychological state of the patient must be identified. In addition to the treatment of these factors directly, biofeedback, TENS, ultrasound, vapocoolant sprays, exercises, and NSAIDs may be necessary.

As the chronic muscle spasm persists, trigger points can develop within the muscle. These are the focal areas of ischemia that exhibit altered neuronal activity that can keep the entire muscle in a hypertonic state. Trigger points are point-tender, palpable, nodular masses often felt deep within the muscle.

They can develop in any skeletal muscle and are known to exist in both active and latent forms, often lasting for years. Injection of trigger points with local anesthetics devoid of vasoconstrictor in addition to physical therapy manual techniques and modalities has proved effective in relieving pain in most patients.

Dental Malocclusion

Neurologically, the act of chewing involves an extremely complex system of motor stimulation of various muscle groups. During mastication, the bolus of food on the occlusal surfaces of the teeth is a fulcrum around which the mandible acts as a class II or class III lever. Periodontal ligament receptors supply the CNS with information about the changing position of the fulcrum and the pressures being generated. This information is used to control the necessary changes in the muscle contraction very rapidly during the chewing stroke to protect the teeth and the joints from damage and is accomplished through a system of reflex inhibition of muscles and muscle groups. The presence, absence, and position of the teeth are a major influencing factor in the resultant load to the joints and to the muscle patterns that develop.

At times other than during the power strokes of chewing, dental occlusion still exerts a great influence on the stomatognathic system. When one considers that total actual chewing time may last no longer than 1 hour a day, the effect of the dental occlusion on the resting position of the mandible during non-chewing time acquires greater significance as a factor in head and neck musculoskeletal harmony.

The mandible is said to be in centric relation (CR) to the maxilla when the TMJ are centered. This is a muscularly determined position where the muscles are at their most relaxed position. Centric occlusion (CO) is the tooth contact that exists when the mandible is placed in CR and closed until tooth contact occurs. Maximum intercuspation dictates the final position of the TMJs as the endpoint of chewing and at the endpoint of empty mouth closure (Fig. 6-7). When the teeth are in maximum intercuspation, the position of the mandible relative to the maxilla may be the CR position. Methods of positioning the mandible in a CR position may differ from dentist to dentist, and various techniques are described in the literature. Difficulty in passively attaining this position may be related to the force applied, the velocity and rhythm in which the mandible is manipulated, and the distance through which it is moved to closure.

If the maximum intercuspation does not exist in the CR position and a shift or slide is detected as the mandible moves from its initial point of tooth contact into maximum intercuspation, a malocclusion is said to exist. Other types of malocclusion are based on missing teeth or vertical dimension of the occlusion and on the contact of the teeth when the mandible moves laterally or protrusively while maintaining tooth contact. A detailed discussion of these many facets is beyond the scope of this text. When the occlusion of the teeth

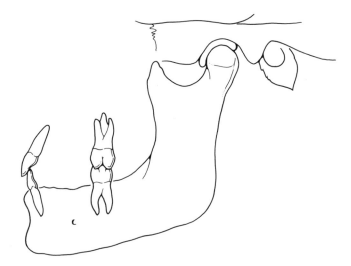

Fig. 6-7. Normal relationship of disc–condyle assembly in the CR position with maximum intercuspation coincidental with CO.

is not in harmony with masticatory muscle function and TMJ function, either the teeth, joints, or muscles separately or in combination will change in form, function, or position to a new point of equilibrium. If a malocclusion exists and the patient is asymptomatic with no physical findings of pathology in the dentition, muscles, and joints, adaptation has occurred and the malocclusion must be considered normal for that person. If the changes necessary are beyond the range of physiologic adaptability, degeneration or pathology will occur. This may appear as tooth mobility or wear, muscle hyperactivity associated with fatigue and pain, or degeneration of the hard or soft tissues in the TMJs.

If a malocclusion exists in the symptomatic patient, its elimination is often helpful in treatment. Occlusal disharmony is often the sustaining factor in masticatory muscle and TMJ dysfunction. Clinical observation has shown certain occlusal conditions to be either the initiating and/or perpetuating factor responsible for disharmony in the masticatory system. The available scientific evidence confirms, in general, the clinical concepts that the following dental conditions are often etiologic factors in TMJ and masticatory muscle dysfunction. However, there are no data that irrefutably define the affects of malocclusion in the individual patient.

Lack of Posterior Support. A lack of posterior support resulting from either missing teeth or underoccluded teeth and restorations will increase mandibular elevator muscle activity and TMJ loading. A statistical relationship exists between the lack of posterior support and the remodeling and degenerative changes within the TMJs. It must be stressed that these joint changes do not relate in a one-to-one relationship with the presence of pain or decrease in mandibular opening. Wear, mobility, and splaying of the upper anterior teeth often occur as the occlusal load is shifted to them. The spaces or diastema resulting from tooth splaying, which in some patients occurs slowly over long periods, can indicate a collapse in the vertical dimension of occlusion. In deep vertical overbite cases, characteristically angle class II division 2 malocclusions, the barrier imposed by the upper maxillary teeth force the mandible into a retruded position. Improper anterior coupling causes the intrusive force delivered by the masseters to become proportionately greater and is responsible for the loss of intermaxillary height and the production of a deep overbite. The reason for this phenomenon rests in the analysis of the lever system of jaw mechanics. The incisors are the farthest from the force vectors and fulcrum and thus receive a comparatively light closing force. The molars, being closer to the fulcrum and force, receive a heavy intrusive force. The anterior teeth are thus able to maintain the vertical dimension with contact while the molars alone would be intruded. A lack of coupling of the anterior teeth results in a large curve of Spee as the anterior teeth extrude and the posterior teeth intrude.

Functional retrusion occurs as the patient closes into CO. The lower incisors contacting the steep lingual guide plane of the upper incisors are forced more distal and cervical along its lingual surface than ideal. This acts to drive the condyle distally in the fossa and impinge on the bilaminar zone. As the condyle assumes a retroposition in the joint, the superior head of the lateral pterygoid muscle stretches. Reflex action can lead the premature contraction of the muscle and anterior disc displacement. This action may stimulate spasms associated with other masticatory muscles and cause pain and discomfort to the patient.

In mandibular opening, any degree of pure rotation without translation is uncommon and is only expected in the early phase of opening. In deep bite cases, forward translation of the condyle is limited by incisor contact, and until the rotation has reached such an extent that the incisors disclude, no translation is possible. Under these conditions, there is some risk that the insertion of the upper head of the lateral pterygoid to the disc may be stretched as the condylar head rotates slightly distal. The larger the degree of overbite, the more pure rotation is needed and the more likely is the chance of damage to the insertion of the lateral pterygoid muscle. The damage may influence and disrupt the correctly timed contraction of the upper head of the lateral pterygoid muscle. It can then no longer act to stabilize and prevent displacement of the disc during forward movement resulting in "clicking."

The above situation may also be produced iatrogenically. Although good orthodontics and good dentistry do not cause TMJ dysfunction, poor orthodontics or improper anterior crowns, which result in premature anterior contact or under torquing of the upper incisors, may contribute to functional mandibular retrusion. This condition is often observed with prolonged use of intermaxillary traction and incisor extrusion. Berry and Watkins[5] reported symptoms of mandibular dysfunction in 18 patients who had undergone orthodontic treatment an average of 7.3 years previously. In all but two of the cases, upper premolars were extracted and the incisors were retroinclined, producing an increase in overbite. They concluded that retraction and retroinclination of the upper anterior teeth in young children may predispose the child to mandibular dysfunction. In growing individuals, the deep bite not only restricts the mandibular movements but also may have a retarding effect on mandibular growth and "hold back" its horizontal expression, resulting in a class II malocclusion. This situation is most often observed in low mandibular plane or brachycephalic facial types.

A decrease in the occlusal vertical dimension leading to overclosure also results in a posterior and superior repositioning of the condyle, which results in clicking of the joints and restricted mandibular movements. In a normal, healthy state, the condyle is located in the squamous or anterior portion of the fossa, never in the posterior. This contrasts and challenges the previous practice of forcing the condyle back into the superior-most and rear-most position in dental reconstruction.

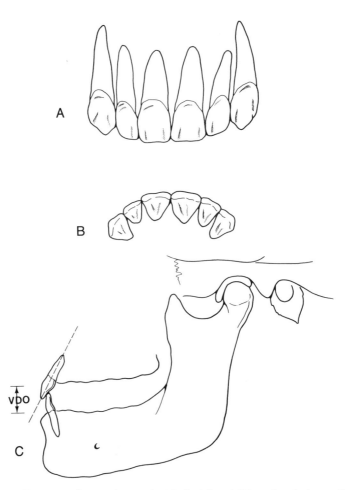

Fig. 6-8.   Maxillary anterior teeth seen in (**A**) facial and (**B**) occlusal views. (**C**) Lateral view of mandible with a lack of posterior tooth support. No collapse of vertical dimension of occlusion is apparent.

Symptomatic patients who lack posterior support and/or who have collapse in the vertical dimension of occlusion (VDO) often exhibit TMJ disc displacements, cervical muscle symptoms, and clinically abnormal head and neck posturing (Figs. 6-8 and 6-9).

Balancing Interferences.   Balancing interferences (tooth contact on the side opposite to which the mandible is moving in a lateral direction with the teeth together) have also been associated with excessive wear and mobility of the posterior teeth, muscle spasm, and joint dysfunction. As the mandible is being guided by and/or is avoiding the balancing interference, the condyle is being

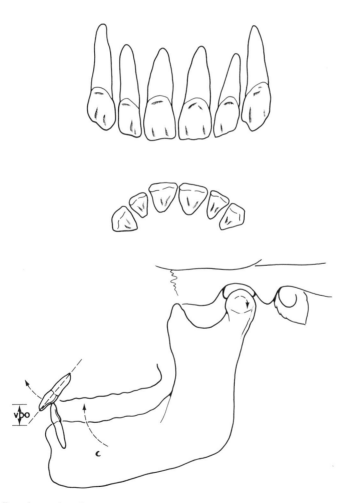

Fig. 6-9.   Resultant development of diastemas and a collapse in vertical dimension of occlusion caused by lack of posterior support.

distracted from the posterior slope of the articular eminence. To maintain joint stability, the disc must remain in intimate contact with the condyle and the eminence. Because the intra-articular space between the condyle and the eminence has increased, the superior head of the lateral pterygoid muscle must bring the disc forward to fill the space with its thicker posterior position. This can lead to muscle fatigue and/or spasm and is believed to be a factor that can lead to disc derangement. Excessive wear of the teeth and bruxism are often believed to be caused by balancing interferences. Gnathologic studies have determined that for proper function of the masticatory complex, the anterior teeth must disclude the posterior teeth during mandibular excursions. This action not only prevents damaging nonphysiologic contact of the posterior teeth, but also maintains the integrity and proper function of the TMJ. Williamson and Lundquist,[6] in a study of anterior guidance using occlusal splints, recorded masticatory muscle activity. They found that only when posterior disclusion is obtained by appropriate anterior guidance can the elevated activity of the temporalis and masseter muscles be reduced. Clinical and scientific observations do not exclusively support this view.

Articulation paper placed between the teeth on one side of the mouth while the patient moves the mandible in the opposite lateral direction will assess the presence of balancing interferences by marking tooth contacts. If they exist, referral to a dentist for evaluation of the occlusion is recommended (Fig. 6-10).

Maximum Intercuspation.   Maximum intercuspation of the teeth determines the final position of the TMJ in the glenoid fossa. It can cause the joints to be slightly distracted from the fossa, it can place the joint posteriorly or grossly anteriorly in the fossa, or it can in some way prevent the disc–condyle complex from maintaining a position of concentricity within the glenoid fossa. The position of the condyle as to its anterior, posterior, and concentric position in the fossa varies in the normal asymptomatic population. Radiographic identification of the condylar position other than as a general reference is not useful as a diagnostic aid or to determine the necessity of treatment (Fig. 6-11).

Detailed evaluation of the occlusion is significant with the disc in its proper position within the TMJ. The occlusal relationships of the teeth can change with alterations in the disc–condyle relationship. The patient who appears to have acceptable occlusal relationships with the disc out of place may have discrepancies in the occlusion when the disc is relocated. Therefore, occlusal evaluation is always made in the light of the existing status of the TMJs.

Scientific correlation between the existence of a malocclusion and mandibular pain and dysfunction does not exit. However, overwhelming clinical experience indicates the need for some form of reversible and/or irreversible occlusal therapy in most patients with pain and dysfunction. Nonetheless, the cornerstone of nonsurgical management of mandibular dysfunction is the use of intraoral orthotic appliances.

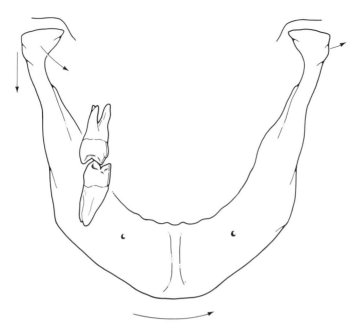

Fig. 6-10. Balancing interference of molar teeth as mandible moves into a left lateral movement. Right condyle is orbiting around left condyle, which is rotating with some lateral movement.

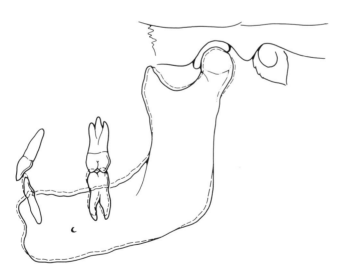

Fig. 6-11. Initial tooth contact CO as mandible maintains a CR position *(solid line).* Movement from CO into maximum intercuspation and the resultant condylar position *(dotted line).*

Orthotic Therapy

Initial treatment involves use of an intraoral orthotic appliance or "splint" to alter the existing occlusal scheme to favor more normal joint stability and muscle function. A variety of splints have been used, ranging from hard acrylic to metal to soft acrylic to fluid-filled appliances that cover all or a portion of the upper or lower teeth. One should select a particular design to fit the individual patient with full knowledge of the effects it may have on the joints, muscles, and teeth. The appliance can thus serve as a diagnostic tool as well as a therapeutic device. Appliances that do not cover or are not in contact with all teeth have the potential for allowing tooth movement and are not considered reversible. For example, a splint that covers the posterior teeth will allow for supereruption of the anterior teeth, thus depending the anterior overbite or creating a condition with a posterior open bite. The appliance can be altered periodically until a stable maxillomandibular relationship is established, with muscle relaxation, pain relief, and a normal disc–condyle–fossa relationship. If necessary, permanent alterations to the dentition using orthodontics, prosthodontics, occlusal equilibration, or surgery can then be made to maintain the position achieved by the appliance. However, to maintain a state of comfort and normal function, it is not always necessary to return a patient to ideal occlusion. Sometimes physical, emotional, or economic factors preclude the immediate transition from the splint to permanent changes in the dentition just described. In such cases, wear of the appliance is tapered to an "as-needed" basis for night time use only.

As mentioned, mandibular positioning can be affected by and can affect cervical structures and position. The alteration of masticatory muscle and joint relationships through orthotic appliances may have an effect on the pain and physical relationships in the cervical area in many patients. Therefore, favorable responses to treatment with the use of an intraoral orthotic appliance *may* or *may not* indicate that the problem is strictly of occlusal origin. Permanent treatment of the dentition in such patients without observing head and neck posture may be fraught with continued complaints of discomfort.

An example of an appliance that fits the criterion of reversibility and that can be used diagnostically as well as therapeutically is the maxillary splint, which covers all the upper teeth and makes contact with all the lower teeth. In patients who do not exhibit a loss of vertical dimension of occlusion and require splint therapy, the appliance is made thin, not to exceed 5 mm measured intraincisally. If the vertical dimension of occlusion is decreased, with the malocclusion showing bite collapse, the appliance is designed to restore the occlusion to a level approximating a normal VDO for the individual. The occlusal surface of the appliance allows for even contact of all teeth simultaneously when the TMJs are in a centric relation position in the glenoid fossa with the disc in place. Disclusion of the posterior teeth during protrusive and lateral movements of the mandible are made off the anterior portion of the splint, with the inclination of the anterior section made as minimal as possible. The inclination of the anterior portion of the splint (and anterior teeth) can restrict the range in which the mandible can rest at any particular time as head posture changes. If the inclination is too vertical or steep, the influence of the occlusion on the rest position of the mandible may not be compatible with the rest position of the mandible during changes in head posture. More freedom in this area will allow more freedom for the mandible to move from a wider variety of rest positions into maximum tooth contact and may decrease masticatory muscle activity (Figs. 6-12 and 6-13). This orthotic essentially provides ideal occlusal guidance in acrylic, thus allowing the muscles to reposition themselves to a relaxed position. The mandibular position is then muscularly determined. Once the relaxed muscle position is established, the occlusion is then analyzed to determine what treatment is required to achieve functional guidance and maximum intercuspation at this position.

The importance of other modalities, such as physical therapy and behavior modification, in combination with the above in certain patients cannot be overstressed. Only when a continuous relief of symptoms is achieved and TMJ function is optimal should permanent changes to the dentition be considered. In achieving this, one should choose the least invasive approach that provides long-term stability in the occlusal relationship established by splint therapy. This may range from occlusal adjustment to orthodontic and prosthodontic treatment to orthognathic surgery, or any combination of treatments.

Articular Disturbances

Disc Derangements

Displacement of the disc within the TMJs has been recognized since the late 1800s. In a case report of two patients, Annandale[7] described the surgical repositioning of the disc in 1884. Many reports and articles have appeared in the literature since then. Not until the mid-1970s was the concept of TMJ disc

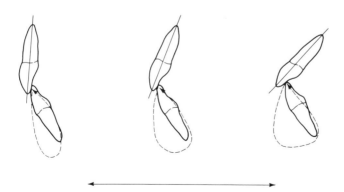

Fig. 6-12. Effect of inclination of anterior teeth on anteroposterior position of rest (posture) of mandible and its movement into intercuspation of the teeth.

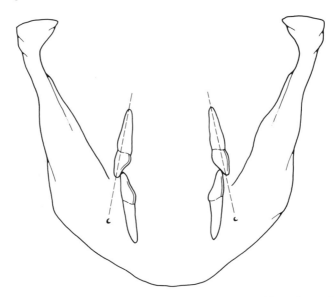

Fig. 6-13. Inclines of posterior teeth affect rest (posture) position of mandible in lateral directions and effect its path of closure into intercuspation of teeth.

displacement and its incidence generally accepted by the dental community. This was largely because of the efforts of Dr. William Farrar of Montgomery, Alabama.

Two general classifications of this disorder are the anteriorly displaced disc that reduces during joint translation and the anteriorly displaced disc without reduction. These clinical entities may exist indefinitely in a single individual or can be only stages in the continuum of a disease process that leads to degenerative joint disease (DJD).

The TMJ are naturally stress-bearing. Degenerative changes are largely influenced by loads applied to the joint in excess of its ability to tolerate or its ability to adapt. Therefore, treatment is directed toward altering forces placed on the joint.

Loading is the result of muscle force. Muscle function that affects the mandible not only involves the masticatory muscles but also muscles controlling cervical spine positioning and tongue function. Clinically, the dental occlusion appears to be the factor that most directly influences masticatory muscle function. Although it is through the occlusion that most of the treatment of TMDs is focused, the importance of cervical involvement in the pain or dysfunction cannot be ignored.

Anterior Repositioning Orthotics.   Treatment of the anteriorly displaced disc with reduction may involve the use of an intraoral appliance to reposition the mandible in a more forward position to restore a normal disc–condyle relationship. The initial forward position is usually an over-corrected position. This is often effective in reducing or eliminating the muscle pain that can accompany disc displacement. However, some patients cannot tolerate the forward repositioning because of muscle pain. In these cases, it may be necessary to treat the muscle condition by using a nonrepositioning splint or physical therapy, or both.

When the disc is reduced by restoring it to its normal relationship to the condyle, the disc–condyle complex is often positioned anteriorly on the posterior slope of the articular eminence (Figs. 6-14 through 6-17). However, in those patients with initial condylar positions that are posterior in the fossa, the forward repositioning to stabilize the disc may return the condyle to a concentric position rather than placing it eccentrically forward in the fossa. The splint is worn continuously except when taken out for cleaning. During this time, efforts are made to eliminate any residual pain the patient may have. Splint therapy may last from several weeks to months as long as the patient shows signs of improvement or increasing joint stability. The ultimate goal is to adjust the appliance so that the disc–condyle complex assumes a concentric position in the glenoid fossa. If this is achieved, the dental relationships are then evaluated to determine how best to restore even tooth contact when the appliance is removed. Dental and maxillomandibular imbalances deemed to be significant can be restored either prosthetically, orthodontically, surgically, with occlusal adjustment, or by any combination of these. Definitive or phase II treatment is necessary for successful treatment to minimize any excessive forces from being placed on the joint structures. Malocclusion, eccentric mandibular movements, and muscle splinting place excessive forces into the TMJs. The ligaments maintaining the integrity of the joint and keeping the disc in position once stretched never regain their full strength, even after successful orthotic therapy. A ligament that was at one time capable of withstanding ex-

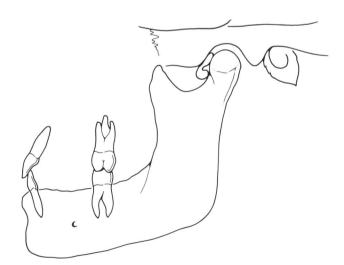

Fig. 6-14. Lateral diagram of a disc displacement.

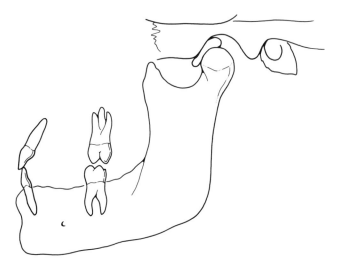

Fig. 6-15. Reduction of disc has occurred by forward and downward advancement of the condyle around posterior band of disc; resultant occlusal relationship from this repositioning.

cessive force is no longer capable. Thus, the occlusal function must be identified to maintain the correction. Application of the basic principles of occlusion is the basis for treatment planning. If the disc–condyle complex cannot be made to return to a concentric position, one should proceed with great caution when considering major changes to the occlusion. No scientific evidence exists to justify occlusal modification to keep the joint in an eccentric position within the glenoid fossa.

Many appliances have been developed to keep the mandible functioning in an anterior position for reduction of disc displacements. These are either of a reversible or irreversible nature and must be used with caution.

Clinical experience has shown that most discs that reduce are amenable to nonsurgical management as described. The degree of displacement or the point at which reduction occurs is a major factor in determining how far the mandible will need to be advanced in splint therapy. If clinical judgment dictates that it will be impossible to return the disc–condyle complex to a concentric position at the end of splint therapy, treatment of this nature should not be initiated. Treatment should then be directed toward pain elimination. It is quite possible to eliminate associated muscle symptoms in many patients while leaving the disc displaced.

If a displaced disc is successfully treated, it should not be assumed that the joint has been made normal and that the damaged or elongated ligaments have shortened or "tightened up." Ligament shortening or tightening has never been shown to exist in any adult joint including the TMJ. It is more likely that success is due to alteration or redistribution of forces to the joint in such a way that they do not violate already damaged structures. Soft and hard tissue re-

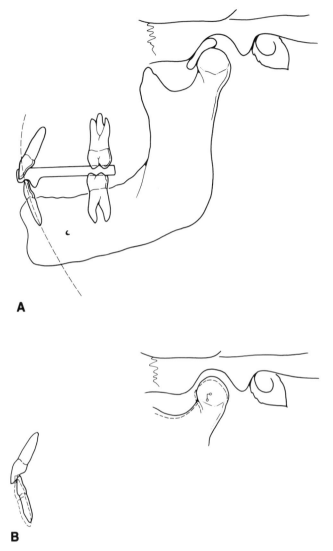

Fig. 6-16. **(A)** Orthotic appliance (splint) in place providing occlusal support at this new position. **(B)** Vertical and horizontal components of forward positioning as seen at level of condyle and anterior teeth. Vertical component represents opening that is created between the posterior teeth.

modeling and resolution of hyperactivity of muscles may also be contributing factors to success.

If the disc remains displaced and the pain and dysfunction are manageable, guidelines to treatment as outlined above for nonarticular disturbances are followed. If the disc remains displaced and an intolerable condition exists that is directly due to the displacement, arthroscopic or open joint surgery should be considered.

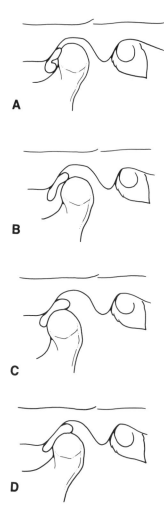

Fig. 6-17. Movement of condyle during disc reduction. **(A)** Disc displacement and resultant function on retrodiscal tissue (not shown). **(B)** Condyle as it passes around posterior band of disc. **(C)** Disc–condyle complex at the initial time of reduction. **(D)** Slight posterior positioning of disc–condyle complex, which often can be achieved immediately; however, disc–condyle complex is not yet in a position of concentricity within glenoid fossa.

    Treatment of the anteriorly displaced disc without reduction differs in the acute and chronic state (Fig. 6-18). In the acute condition, the patient usually has a history of clicking and prior locking and exhibits marked restriction of mandibular opening usually associated with deviation of the affected side. If displacement is not a long-standing condition, one can attempt reduction by manipulation of the condyle, as is discussed in Chapter 7. Intracapsular fluid or local anesthetic injections to alter joint dynamics and muscle injections, vapocoolant sprays, and other modalities to block the muscle splinting may be a useful adjunct to manipulation. To manipulate the mandible, sedation or general anesthesia may also be necessary. If the displacement is successfully reduced, an intraoral appliance must be inserted immediately to keep the mandible from shifting and allowing the disc to displace again. Treatment often follows the course of the anteriorly displaced disc with reduction. If reduction is not successful, traditionally, nonsurgical management would be attempted

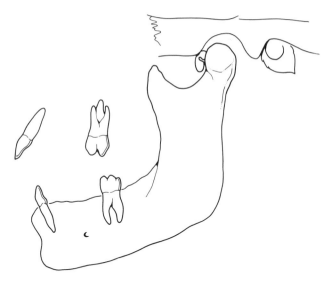

Fig. 6-18. Disc displacement without reduction creating an obstruction to anterior joint translation.

before surgical intervention. However, with the advent of arthroscopic surgery, consideration must be given for early surgical intervention in such cases.

In the chronic condition, the displacement is long-standing, and the patient often gives a history of previous clicking and locking. The patient may have either marked restriction and deviation of mandibular opening or neither. Crepitus within the joint(s) may exist, and degenerative changes may be evident on radiographs; however, this is not always the case. Because the disc cannot be repositioned nonsurgically, treatment is directed toward relief of pain. Splint therapy to eliminate abnormal joint loading and establish normal occlusal relationships is the preferable dental treatment. If the pain is intolerable and cannot be managed through dental treatment, physical therapy, or any of the pain management modalities, surgery may be indicated. In cases in which surgery is not an option and there is limited mouth opening because of a disc displacement that does not reduce, favorable results for increasing the range of motion (ROM) and minimizing masticatory muscle discomfort have been achieved in some patients by applying intraoral stretching techniques that force the disc farther out of position to allow joint translation. This must be attempted with great caution and with the knowledge that it may make the patient more uncomfortable. This is discussed in Chapter 7.

Inflammatory Conditions

The disc and the articulating surfaces of the mandibular condyle and glenoid fossa are nonvascularized and noninnervated and therefore cannot be the primary source of pain. Structures in and around the joint that account for pain from inflammation are the synovial membrane (synovitis), the retrodiscal tissues (retrodiscitis), and the capsule of the TMJ (capsulitis). Often in the clinical setting, all three conditions are concomitant.

Inflammation of the synovial membrane and/or the retrodiscal tissue may be due to local trauma, abuse, or disc displacements or may be secondary to systemic connective tissue disorders. Intracapsular edema and an alteration of joint fluid occur. Pain increases with joint movement and joint loading. Distracting the joint manually or having the patient bite on a separator placed between the teeth on the ipsilateral side should relieve the pain and can be used as a diagnostic test. Undiagnosed systemic disease or locally infectious processes may require laboratory workup or referral. Treatment is based on the etiology of the problem and may involve use of anti-inflammatory medications, a non-chew diet to lessen loading of inflamed tissues, intraoral appliances, or physical therapy modalities such as ultrasound.

Inflammation of the capsule of the TMJ may be due to external trauma or may result from spread of inflammation secondary to the above two conditions. Because the capsule, including the TM ligament, functions to limit mandibular movements, thereby defining border positions, the ligament is passive unless these borders are approached. Therefore, pain will occur during wide opening, chewing of hard foods that can cause joint distraction, or anything that causes posterior displacement of the condyle.

All these conditions may cause temporary repositioning of the mandible, either because of intracapsular edema or as an avoidance phenomenon from nociceptive input into the CNS that alters muscular function. Permanent changes to the occlusion in the acute phase are therefore contraindicated because the mandibular position is artifactual and will change when inflammation resolves. Any of these conditions may evoke a secondary muscle response that may result in muscle pain and spasm. If the problem is long-standing, diagnosing the underlying etiologic factor may be difficult.

Arthritides

Arthritic conditions of the TM articulation are essentially the same as those of other joints, with some modifications caused by specialized anatomic and functional characteristics. Arthritis of any type is a true intra-articular disease and, unlike disc derangements, may exhibit generalized involvement of many joints throughout the body. It is mentioned here for the sake of completeness. Chapter 3 contains a discussion of the classifications and treatment protocol.

Steroids given systemically may produce temporary relief and initiate the reversal of an inflammatory process. However, they also may offer only minor relief of intracapsular pain secondary to an inflammatory condition. The many undesirable side effects associated with chronic use of steroids preclude their use in managing TMJ pain. Intra-articular steroid injections are generally reliable but may be of benefit in isolated cases. Their use is quite limited because of the incidence of aseptic necrosis with multiple injections.

Arthrocentesis of the TMJ, performed under local anesthesia in an office setting, has proved to be an effective modality in the management of some chronic inflammatory states.

Condylar Displacement

The capsule of the TMJ is the structure that determines the limit to which anterior joint translation can occur. Elongation of or damage to the capsular ligament may allow joint translation to occur well anterior to the articular eminence, resulting in joint displacement.

Acute displacement without reduction of the mandibular condyle out of the glenoid fossa demands immediate attention to relieve severe pain and minimize damage to the supporting capsule and internal ligaments of the joint. The condyle is trapped anterior to the articular eminence, and the patient is unable to close the mouth. The clinician manipulates the mandible back into the glenoid fossa by placing the thumbs over the molar teeth or retromolar pad area and applying slow, firm traction in an inferior direction to bring the condyle below the level of the eminence. The force is then directed posteriorly to seat the condyle in the glenoid fossa. Manipulating one side slightly before the other usually facilitates the reduction if bilateral displacements are present. It may be necessary to inject local anesthetic into and around the joint or, in rare cases, to sedate the patient with intravenous medications (Fig. 6-19).

The patient should be advised to avoid wide opening of the mandible (yawning, dental treatment, large boluses of food) for at least 2 weeks. Inter-

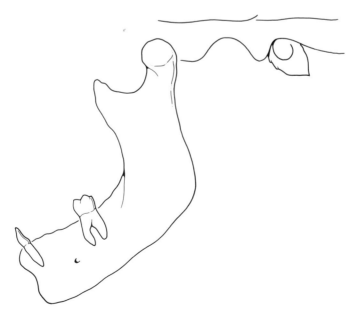

Fig. 6-19. Displaced condyle trapped anterior to articular eminence and often elevated into infratemporal fossa.

maxillary fixation or elastic ligatures may be necessary after reduction if the displacement was particularly difficult to reduce and redisplacement occurs spontaneously. Mild analgesic or NSAIDs may be helpful. Neuromuscular re-education exercises are often helpful to train the patient to avoid another displacement. Nonsurgical management will control most patients with condylar displacements. Surgery is rarely indicated. Nonsurgical management is reviewed in Chapter 7.

Sequence of Treatment

Once a working diagnosis is made, the modalities deemed necessary for treatment will depend largely on the nature of the pain the patient is experiencing. Other than the history and physical findings, few objective tests are available to aid in diagnosing mandibular-related problems. Therapeutic tools should be used in a manner that will offer diagnostic information. The physiologic effects of all modalities described previously must be understood if they are to serve the dual role of having diagnostic and therapeutic value. If a specific treatment is successful, it is not only therapeutic to the patient but also confirms the diagnosis. If the modality is ineffective in alleviating pain or restoring function, it still offers valuable diagnostic information and will help guide further treatment. The efficacy of certain modalities often lies in the clinician's skill and judgment. The shotgun approach of offering many types of therapy at the same time may be temporarily successful, but the tendency to overtreat and the lack of confirmation of the original diagnosis often outweigh short-term gains.

The treatment of TMJ, masticatory, and cervical dysfunction problems is not technique-oriented. Treatment must be tailored to the individual patient. Patients should understand that the treatment is aimed at helping them manage their problem to a level of tolerance and that "cures" rarely exist. Ideally, the level reached is one of normal function and total comfort. Such a favorable result should still be interpreted as a level of management and not cure, because relapses can and do occur.

The need for a comprehensive diagnosis and coordinated treatment plan for the patient with involvement of more than one aspect of head and neck musculoskeletal dysfunction cannot be overstressed. Muscle is the common denominator to the dentist and physical therapist, and an understanding of each other's treatment principles is imperative.

The sequence of treatment for the patient with significant muscle involvement of both neck and jaw muscles often varies depending on the location of the pain and the degree of muscle involvement. For example, a patient with an anteriorly displaced disc with the reduction may not tolerate forward repositioning of the mandible if there is concomitant severe muscle spasm in the neck or face. It may then be necessary to delay treatment of the intracuspular problem and treat the muscle condition by physical therapy or splint therapy aimed at temporary stabilization of the occlusion. Once this is accomplished, treatment of the displaced disc may then be tolerated. Another example is the patient who is initially under the care of the physical therapist for significant cervical muscle pain but who also has a marked malocclusion. Physical therapy may offer limited relief until maxillomandibular relationships are addressed, at which time further physical therapy becomes significantly more effective.

A general rule of thumb for sequencing treatment of patients with multiple areas of involvement is to treat the area of the greatest pain first. This may require temporary disregard to physical imbalances such as malocclusions or aberrant head positioning until a more appropriate time. The sequence of treatment modalities and the manner in which they are applied to such patients requires considerable skill and communication between the clinicians involved. If the diagnosis is correct, failure to gain relief of symptoms is not necessarily the result of an inappropriate choice of modalities. Instead, it can be the result of an error in the sequence of manner in which they are applied. Occasionally, after several physiologic attempts at treatment have been unsuccessful, a referral will be made for stress management through autosuggestion, biofeedback, psychological counseling, or psychotherapy.

A psychological referral is not an effort to dismiss the patient's symptoms as imaginary. On the contrary, the patient's condition is understood to be quite real and may become more serious if the problem is not resolved. TMJ dysfunction is a real physical problem that may have a psychological origin. A decision for a psychological referral is based on an understanding that there are times when emotional tensions become an overriding factor and other physical measures do not provide relief. Often such patients are coping well with life's challenges and are using their teeth as a release, thus they may be quite unaware that they are tense. It is long known that the teeth and jaws are used in coping with unpleasant or unavoidable situations. Implicit in such popular sayings as "we'll have to bite the bullet" or "you'll just have to grit your teeth and bear it" is the assumption that clenching and grinding are common coping mechanisms. These coping mechanisms are not a recent discovery of our modern technical age. Biblical accounts refer to the wailing and gnashing of teeth of the suffering. It is not surprising, then, that investigators find elevated levels of emotional tension and associate clenching and grinding behavior in some patients with TMJ dysfunction. Appropriate psychological intervention may provide the only successful avenue for achieving relief from the cycle of facial muscle spasm and pain.

CONCLUSION

TMJ dysfunction is a complex disorder involving the function of the jaw joint, teeth, and facial muscles. The TMJ is also closely related to body posture and functioning of the muscles connecting the head, neck, and shoulders. There is no one simple solution or treatment that can be applied to every case of TMJ dysfunction. Each patient must be individually assessed, and treatment and appliances must be custom-designed for that individual. The progress of treatment is based on an ongoing re-evaluation of the patient's response to treatment. Decisions to proceed with our original treatment plan, modify it, or refer the patient to other specialists for evaluation are made based on the individual patient's response to the course of treatment. Treatment may involve specialists in the fields of manual therapy, oral surgery, neurology, internal medicine, or psychology.

The overall goals of treatment, regardless of the means of treatment, are to achieve a normal full ROM of the jaw with an absence of pain. After active treatment, we would ideally like to see the patient's own teeth, or prosthetic replacements, function properly at the muscle relaxed position. Excessive force on the joint structures has been eliminated, and the correction is stabilized.

Successful treatment requires long-term stabilization and management of the condition. Once a joint or ligament is damaged, it is always susceptible to reinjury. Total management and care are essential as there is unfortunately no simple cure for TMJ dysfunction.

Many facets of pain, pain behavior, and musculoskeletal disturbances remain unknown. Population norms for many of the clinical guidelines to treatment now in vogue have not been established. Much information can be gleaned from the treatment of other muscle–joint systems in the body and from open dialogue among the several disciplines involved in the treatment of pain. A multidisciplinary approach to such complex issues appears mandatory.

REFERENCES

1. Harvold EP, Chierici G, Vargervik K: Experiments on the development of dental malocclusion. Am J Orthod 61:38, 1972
2. Harvold EP: Neuromuscular and morphological adaptations in experimentally induced oral respiration. In McNamara JA (ed): Naso-Respiration Function and Craniofacial Growth, Craniofacial Growth Series, Monograph No. 9. Center for Growth and Development, The University of Michigan, Ann Arbor, 1979
3. Harvold EP, Experiments on Mandibular Morphogenesis. In McNamara JA (ed): Determinents of Mandibular Form and Growth, Craniofacial Growth Series, Monograph No. 4. Center for Human Growth and Development, The University of Michigan, Ann Arbor, 1975
4. Linder-Aronson S, Woodside DG: The growth in the sagittal depth of the bony nasopharynx in relation to some other facial variables. In McNamara JA (ed): Naso-Respiratory Function and Craniofacial Growth, Monograph No. 9. Center for Human Growth and Development, The University of Michigan, Ann Arbor, 1979
5. Berry DC, Watkins AC: Mandibular dysfunction and incisor relationship. Br Dent J 74:144, 1978
6. Williamson EH, Lundquist DO: Anterior guidance: its effect of electromyographic activity of the temporal and masseter muscle. J Prosth Dent 49:816, 1983
7. Annandale T: On displacement of the interarticular cartilage of the lower jaw and its treatment by operation. Lancet 1:411, 1887
8. Ricketts R: A study of changes in temporomandibular relations associated with treatment of class II malocclusion. Am J Orthod 38:919, 1952

9. Lawrence E, Lawrence K: The clinical and radiographic recognition of nasal airway distraction and its effect on facial growth. J Clev Dent Soc 44: 1988

SUGGESTED READINGS

Academy of Denture Prosthetics (ADP): Glossary of prosthodontic terms. 3rd Ed. J Prosthet Dent 20:443, 1968

Atwood DA: A critique of research of the rest position of the mandible. J Prosthet Dent 16:848, 1966

Balyeat R, Bowen R: Facial and dental deformities due to perennial nasal allergy in childhood. Int J Orthod 20:445, 1934

Beard CC, Clayton JA: Effects of occlusal therapy on TMJ dysfunction. J Prosthet Dent 44:324, 1980

Bell W: Orofacial Pains: Differential Diagnosis. Year Book Medical, Chicago, 1979

Carlsson GE: Mandibular dysfunction and temporomandibular joint pathosis. J Prosthet Dent 43:658, 1980

Catlin G: Breath of Life or Malrespiration and Its Effect upon the Enjoyment and Life of Man. John Wiley, New York, 1861

Darnell M: A proposed chronology of events for forward head posture. J Craniomandib Pract 1: 1983

Farrar WB: Diagnosis and treatment of anterior dislocation of the articular disc. NY J Dent 41:348, 1972

Graber TM: Overbite—The Dentist's Challenge. J Am Dent Assoc 79: 1969

Guichet NF: Biological laws governing functions of muscular that move the mandible. Part II: condylar position. J Prosthet Dent 38:35, 1977

Harvold EP: In search of understanding basic mechanisms of orthodontic treatment. Ann Br Soc Study Orthod Torquay, 1981

Hellman M: A preliminary study as it affects the human face. Dent Cosmos 69: 250, 1927

Isberg-Holm A: Temporomandibular Joint Clicking. Department of Oral Radiation, Karolinska Institute, Stockholm, Sweden, 1980

Goldstein DF, Kraus SL, Williams WB: Influence of cervical posture on mandibular movement. J Prosthet Dent 52:421, 1984

Joseph R: The effect of airway interference on the growth and development of the face, jaws and dentition. Int J Orofac Myol 1982

Kreutziger KL, Mahan PE: Temporomandibular degenerative joint disease. Part I. Anatomy, pathophysiology and clinical description. Oral Surg 40:165, 1975

Lanier B, Tremblay N: An approach to the medical management of chronic mouthbreathing. In McNamara JA (ed): NasoRespiratory Function and Craniofacial Growth. Craniofacial Growth Series. Monograph No. 9. The University of Michigan, Ann Arbor, 1979

Laskin DM: Etiology of the pain-dysfunction syndrome. J Am Dent Assoc 79:147, 1969

Levy P: Physiologic Response to Dental Malocclusion and Misplaced Mandibular Posture: The Keys to Temporomandibular Joint and Associated Neuromuscular Disorders. Basal Facts 4:103, 1977

McNeil C, Danzig WM, Farrar WB et al: Cranomandibular (TMJ) disorders. The state of the art. J Prosthet Dent 44:434, 1980

Meyer RA, Merrill RG, Razook SJ et al: Temporomandibular Joint Disorders: Update 1982. Continuing education course material, Emory University School of Dentistry

Mohl ND: Head posture and its role in occlusion. NY State Dent J 42:17, 1976

Mohl ND: The role of head posture in mandibular function. p. 97. In Solberg WK, Clark G (eds): Abnormal Jaw Mechanics Diagnosis and Treatment. Quintessence, Chicago, 1984

Posselt U: Studies on the mobility of the human mandible. Acta Ondont Scand 10: 1, 1952

Quinn G: Airway interferences and its effect upon the growth and development of the face, jaws, dentition and associated parts. The portal of life. NC Dent J Winter–Spring, 1978

Quinn GW, Pickrell KL: Mandibular hypoplasia and airway interference. NC Dent J 61:19, 1978

Ramjford SP, Ash MM: Occlusion. 3rd Ed. WB Saunders, Philadelphia, 1983

Ricketts R: Laminography in the diagnosis of temporomandibular joint disorders. J Am Dent Assoc 79:118, 1953

Ricketts R: Respiratory obstruction syndrome. Am J Orthod 54:495, 1968

Ricketts RM: The interdependence of the nasal and oral capsules. In McNamara JA (ed): Naso-Respiratory Function and Craniofacial Growth, Craniofacial Growth Series, Monograph No. 9. Center for Human Growth and Development, The University of Michigan, Ann Arbor, 1979

Ritter F: Physiology of the nose, paranasal sinuses and middle ear. In Middeton E (ed): Allergy: Principles and Practice. Vol. 1. CV Mosby, St. Louis, 1978

Root GR, Kraus SL, Razook SJ, Samson GS: Effect of an intraoral splint on head and neck posture. J Prosthet Dent 58:90, 1987

Sicher H: Structural and functional basis for disorders of the temporomandibular articulation. J Oral Surg 13:275, 1955

Sicher H: Oral Anatomy. CV Mosby, St. Louis, 1965

Subtenly J: Effects of disease of tonsils and adenoids in dentofacial morphology. Ann Otol Rhinol Laryngol, suppl. 19:50, 1975

Subtenly JD: The significance of adenoid tissue. Angle Orthod 20:59, 1954

Todd TW, Cohen MD, Broadbent B: The role of allergy in the etiology of orthodontics deformity. J Allergy 10:246, 1939

Toller PA: The Synovial Apparatus and Temporomandibular Joint Dysfunction. Br Dent J 111:355, 1961

Travell J: Temporomandibular joint pain referred from the muscles of the head and neck. J Prosthet Dent 10:745, 1960

Travell J, Simons D: Myofascial Pain and Dysfunction: The Trigger Point Manual. Williams & Wilkins, Baltimore, 1983

Van Sickels J, Ivey D: Myofacial pain dysfunction: a manifestation of the short face syndrome. J Prosth Dent 42: 1979

Vig PS: Experimental manipulation of head posture. Am J Orthod 77:258, 1980

Watson W: The symposium through the eyes of the editor. Am J Ortho 80: 1981

7 | Physical Therapy Management of TMD

Steven L. Kraus

Physical therapy in the management of TMD "is well recognized as an effective, conservative method of treatment for TMD"[1] and should be routinely used in TMD therapy.[2] Some studies suggest, however, that physical therapy provides only minimal, if any, therapeutic value in the treatment of TMD.[3,4] There are several basic explanations for differing conclusions on the effectiveness of physical therapy for TMD. The first and most apparent explanation is the misuse and abuse of the term *physical therapy*. Health professionals and lay practitioners who are not physical therapists should not suggest that exercises, ice packs, and moist heat treatment are physical therapy.[4] Patients who are told to purchase a sporting goods mouth appliance or told to purchase an over-the-counter medication are not misled that they are receiving dentistry or medicine. There should be no doubt by the patient or insurance companies that when physical therapy is administered for TMD or for other musculoskeletal disorders, a licensed professional physical therapist is providing evaluation and treatment. If treatment is not offered by a physical therapist, then said treatment should be referred to as simply a modality or an exercise, nothing more.

Physical therapists, specialized in musculoskeletal dysfunction, offer patients a thorough evaluation and comprehensive treatment plan. Treatment may focus on instructions in specific exercises or application of modalities and manual procedures. The physical therapist will be able to assess and modify the treatments based on the change in the patient's signs and symptoms. Physical therapy management of TMD provides a therapeutic and cost-effective approach. Physical therapy will be a primary source of treatment for most patients experiencing TMD. For other patients, physical therapy may be an important adjunct to treatment(s) such as occlusal appliances and nonsteroidal anti-inflammatory medication.

Criteria used for "patient selection" offer a second explanation for differences in physical therapy efficacy in the management of TMD. Let us assume that the objectives of a research paper were to investigate the effectiveness of a particular treatment on a TMJ patient population. After reading the methodology section of this research paper, it was clear that the authors used inaccurate criteria to establish a TMJ patient population. The conclusions reached in this paper as to the effectiveness of a treatment(s) would not be valid for the true TMJ population. Also, if criteria used for patient selection are not the same for all studies, any attempt to compare treatment outcomes between studies would be difficult.[5,6] Signs and symptoms of what constitute the TMD patient population have reached a level of general acceptance only quite recently.[1,5,6] A great deal of work is needed to repeat past research on the effectiveness of different treatments because we now have a better understanding as to what disorders of the TMJ we are treating. Furthermore, studies investigating the effectiveness of physical therapy in the treatment of TMD should clearly state whether a licensed physical therapist is actually involved in the administration of such modalities or procedures if the effectiveness of physical therapy is to be validated or rebuked.

To be able to classify a patient into any one or combination of the various categories of TMD, the clinician will need to acquire an understanding of the subset diagnostic classification system of TMD that is endorsed by the American Academy of Orofacial Pain.[1,5,7] The reader is referred to Chapter 3 as well as to the References[1,8] to develop an insight into understanding the diagnostic classifications for TMD.

When treatments are discussed for TMD, the reader must not be misled into thinking this is a "cookbook" approach. Treatments are for a specific condition and not for a specific patient with a condition. Patients often present with disorders of the TMJ but with involvement in adjacent areas. Disorders involving the muscles of mastication, occlusion, and cervical spine are frequently additional sources for the patient's signs and symptoms. Sequencing of treatments for patients with multiple functional disorders and emotional disturbances that accompany pain (see Ch. 13) is beyond the scope and objectives of this chapter.

Whether treatments offered for TMD include a home exercise program, use of an occlusal appliance, or medication, patient education and patient compliance are essential. In a recent study, a critical factor in promoting patient compliance was the patient–clinician relationship. The most frequently cited reason for noncompliance was the patient's dislike of the clinician.[9] Patient education is inherently connected with physical therapy and is an essential part of most treatment regimes.[10] The kind, quantity, and quality of patient education along with patient attitude and therapist behavior are all related to therapeutic results of treatment and patient compliance.[10]

The subset diagnostic categories of TMD that are best managed by a physical therapist are *inflammation, hypermobility,* and *hypomobility.* These classifications provide a means of focusing the reader's attention on three broad conditions of the TMJ from which a physical therapy treatment program can be formulated. It does not intend to replace existing classification systems.

Progression from one treatment to the next is based on the degree of inflammation, hypermobility, and hypomobility and the patient's response (signs and symptoms) to the previous treatment(s). When possible, the patient should be encouraged to continue those exercises that can be included in a home exercise program. Questions pertaining to the frequency and repetitions of a procedure or exercise are dependent on the patient's condition and life style.

INFLAMMATION

Of the various disorders associated with the TMJ, I believe that inflammation is the most common source for patient symptoms and should be addressed first. Although inflammation often accompanies conditions such as hypermobility and hypomobility, one should not assume these other conditions are the primary cause for the inflammation. Hypermobility and hypomobility have a high occurrence in the nonpatient population.

Tissues subject to inflammation are the synovium (synovitis), which includes the retrodiscal tissue, and the capsule (capsulitis).[1] These tissues can become inflamed secondary to blunt trauma to the mandible or secondary to maintaining an open-mouth position as in various dental procedures. A less obvious cause but perhaps the most common cause is excessive or prolonged loading to the joint. Although the TMJ is a load-bearing joint,[11] excessive or prolonged loading may occur during functional activities (chewing or talking) and parafunctional activities (clenching or bruxism) and with habits such as fingernail biting, gum or ice chewing, and leaning the chin on hand.

No attempt to distinguish a specific treatment for synovitis or capsulitis will be made because it is difficult to differentiate between the two during physical examination. From the physical therapist's perspective, treatments for inflammation related to polyarthritides[1] (i.e., rheumatoid arthritis [RA], juvenile rheumatoid arthritis, spondyloarthropathies, and crystal-induced disease) do not differ from treatment for common inflammatory conditions. Such polyarthritides will require additional dental and/or medical input. The reader is referred to the References for additional information on treatment related to rheumatologic diseases.[12]

Treatment

Habit Awareness and Oral Modification

Treatment for inflammation of the TMJ will center on the avoidance of unnecessary or excessive loading to the joint. Habit modification of fingernail biting, gum or ice chewing, leaning the chin on hand, or any other activities that do not involve talking, chewing food, and drinking fluid is strongly encouraged. The patient should avoid excessive talking and should consider a soft food diet. In a study that examined the relationship between treatment outcome and diverse psychological factors for patients with TMD,[13] the authors concluded that "the patient's awareness of the dysfunction as a problem over which he or she has some degree of control may be one of the essential and common ingredients for successful outcome." They suggest that educating patients about exacerbating factors (i.e., fingernail biting, gum chewing, etc.) may be enough to relieve pain if the patient makes a concerted effort to control these same factors. Controlling parafunctional activity that contributes to excessive loading of the TMJ will be covered next.

Tongue Up/Teeth Apart/Breath/Swallow

Muscle hyperactivity plays a perpetuating if not a predisposing and precipitating role in inflammation and other disorders of the TMJ.[14] Masticatory muscle hyperactivity causes excessive loading to the joint. Parafunctional activity involves masticatory muscle hyperactivity. Parafunction can be defined as repetitive activity, frequently contributing to dental, periodontal, or *neuromuscular damage*.[15] Parafunction consists of repetitive activity involving clenching and/or bruxism (tooth grinding). Most patients are unaware of the nature, intensity, and frequency of their parafunctional activity. Parafunction may occur as diurnal or nocturnal or both. Diurnal activity is best controlled through the exercises that will be discussed below.

Diurnal parafunction usually results from stressful situations such as office or home conflicts or is related to "type A" behavior (hurried, pressured, controlling, demanding). Whatever the environmental and/or emotional cause, diurnal parafunction does not have to occur if emphasis is placed on "self-awareness." An informed patient who feels some degree of control over parafunction can take appropriate action as to how to respond to stress. The neuromuscular re-education exercise consisting of tongue up/teeth apart/breath/swallow (TTBS) should be instructed to the patient as a means of controlling diurnal parafunction. TTBS is a way of initiating cortical awareness and control toward "normal" muscle activity of the jaw at rest or moving. Once a harmful activity is recognized consciously, steps can be taken to replace it with a therapeutic activity. TTBS provides the patient a tool to "self-correct." Motivation by the patient to perform TTBS is essential. Motivation is largely fueled by the clinician's understanding of the physiology behind TTBS and the ability to demonstrate and communicate the application of this and other neuromuscular re-educational exercises in a meaningful way.

TTB aims to achieve a rest position of the mandible known as the upright postural position of the mandible.[16] A rest position of the mandible is one of minimal masticatory muscle activity. It is identified by an absence of movement of the mandible and by positioning the teeth of the upper and lower arches apart. The purpose of educating the patient on the normal sequence of swallowing (S) is to ensure that the patient is not using unnecessary/excessive muscle activity during swallowing and that swallowing is performed with teeth apart.

Tongue Up. The tongue is active during most oral-mandibular functions. The tongue assists in mixing food and in delivery of food into the posterior part of the mouth for swallowing, and it plays an important role in the action of swallowing. The tongue not only has many sensory functions but also acts efficiently in discriminating the characteristics of food as well as contributing to speech. The very fact that we seldom bite our tongues during normal oral function is due to the highly developed, skillfully coordinated neurofunctions operating between the tongue and the mandibular muscles. The coordination between the tongue and mandibular muscles is dependent on the jaw–tongue reflex.[17,18]

The tongue is composed of various intrinsic and extrinsic muscles. The genioglossus is the main muscle responsible for positioning the tongue in the oral cavity. The genioglossus muscle is primarily responsible for establishing and maintaining the rest position of the tongue and is active in elevating and protruding the tongue.[19,20] "Tongue up" refers to the position of the tongue when at rest. The rest position of the tongue or "postural position" is up against the palate of the mouth[19] (Fig. 7-1). The most anterosuperior tip of the tongue will lie in an area against the palate just posteriorly to the back side of the upper central incisors. No pressure by the tongue should be made against the back side of the upper central incisors. The remaining portion of the tongue, at least the first half of the tongue, will be against the palate. To be sure the

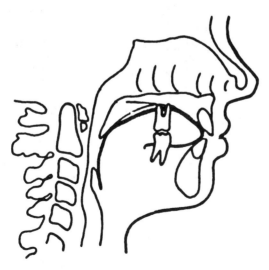

Fig. 7-1. Rest position of the tongue. The anterorsuperior tip of the tongue lies against the palate just posterior to the upper central incisors. In this position, the teeth of the upper and lower arches are apart. (From Kraus,[163] with permission.)

patient does not "poke" the tongue into this position, instruct the patient to let the tongue "flatten out from side to side" as it lies against the palate. In this position, the most posterior part of the tongue will form the anterior wall of the pharynx.[21]

The position of the tongue at rest not only encourages the tongue muscles to maintain a resting muscle tone but also encourages the muscles that elevate the mandible (temporalis, masseter, internal pterygoid) to maintain a resting muscle tone (jaw–tongue reflex).[17,18,22] Unless the patient is chewing, talking, coughing, swallowing, or licking their lips, their tongue should be in the rest position at all times. If the patient has a maxillary occlusal appliance, the appliance, if possible, should not cover the palate of the mouth. Palatal coverage by the appliance could interfere with the rest position of the tongue. Patients who are sensitive to a proper tongue position at rest would respond best to an occlusal appliance that does not cover the palate.

Teeth Apart.   Informing the patient of the simple fact that the back teeth should be apart, is at times, all that is needed to be therapeutic in reducing masticatory muscle hyperactivity. Instructing the patient on the rest position of the tongue will assist the patient in self-awareness of keeping teeth apart. Have the patient focus on the tongue position at rest. Then ask the patient to bring the back teeth together. The patient will do one of two things. The patient will have to pull the tongue back out of the way or end up biting the tongue.

Patients who have either a maxillary or mandibular appliance should be told that the appliance is not there for them to "bite" into even if it is referred to as a "bite appliance." Reason with patients by telling them that the appliance is not to stop them from doing parafunctional activities. Instead a properly "balanced" appliance is to minimize the harmful effects of parafunctional activities on the teeth, TMJ and associated muscles of mastication, and cervical spine. Patients must become aware of tongue up and teeth apart with or without an appliance.

Comments on Nocturnal Parafunction: Nocturnal parafunction is more difficult to control than diurnal parafunction. Because the etiology of nocturnal parafunction is still being investigated, this author would offer the following suggestions from the physical therapist's perspective. Nocturnal parafunction is usually suspected with patients who, on awakening during the night or morning, report headaches, facial, jaw, and tooth/teeth symptoms. It has been my observation that nocturnal parafunction can be influenced in a positive way by addressing the presence of a symptomatic cervical spine disorder (see Ch. 11) along with educating the patient in proper sleeping postures to include the use of proper cervical support for the neck. Attention given to the cervical spine has appeared to decrease nocturnal parafunction as identified by symptomatic improvement in the morning. I would suggest as a topic for future research the relationship of a symptomatic or asymptomatic cervical spine disorder and nocturnal parafunction.

Breathing. "Nasal breathing is essential to the normal well being of the body."[23] Nasal breathing permits the air to be warmed, moistened, and cleansed before it reaches the lungs. Nasal breathing will call on a more ideal use of the diaphragm, the principal driver of respiration. Proper use of the diaphragm allows ideal ventilation of the lungs. Diaphragmatic breathing is an excellent way to promote general relaxation of the body.

Diaphragmatic breathing occurs more easily by breathing through the nose. A correct rest position of the tongue forces nasal-diaphragmatic breathing. This occurs more easily in the absence of any resistance in the upper airway cavity (i.e., colds, allergies, nasal septum deviations, etc.).

Breathing through the mouth decreases the effects of diaphragmatic breathing and increases use of accessory muscles of breathing. Primary accessory muscles are the scalenes and the sternocleidomastoid (SCM).[24] The physical therapist may need to apply various manual techniques to enhance proper use of the diaphragm. Rib cage and thoracic spine mobility will also need to be evaluated because these factors influence diaphragmatic breathing.

Swallowing. The act of swallowing food, liquid, and saliva occurs throughout the day. Excessive masticatory muscle activity is suggested to occur in patients who acquire an altered sequence of swallowing in which a tongue thrust occurs. The most frequently cited signs of tongue thrust activity during swallowing include protrusion of the tongue against or between the anterior teeth and excessive circumoral muscle activity.[25] A strong relationship does appear to exist between a tongue thrust and pediatric anterior open bites.[26,27] However, in the absence of a pediatric tongue thrust and the frequently associated dental and skeletal changes, I have observed that an adult can acquire a tongue thrust, which is here referred to as "an acquired adult tongue thrust." It is theorized that tongue movement and positioning in the oral cavity are influenced by dysfunctional mobility and positioning of the cervical spine.[28] A recent paper suggests that positional changes of the head may have an effect on genioglossus muscle activation thresholds.[29] The genioglossus muscle is the primary muscle that protrudes the tongue.[19] Attempt to look up at the ceiling and swallow. Not only is it difficult to swallow with such an extended head position, but to complete the swallowing cycle, the teeth will be brought together firmly.

The literature is not clear in clarifying whether humans swallow with the teeth together or apart. This debate may occur because cervical spine mobility and positioning have not been a variable that has been fully recognized and controlled in past studies.[30] This author observes that in the presence of good mobility and positioning of the cervical spine, swallowing occurs with teeth out of contact. In the presence of a cervical spine disorder contributing to an acquired adult tongue thrust, not only is it suggested that tooth contact occurs but an increase in duration of the teeth in occlusion occurs. An acquired adult tongue thrust may therefore contribute to masticatory muscle hyperactivity but may also contribute to symptoms such as difficulty in swallowing, scratching sensations in the throat that do not become a sore throat, and shortness of breath.[28]

The evaluation used by Barrett and Hanson[31] to determine the presence of a pediatric anterior tongue thrust is not helpful in determining the presence of an acquired adult tongue thrust. Barrett and Hanson appear to rely on dental and skeletal changes when deciding if a tongue thrust is present. The following evaluation is recommended by this author to help in determining the presence of an "acquired adult tongue thrust":

1.   Have the patient swallow water two to four times, pausing briefly between each swallow. During each swallow, palpate the hyoid bone (Fig. 7-2). A quick up and down movement of the hyoid bone (like a flicker) should normally be felt. With an acquired adult tongue thrust, a slow up and down movement of the hyoid bone is felt.

2.   Palpation of the suboccipital muscles is performed simultaneously with step 1 (Fig. 7-2). As the patient swallows, little if any contractions should be felt to occur in the suboccipital muscles. With an acquired adult tongue thrust, suboccipital muscle contractions will occur.

3.   During a normal swallow, no head movement should be observed. With an acquired adult tongue thrust extension of the head on the neck and, in more

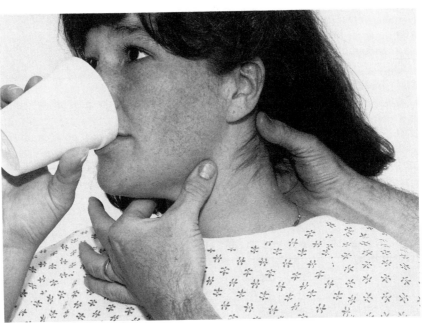

Fig. 7-2.   Evaluation for the presence of an acquired adult tongue thrust. The clinician's left hand is palpating hyoid bone movement while the right hand is palpating suboccipital muscle contraction. Head and neck movement along with lip activity are observed for by the clinician.

severe cases, an actual forward craning movement of the entire head and neck will be observed.

4. During a normal swallow, no excessive lip activity should be observed. Lip activity will be seen with the acquired adult tongue thrust. This is the least observable activity with the acquired adult tongue thrust.

5. While the patient swallows, have the patient become aware of the tongue movement and position during swallowing, especially the anterior tip of the tongue. During normal swallowing, the patient should not be aware of the tip of the tongue pressing forward. With an acquired adult tongue thrust, the patient will typically state that the tip of the tongue presses firmly against the back side of his front teeth or straight forward or down against the back side of his bottom teeth.

Treatment of acquired adult tongue thrust consists of treatment of cervical spine disorder. Chapter 11 provides an overview of treatment for a cervical spine disorder. In addition to the cervical spine treatment, the patient will need to be instructed on the normal sequence of swallowing (Fig. 7-3):

Stage 1. Instruct the patient where the tongue should be positioned at rest (Fig. 7-3, stage 1).

Stage 2. When water enters the oral cavity, the tongue will have dropped down from the rest position (Fig. 7-3, stage 2).

Stage 3. The initial phase of swallowing occurs when the tip of the tongue goes back to its rest position (Fig. 7-3, stage 3). From that point on, no pressure should be felt with the tip of the tongue pressing against the teeth.

Stage 4. The main force of swallowing will occur with the middle one-third of the tongue (Fig. 7-3, stage 4). The tongue should be perceived as moving like a "wave." Although the wave will start at the tip of the tongue, its main force will occur with the middle one-third of the tongue. Inform the patient that the posterior teeth should not come into contact while swallowing.

Stage 5. The tongue returns to its rest position, completing the swallowing cycle (Fig. 7-3, stage 5).

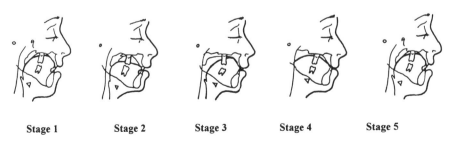

Stage 1   Stage 2   Stage 3   Stage 4   Stage 5

Fig. 7-3.   Normal sequence of swallowing. (From Kraus,[163] with permission.)

Tongue Up and Wiggle

Tongue up and wiggle is an exercise to be performed when the patient is suspected of "bracing" their mandible with their muscles. Bracing would be defined as masticatory muscle hyperactivity but with teeth out of occlusion.

Patients who brace their mandible would be identified by:

Palpation to determine the presence of masticatory muscle hyperactivity
Minimal or no occlusal wear
Patient denial of diurnal parafunction
Reports of no symptoms on awakening to suggest the absence of nocturnal parafunction
Minimal therapeutic value received from habit awareness, oral modification, and TTBS

The patient is instructed on the rest position of the tongue. From this tongue up position and teeth apart position, the patient is asked to oscillate or "wiggle" the jaw from side to side. Great care is taken not to have the patient oscillate the mandible through a large range of lateral motion for two reasons. First, excessive lateral excursions mean the joint contralateral to the side of movement is translating. If the joint is inflamed, translation may further increase inflammation. Second, if the patient has a disc displacement that reduces, large lateral excursions may produce joint noises related to the disc displacement. Repetitively reproducing joint noises associated with a disc displacement with reduction may cause an asymptomatic disc displacement to become painful.

To control for excessive lateral excursion that may occur with this exercise, the patient is asked to place the tips of the index fingers to each side of the chin, approximately 1 mm from the skin (Fig. 7-4). When the patient oscillates the mandible from side to side, the index fingers will provide proprioceptive feedback to control excessive lateral excursions. Once the importance of limiting the amount of movement is understood by the patient, speed of the movement may be increased. The objective of mandibular oscillations is to teach an exercise that counters habitual jaw bracing.

Tongue Up and Open and Close With Speed

Hypomobility may be associated with inflammation because the patient is reluctant to open the mouth. The objective of this exercise is to avoid immobility by encouraging movement that avoids translation.

This exercise involves having the patient open and close the mouth wide while keeping the tongue in its rest position (Fig. 7-5). Tongue up while opening allows the condyles to rotate but not to translate. It is the translation of the condyle that often perpetuates inflammation. Tongue up while opening permits at least 20 to 25 mm of mandibular opening. Once controlled opening is under-

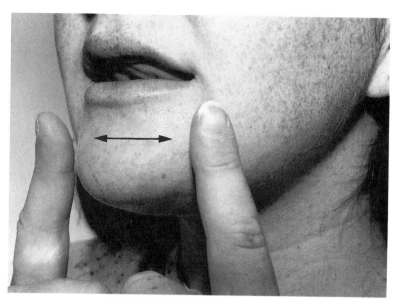

Fig. 7-4. Tongue up and wiggle. This exercise is instructed when the patient is suspected of bracing the mandible with teeth out of occlusion. Note the rest position of the tongue and the minimal space between the tip of the index fingers and the chin as appreciated with the patient's right index finger.

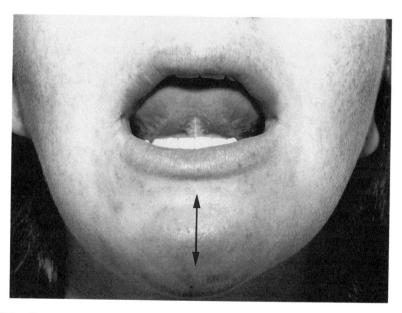

Fig. 7-5. Tongue up and open and close with speed. Exercise allows for condylar rotation while controlling translation. This exercise would primarily be performed for inflammation or for inflammation secondary to arthroscopy or arthrotomy. When yawning, tongue up is performed to restrict mandibular opening.

stood by the patient, the patient can increase the speed of movement. Increasing the speed of opening and closing would be similar to oscillating, which may provide a secondary benefit of enhancing relaxation of the muscles of mastication. A patient who becomes used to opening to 20 to 25 mm will be less reluctant to increase the opening beyond 20 to 25 mm when it is time to do so.

Cervical Spine Disorders

The role of the cervical spine in the management of TMD is covered in Chapter 11. A cervical spine disorder can cause masticatory muscle hyperactivity. As with TMD, there are many subset diagnostic categories of cervical spine disorders. One common category is cervical spine muscle hyperactivity. Cervical spine muscle hyperactivity can cause masticatory muscle hyperactivity, which, in turn, can cause or perpetuate TMJ inflammation. Treatment offered for TMJ inflammation may be indirect through treatment of the cervical spine, which will often relax the muscles of mastication.

Intraoral and Extraoral Massage/Stretching

As mentioned earlier, decreasing masticatory muscle hyperactivity can provide a significant therapeutic outcome in controlling inflammation. Decreasing the "tone" of certain muscles of mastication that may be hyperactive or tight may require intraoral and extraoral massage or stretching techniques by the physical therapist. Direction, force, duration, and movement of a massage or stretch along with the clinician's skill and knowledge of anatomy may influence the therapeutic outcome of such techniques. No effort will be made in this chapter to discuss a particular massage or stretching technique that enhances masticatory muscle hyperactivity. As with many manual techniques, it is not so much the "technique" but more the attention and skill of the clinician that makes the technique therapeutic.

Modalities

The modalities I most commonly use for controlling inflammation are cold, nonthermal ultrasound, phonophoresis, and iontophoresis. Management of masticatory muscle hyperactivity usually involves modalities. Heat/cold, thermal ultrasound, various electrical stimulation parameters, and flourimethane spray are those I most commonly select.

It is a matter of clinical judgment and experience as to the sequence and choice of modalities. As a means of cost containment, I typically use mandibular exercises and manual therapy before escalating to the use of modalities other than those a patient can use at home (i.e., heat and ice). Patient education regarding condition along with a home exercise program plus manual treatments offered to the cervical spine and muscles of mastication have produced a greater predictable benefit than the use of modalities. The therapeutic value of the modalities in the treatment of inflammation as well as for masticatory muscle hyperactivity should not be underestimated. If a patient is receiving only modalities with no other treatment, it should be of great concern to patients, physicians, and insurance companies. The reader is referred to reference 32 as well as to Chapter 10 *(Postarthroscopic Surgery)* of this text for additional information on modalities.

Summary

In the vast majority of uninvolved patients (i.e., multiple surgeries, multiple diagnoses, high stress, etc) who receive the above treatments, inflammation will be resolved within the first 4 to 6 weeks. Masticatory muscle hyperactivity is considered to play a perpetuating if not a predisposing and precipitating role in inflammation. Treatment for masticatory muscle hyperactivity will usually be offered during this 4 to 6 week time period. Treatments will concentrate on awareness exercises, treatment of cervical spine disorder(s), and modalities. This author places a great deal of emphasis on patient education and the management of the symptomatic cervical spine for controlling masticatory muscle hyperactivity (see Ch. 11). If a patient continues to demonstrate signs and symptoms of inflammation after 4 to 6 weeks of treatment, it is usually due to uncontrolled masticatory muscle hyperactivity that is perpetuating the inflammatory process. In the presence of inflammation and/or muscle hyperactivity that continues beyond 4 to 6 weeks, the patient will need to consult with a dentist. At this stage, the dentist will often offer an appropriate occlusal appliance and nonsteroidal anti-inflammatory medication (see Ch. 6).

HYPERMOBILITY

Hypermobility is identified when the condyle functions beyond the articular crest onto the articular tubercle. The condyle when functioning onto the articular tubercle can be said to be functioning outside its physiologic range but within its anatomic range. Through the contraction of muscles that elevate the mandible, it is possible for the condyle to return to the articular eminence. If the condyle(s) cannot return to the articular eminence by the contraction of muscles but instead remains within the area of the articular tubercle, condylar dislocation is present. Dislocation occurs when the condyle is outside both its physiologic and anatomic boundaries.

The diagnosis of hypermobility can be made by taking radiographs of the TMJ with the patient's mouth fully opened. Hypermobility is such a benign condition that the expense and exposure to radiation does not justify radiographs for the sole purpose of identifying hypermobility. Evaluation of hypermobility can be performed instead when the clinician palpates the lateral pole(s) and feels excessive excursion of the lateral poles during mandibular opening.[8] Often associated with excessive lateral pole excursion is a combination of mandibular deflection away from the side of hypermobility, possible joint noises, and opening in excess of 40 mm.[8]

The etiology of TMJ hypermobility is unknown. Potential predisposing factors have been suggested that range from joint laxity to psychiatric disorders to skeletal abnormalities.[33] A recent investigation suggests systemic hypermobility (ligament laxity) may be closely related to TMJ hypermobility.[34] However, most studies on systemic hypermobility have investigated whether a correlation exists between systemic hypermobility and disc displacements/osteoarthrosis of the TMJ.[35,36] In one study, the authors concluded that disc displacements of the TMJ are a symptom of "joint hypermobility syndrome" (articular complaints in hypermobile subjects who have no diagnosed rheumatic disease).[35] However, another study showed that generalized joint hypermobility was not a predisposing factor to TMJ disc displacements and osteoarthrosis.[36] Regardless of the proposed etiologic factors to TMJ hypermobility, the only way the condyle can translate sufficiently enough to achieve an anterior position on the articular tubercle is through the contraction of the muscles that depress the mandible.

The occurrence of hypermobility is seen frequently with asymptomatic patients. Because hypermobility is as common as disc displacements, one can conclude such conditions may be a variation of the normal. Knowing that hypermobility is going to be present with many patients, the question is, when is it important to treat hypermobility? *Hypermobility is important to treat when inflammation is present or when the patient has pain with full opening.*

Treatment

In the presence of inflammation, if the patient were to open the mouth wide, such as during periods of yawning, excessive translation may perpetuate the inflammatory condition. However, repetitive excessive opening during acts of singing, yelling, etc., or prolonged full opening that occurs during various dental procedures or intubation performed for general anesthesia may be sufficient force to cause inflammation or some other subset diagnostic category of TMD in a previously asymptomatic TMJ.[37] If the clinician diagnoses a patient as having an asymptomatic hypermobile joint, it would be appropriate to educate the patient on the recommended treatment for hypermobility for the purpose of prevention. If a prolonged dental procedure is required, the patient should be given frequent rest periods from the open-mouth position.

Treatment for hypermobility should fall way short of surgery for the vast majority of patients. Surgeries such as eminectomy, condylotomy, sectioning of the lateral pterygoid muscle, intracapsular injection of sclerosing solutions, and increasing the height of the articular eminence to block anterior movement of the condyle are suggested surgical treatments for hypermobility.[38,39] Surgery performed for hypermobility should only be performed when all other conservative care has been tried.

The following are treatments for hypermobility listed in the order I follow. How far the clinician escalates in the instruction of the exercise depends on the needs of the individual patient. Treatments focus on patient self-awareness and neuromuscular re-educational exercises used to control excessive translation associated with hypermobility. If inflammation is present, one would pursue the course of treatment discussed in the section on inflammation.

Do Not Open Wide

The patient is instructed to avoid opening the mouth so wide. Help the patient to identify activities that encourage wide opening such as yawning, singing, yelling, eating a large sandwich, or dental work. Should a patient require intubation for general anesthesia, the patient should inform the anesthesiologist to take the necessary precautions during intubation. Of the activities listed above, yawning occurs most frequently at a subconscious level and is thus more difficult to control.

Yawn With Tongue Up

Instruct the patient on the rest position of the tongue. The inferior surface of the tongue is connected with the mandible by a mucous membrane that lies over the floor of the mouth to the lingual surface of the gum.[40] The mucous membrane in its midline forms a distinct vertical fold, the frenulum. By keeping the tongue up during yawning, the frenulum (mucous membrane) is responsible for restricting the amount of mouth opening. Tongue up during mouth opening allows only rotation of the condyles and minimal if any translation of the condyles (Fig. 7-5). The clinician will need to reason with the patient that yawning in this manner may lack some of the satisfaction associated with a wide yawn but avoids the potential for pain.

Lateral Pole Palpation

In this exercise, the patient touches the lateral poles of the condyles with the middle or index fingers. The patient then places the tongue flat against the palate of the mouth. The patient is asked to open the mouth, keeping the tongue against the palate. While opening, the patient palpates the lateral poles (Fig. 7-6). During opening, the patient is asked to keep the lateral poles from moving forward, which should not occur if performed with tongue up. Proprioceptive feedback of the tongue against the palate while monitoring the lateral pole movement with the fingers will promote condylar rotation.

Once the patient can perform this exercise correctly, the patient drops the

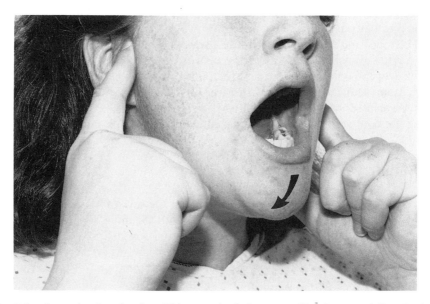

Fig. 7-6. Lateral pole palpation. This exercise is for controlling hypermobility. Patient in this photograph has already dropped the tongue from its rest position. The necessary amount of translation may be identified by the patient palpating for a small impression posterior to the lateral poles, as shown by the patient's right index finger.

tongue away from the palate to allow translation. This time, however, the translation is controlled. The goal is to have the patient achieve 40 mm of mandibular opening. The necessary amount of translation may be identified by the patient palpating for a small impression posterior to the lateral pole, indicating controlled translation has occurred (Fig. 7-6). As with any exercise, repetition and the patient's conscious effort will determine the success of treatment in achieving neuromuscular control during mandibular opening.

Isometric Exercise

Isometric exercises classically involve resisting opening, closing, lateral, protrusive, and retrusive movements of the mandible.[41] The resistance is usually offered by the patient's hand or fingers placed on the mandible. Isometric exercises have been prescribed to help with hypermobility but also to aid in "minimizing clicking, retraining muscles to contract symmetrically, overcoming zigzag opening patterns, and increasing mouth opening when it is restricted by muscle spasm."[42]

Isometric muscular contraction occurs when muscle(s) are contracted against an unyielding resistance in which the proximal and distal attachments neither separate nor approximate (i.e., no physiologic joint motion is produced). The amount of muscle contraction (force) depends on the number of motor units recruited. A motor unit consists of all the muscle fibers innervated by a single motor nerve fiber.[43] For the best results in treating hypermobility using isometrics, this author would suggest using *minimal* muscle contraction.

Isometric contraction of the elevator muscles of the mandible offers a good starting point to gain control over hypermobility. Hypermobility may also be controlled by resisting those muscles involved with mandibular depression, lateral excursion, and protrusion. Contraction of the muscles responsible for all mandibular movement may help in appropriately retraining (rhythmic stabilization) a very detailed, reflexly coordinated neuromuscular system. Isometrics for the purpose of controlling hypermobility of the TMJ are not so much for strengthening purposes but for the *control of movement*. Control of movement can also be implemented with isotonic contractions as well. Isotonic muscular contraction allows the proximal and distal attachments to either approximate (muscle shortening or concentric contraction) or separate (muscle lengthening or eccentric mode).

The patient is instructed to place the tongue in the rest position with teeth apart and place the tip of each index finger against the side of the jaw (Fig. 7-7). The patient commands him- or herself to "hold, do not let the jaw move," thereby making it a hold–relax technique versus a contract–relax technique. A hold–relax technique gives the patient more finesse in controlling the amount of pressure being applied to the jaw. The force of the isometric exercises is minimal. The direction of force applied to the mandible will be in various planes (i.e., sagittal, horizontal, frontal, and oblique), thereby contracting all muscles

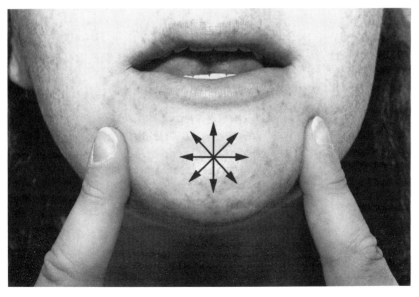

Fig. 7-7. Isometric exercise. This hold–relax isometric exercise is performed for controlling hypermobility. The direction of force can be applied in various planes (i.e., sagittal, horizontal, frontal, and oblique).

used in positioning and movement of the mandible. The duration of resistance in any one plane is for only a short period of time.

Isometric exercises for conditions other than for hypermobility are listed below.

Joint Noises (the Reciprocal Click) Related to a Disk Displacement With Reduction. If isometric exercises are instructed with the intention of treating joint noises related to a disc displacement with reduction, such exercises should be performed with the disc in "proper" position. Proper disc position is assumed to have occurred once the patient opens the mouth wide enough for both the clinician and the patient to feel/hear the opening click. For isometric exercises to maintain the disc in proper position through muscle re-education and/or strengthening, the disc must first be in the reduced position. Clinically, this author would only attempt such a feat if the patient was very young, with a disc displaced for only a relatively short time and with the patient wearing an occlusal appliance.

The patient and the clinician should not assume that the absence of joint noises during opening and closing signifies the permanent reduction of a disc displacement regardless of the treatment offered. Patients with a disc displacement with reduction can rotate their condyles up to 20 to 25 mm of mandibular opening without eliciting any opening joint noise. Clinicians may think the treatment using isometrics or isotonics is treating joint noises related to a disc displacement with reduction, when in fact such exercises are simply not allowing for full mandibular opening to occur to expose the opening noise.[44] More discussion on disc displacements is covered later in this chapter.

Asymmetries of Mandibular Movement. Asymmetries of mandibular movement (deviation/deflection) are frequently seen during mandibular opening and closing as well as protrusion and to some extent during lateral excursions. When the TMJ evaluation is negative for etiologies that are known to be associated with mandibular deviations and deflections, the aberrant movement may be normal and may not require any form of treatment. Pantomographs of 200 asymptomatic female subjects showed the appearance of the TMJ varied widely.[45] There was at least some evidence of remodeling in nearly every joint. Condylar flattening and sclerosis were the more common changes. Age was a factor in the degree of remolding. Another study raised the possibility that aberrant muscle attachments may be primarily or secondarily responsible for deviations in opening and closing movements of the mandible.[46] Instructing the patient on isometric exercises to correct mandibular deflections and/or deviations related to remolding or aberrant muscle attachments would be unproductive. If mandibular dynamics are asymmetrical yet *functional and pain-free,* then no treatment is necessary.

Mandibular Muscle Weakness. I find that weakness of jaw muscles is the exception rather than the rule. The idea that a jaw muscle can be isolated to "test" the muscle to see if it is weak is difficult to accept. Even if the muscle can be isolated, false-positive muscle testing can occur due to (1) the patient's unwillingness to contract maximally, (2) pain-limiting maximum contraction, and (3) pseudo-weakness secondary to reflex inhibition.[47,48] Isometric exercise for the purpose of strengthening suspected jaw muscle weakness needs to be re-evaluated. Only muscle weakness related to prolonged immobility (i.e., intermaxillary fixation postorthognathic surgery or trauma) would require me to instruct the patient in isometric strengthening exercises.

Mandibular Muscle Relaxation.   Contracting one muscle or group of muscles causes reflex inhibition of the antagonist muscle or group of muscles. In the jaw, an example is to contract the depressor muscles of the mandible to cause a reciprocal inhibition of the elevator (antagonist) muscles. Questions of duration and what amount of resistance is needed to initiate inhibition of the antagonist muscles in a dysfunctional state remain unanswered.[49,50]

An isometric contraction of a muscle(s) producing a specific movement may induce relaxation of the muscle(s). Muscles that elevate the mandible (i.e., temporalis, masseter, and internal pterygoid) are often in need of inhibition. For effective inhibition, the elevator muscles should be in a position of slight stretch. The patient contracts the elevator muscles maximally against an unyielding force (patient's fingers draped over the lower incisors). For the elevator muscles to relax reflexly, a great amount of tension is required to stimulate the Golgi tendon organs (GTOs). No physiologic information is available as to how long this inhibition persists.[51] The concern I have is the effects that a maximum isometric contraction has on the presence of symptomatic muscles (elevator muscle of the mandible) and TMJ(s). I prefer not to overcontract muscles or overload joints that are symptomatic. Good clinical decision making is mandated in this instance. I prefer minimal isometric contraction. Minimal contraction will give the patient cortical awareness of the muscle contracting and then relaxing. Over time, this form of light isometric contraction may provide relaxation if performed in conjunction with other forms of treatment. Isometric exercises for the purpose of encouraging relaxation of the elevator muscle of the mandible are applied in a similar way as isometrics for controlling hypermobility (Fig. 7-7).

HYPOMOBILITY

Hypomobility is defined here as a limitation in functional movements of the mandible. Mandibular hypomobility may result from disorders of the mandible or cranial bones that include aplasia, hypoplasia, hyperplasia, dysplasia, neoplasia, and fracture.[1] Masticatory muscle disorders such as myofascial pain, myositis, spasm, protective splinting, contracture, and neoplasia may also contribute to hypomobility.[1] TMDs that can contribute to mandibular hypomobility are ankylosis (bony or fibrosis); arthritides, especially polyarthritides involving the periarticular tissue (capsule) and structural bony changes; disc displacement (acute disc displacement that does not reduce); and inflammation (i.e., joint effusion).

Disorders of the mandible/cranial bones are managed by the dental and medical professions. Disorders of the masticatory muscles are managed by any one or combination of the dental, physical therapy, or psychological professions. Other than inflammation addressed earlier, the tissue conditions contributing to hypomobility for which physical therapy is most helpful are *periarticular tissue tightness* and acute disc displacement that does not reduce.

The physiologic and neurophysiologic sequelae of TMJ hypomobility and response to treatments are not well documented. The physiologic and neurophysiologic effects that hypomobility has on other diarthrodial joints of the body are well documented.[52-57] The effects of hypomobility/immobility on the immediate tissues associated with the TMJ will be extrapolated from what is known about other joints and applied to the TMJ. The following discussion of the effects of hypomobility does not purport to be comprehensive but only to highlight the clinical need for treatment of TMJ hypomobility.

Hypomobility Affecting Kinematics

The nature of movement or kinematics at any joint is largely determined by the joint structure, including the shape of the joint surfaces. The traditional structural classification of the TMJ is ginglymoarthrodial. *Ginglymus* means a simple hinge joint. *Arthrodia* means a joint in which the articular surfaces are flat and glide over or against each other during movements.[58] The traditional classification of joint movement includes the following[59]:

1. *Angled*—indicating an increase or decrease in the angle formed between two bones (e.g., flexion–extension at the elbow).
2. *Circumduction*—the movement of a bone circumscribing a cone (e.g., circumduction at the hip or shoulder)
3. *Rotation*—movement occurring about the longitudinal axis of a bone (e.g., internal–external rotation at the shoulder)
4. *Sliding*—one bone sliding over another with little or no appreciable rotation or angular movement (e.g., movement occurring between carpals)

This type of movement classification describes osteokinematic movement. Osteokinematics[60,61] deals primarily with the overall movement of bones (mandible), with little reference to their related joints. An analogy of this would be describing the movement of a door (the mandible) without consideration of its hinges (the joints). Arthrokinematics,[60,61] however, is concerned with the intimate mechanics of the movements occurring between joint surfaces (condyle-articular eminence).

Osteokinematics

Three basic mandibular movements exist within the mandible. The motions can be described as (1) depression, (2) protrusion, and (3) lateral excursions.[62] These three basic movements can be combined to produce an infinite variety of mandibular movements. Closing or retrusion are not osteokinematic movements that are evaluated in the same way as other movements. Restriction in closing or retrusion may occur in the last few degrees of jaw closing, when the patient is unable to bring the back teeth together. This usually is due to, but not limited to, any one or combination of joint effusion, hyperactivity of the lower head of the external pterygoid, prolonged use of an appliance such as an anterior repositioning appliance, posterior disc displacement (uncommon), or a malocclusion.

Hypomobility can hinder the patient's ability to function during acts of chewing (involving lateral excursions), talking, yawning, etc. The goals of treatment of hypomobility are to restore osteokinematics as follows:

Depression: Functional depression describes the ability to open the mouth actively to 40 mm measured by placing a millimeter ruler between the tips of the right or left maxillary and mandibular central incisors. Ideally no deflection or deviation should be present.

Protrusion: Functional protrusion is the ability to actively protrude the mandible so that at least an edge-to-edge position can be achieved between maxillary and mandibular central incisors. Ideally, the mandibular central incisors should move past the maxillary central incisors by several millimeters. Ideally, no deflection or deviation should be present.

Lateral excursion: Functional lateral excursion is the ability to actively move the mandible laterally so that at least the mandibular canine achieves an end-to-end position in relation to the maxillary canine. Ideally, the mandibular canine should move past the maxillary canine by several millimeters.

Arthrokinematics

As stated earlier, arthrokinematics are concerned with the intimate mechanics of the movements occurring between joint surfaces (condyle–articular eminence). In orthopaedic physical therapy, a particular jargon has evolved in the area of arthrokinematics. Unfortunately, the use of certain terms is often inconsistent.

Accessory Movements.   Arthrokinematics of any joint involves a study of accessory joint movements. Accessory movements are those motions available between joint surfaces that allow for a full, pain-free osteokinematic movement to be present. Accessory movements can consist of either active or passive accessory movements.

Active Accessory Movements.   Active accessory movements occur in response to muscle contractions but are guided by the shape of the articulating surfaces and by the periarticular tissues. Active accessory movements include[63–65] *spin, roll* (rotation), *slide* (translation), *distraction,* and *compression.*

Active accessory movements occur largely in response to muscle contractions. It would follow that treatments would center on actively moving the mandible into the identified restricted active accessory motion. If, for example, the active accessory movement of translation is restricted, the patient can actively protrude the mandible. By actively protruding the mandible, the active accessory movement of translation of the condylar head is restored and thus the osteokinematic movement of protrusion. However, if osteokinematic movement requires a combination of two or more active accessory movements, a slightly different approach to treatment is needed. For example, the osteokinematic movement of depression involves a combination of the active accessory movements of rotation and translation of the condylar head. If depression is restricted and the clinician actively forces the mouth open, he or she is disregarding the importance of accessory movements. Instead, the clinician will need to address separately the active accessory rotation and translation movements of the condylar head. The patient can be told to protrude the mandible first to regain condylar translation. Once condylar translation is improving, active opening of the mouth can follow.

Restricted accessory movements may also be restored passively through the application of intraoral techniques addressing passive accessory movements. The choice of using active or passive accessory movements or both is entirely based on the clinical presentation of the patient and the etiology of the hypomobility.

Passive Accessory Movements.   Accessory movements of a joint that cannot be produced by the action of muscle contractions but instead are produced passively in response to an outside force are referred to as *passive accessory movements* or *joint play movements.*[66] Joint play movements include any one or combination of spin, rotation, translation, distraction, and compression, as described for active accessory movements. An additional joint play movement that does not double as an active accessory movement is lateral glide.

Joint play movements can occur in any particular joint position. Joint play movements are the inherent quality of the joint to "give." The "built-in" factor of joint play is critical to promote efficient functional movements.[67] An analogy is a hinge on a door that has play between its components to allow the door to open and close smoothly and easily. A loss or decrease in the joint play movement(s) of the TMJ may be a primary restricting factor to osteokinematic movements of the mandible as well as to active accessory movements.

Summary of Accessory Movements.   Five active accessory movements (spin, rotation, translation, distraction, and compression) and six passive accessory movements (spin, rotation, translation, distraction, compression, and lateral glide) may seem overwhelming to evaluate and treat when osteokinematic movement is restricted. Without oversimplifying the kinematics of the TMJ, this author finds certain accessory movements to be more restricted than others. Accessory movements restricted secondary to periarticular tissue tightness and disc displacements are active and passive accessory movements of *translation* and *distraction* and the passive accessory movement of *lateral glide*. Of these three accessory movements, *translation* is the primary accessory movement that causes the most limitation in osteokinematic movement of the mandible and the more difficult one to restore.

Hypomobility Affecting Articular Cartilage

Joints lacking full range of motion (ROM) have a distinct reduction in supply of blood to the joint capsule.[68] A reduction in blood supply decreases nutrients going to the cells that make up the synovial membrane, which, in turn, produces synovial fluid.[69] Synovial fluid supplies oxygen and nutrients to the articular cartilage. Without full range of joint movement, there will be inadequate mixing of the synovial fluid. Waste products of metabolism will accumulate on the surfaces of the cartilage causing cartilage cell dystrophy. Joint immobilization can therefore initiate an arthritic process.[68]

Articular cartilage's main function is to distribute compressive forces to the underlying subchondral bone.[53,70] Hypomobility alters the biomechanics of the joint, resulting in improper loading of articular cartilage. Hypomobility will cause certain areas of the articular cartilage to receive higher than normal impact loads, leading to potential fatigue failure and arthritic changes in the articular cartilage. The effects hypomobility has on articular cartilage are dependent on the amplitudes, frequency, duration, and rate of application of loading.[71]

Research on the effects of immobilization on the primate TMJ[72] concluded that prolonged immobilization of the TMJ results in degenerative changes in the articular cartilage. The degenerative changes of immobilization may be reversed once remobilization is established.

Hypomobility Affecting Mechanoreceptor Activity

Clinicians need to acknowledge the importance of the mechanoreceptors of the TMJ and how mechanoreceptor activity can be affected by hypomobility. The TMJ, as with all mammalian synovial joints, contains four types of receptor nerve endings, which can be differentiated on the basis of morphologic and functional characteristics.[73,74] TMJ synovial receptors are located in the fibrous joint capsule, the lateral ligament, and the posterior articular pad but are absent from the intra-articular disc (central portion) and synovial tissues. Terminating on the receptors are the deep temporal, masseter, and auriculotemporal nerves, which originate from the mandibular division of cranial V.[75,76] For clarity purposes, emphasis will be placed on hypomobility affecting the joint capsule (periarticular tissue), which contains an abundance of type I, II, III, and IV receptors.

Type I receptors are continuously discharging because of their low-threshold and slow-adapting characteristics. Continuous discharging occurs, even when the mandible is at rest. The type I receptors provide continuous kinesthetic and postural perception of the mandible. Type I receptors also exert powerful reciprocally coordinated, facilitory, and inhibitory reflex effects on motor unit activity to the mandibular muscles.[74]

Type II receptors have low-threshold and rapid-adapting characteristics. They fire briefly as mandibular movements are initiated and exert transient coordinated reflex effects on the related musculature.[74]

Type III receptors are high-threshold and slow-adapting receptors, which do not fire under normal circumstances but become active only when excessive tension is developed in the lateral TMJ ligament. Type III activation has been demonstrated to result reflexively in pterygoid and mylohyoid muscle spasms and temporalis and masseter muscle inhibition.[74]

Type IV receptors constitute the pain receptor system of the articular tissues and are entirely inactive in normal circumstances. They become active when the TMJ articular tissues (joint capsule, posterior pad, and TMJ ligament) are subjected to marked mechanical deformation, tension, or direct chemical irritation.[77]

Afferent discharges from types I, II, and III, as well as other receptors in the skin, subcutaneous tissue, and muscles about the synovial joints, all converge on inhibitory interneurons, segmentally and intersegmentally. This convergence modulates the centripetal flow of nociceptive afferent activity derived from the joint tissues having type IV receptors. The degree of joint (TMJ) pain experienced by a patient depends not only on the intensity of type IV irritation but also on the frequency of ongoing afferent discharges from the various types of mechanoreceptors embedded in the same joint capsule (TMJ), related soft tissues, and muscles.[78] Deliberate stimulation of the type I, II, and III mechanoreceptors in the TMJ capsule and adjacent tissues by the use of transcutaneous electrical nerve stimulation (TENS) or intraoral manual oscillatory techniques may help enhance the modulating effect of the primary afferent activity on the type IV receptors of the TMJ. If capsular tightness (fibrosis) is the primary cause of type IV activation, complete alleviation of pain may occur when proper intraoral arthrokinematic techniques are applied and capsular extensibility is restored.

Clinical Implications

Capsular tightness affecting mechanoreceptor activity needs to be investigated when the patient perceives that the "bite is off." Patient perception of an "uneven bite" may be due to a malocclusion. If the attending dentist cannot identify occlusal factors contributing to the patient's bite "not feeling right," altered mechanoreceptor activity needs to be considered. Altered mechano-receptor activity contributing to improper proprioceptive feedback along with muscle activity may contribute to the patient's perception of a "pseudo" mal-occlusion. If capsular tightness was identified and treated, the patient's per-ception of the initial tooth/teeth contact during jaw closing may then be per-ceived as being "normal."

Dental procedures that place the condyle in a position that "strains" the capsule may need to be re-examined. The condyle position for recapturing a disc displacement with an anterior repositioning appliance (ARA) illustrates the potential for capsular strain. The ARA often places the condyle in an overcorrected position anteriorly and could be considered a strained position for the joint capsule. An overcorrected position may not be conducive to the articular receptor system of the TMJ capsule. This may especially be true when it appears that the mechanoreceptors located in the anterior region of the joint capsule make a facilitory contribution to supramandibular muscle activity.[79]

An acute disc displacement without reduction is a hypomobile condition. Capsular tightness secondary to a loss of full joint mobility may occur. Pro-cedures performed that are successful at reducing the disc may be followed by an ARA to maintain disc position. Poor tolerance to the appliance may occur for reasons mentioned above. Exacerbation of symptoms may result from an untreated capsular restriction in response to hypomobility secondary to an acute disc displacement without reduction.

Certain techniques used by dentists to establish centric relation (CR) may be a strained position for the capsule. CR is a clinical concept intended to provide a reproducible jaw relationship during occlusal adjustments and re-construction. There is controversy over the exact definition, condylar position, and technique used for CR.[80] The basic objective for achieving CR is to arrive at an occlusal relationship that will promote neuromuscular harmony of the muscles of mastication. Capsular tightness affects mechanoreceptor activity, which in turn influences mandibular muscle activity. The objective of achieving neuromuscular harmony may be better accomplished if capsular tightness as well as cervical spine disorders, which can also affect mandibular muscle ac-tivity (see Ch. 11), are dealt with before establishing CR through irreversible occlusal adjustments and/or reconstruction.

Treatment

Dysfunctional osteokinematic movements of the mandible secondary to periarticular tissue tightness and an acute disc displacement that does not re-duce are discussed. If functional mandibular movements are restored, thera-peutic effects of increased mobility on kinematics, articular cartilage, and mechanoreceptors of the TMJ will occur.

Hypomobility Caused by Periarticular Tissue Tightness

Periarticular tissue refers to the capsular-ligamentous tissue of joints. The entire lateral aspect of the TMJ capsule is thickened, forming the temporomandibular (TM) ligament, and the TMJ ligament should thus be regarded as part of and inseparable from the capsule.[81] A capsule is a "sac-like envelope which encloses the cavity of a synovial joint by attaching to the circumference of the articular end of each involved bone."[82] The capsule of the TMJ, although somewhat deficient anteriorly, is circumferentially attached to the rim of the glenoid fossa and articular eminence of the temporal bone above and to the neck of the condyle below. The capsule is dense, irregular connective tissue with two layers. The outer fibrous layer consists mostly of collagen, and the inner layer is the synovial lining.

Etiology of Capsular Tightness. Biochemical and biomechanical changes occur in the capsule when normal ROM of the joint is decreased. Changes of this type have been documented in the literature.[83–85] Biochemically, a reduction in water and glycosaminoglycans (GAG) results. GAG and water form a semifluid viscous gel that acts as a lubricant between collagen fibers making up the outer layer of the capsule. Free gliding of collagen fibers over one another is essential for the extensibility of a joint capsule. Biomechanically, when there is a reduction in water and GAG, the capsule becomes tight because of loss of free gliding of collagen fibers. The following is a list of common etiologies that can contribute to capsular tightness of the TMJ.

Macrotrauma. The human body's response to injury is always the same regardless of the location or the type of injury (i.e., a direct blow or surgical intervention).[86] The response to trauma is vasodilation (*redness*), swelling (*exudate and bleeding from torn vessels*), increase in blood flow and/or chemical and metabolic activity (*heat*), and irritation of nerve endings (*pain*). Hypomobility that follows trauma is due to pain, reflex muscle guarding, and joint effusion. Subsequent loss of function may result from a combination of active destruction of tissue and dense scar formation in the injured joint capsule and other involved soft tissue.[86]

Direct trauma to the joint capsule would also involve **joint effusion,** especially if the joint capsule was torn or stretched. Joint effusion can cause the appearance of capsular tightness due to distention of the joint capsule. Parts of the capsule that are normally lax to allow for a specific ROM are no longer lax because of capsular distention. It is important for the clinician to recognize that significant joint effusion can cause hypomobility. Stretching the joint capsule would be contraindicated in the presence of joint effusion. Instead, the clinician should assist in the resolution of the acute intracapsular inflammatory process (see Inflammation). Once the inflammation is controlled, treatment for capsular tightness, including stretching, may be necessary.

Adhesions, which develop secondary to joint effusion, may develop between the collagen fibrils of the capsule as well as between the joint surfaces and the intra-articular disc. The potential for adhesions to follow trauma or open joint surgery for various joint disorders is likely unless proper kinematics of the joint are restored soon. Adhesions unrelated to trauma may also occur in the upper joint space secondary to an acute disc displacement without reduction.[87,88]

Microtrauma.   Microtrauma may occur with a "malocclusion of the teeth resulting in a change of the maxillo-mandibular relationship and therefore in a change in joint position and in the pattern of capsular stress."[89] Habits can be an additional source of microtrauma to the capsule. Gum chewing, biting on pencils, and leaning the jaw on the hands need to be avoided to prevent unnecessary stress to the capsule.

Postarthrotomy.   During an open joint procedure, it is clear that the capsule will have been traumatized. Physical therapy treatments for rehabilitating the TMJ after arthrotomy will follow procedures discussed in this section and in Chapter 10 *(Postarthrotomy Surgery)* as well as those proposed by Bertolucci.[90] The clinician should not assume that hypomobility postarthrotomy is due only to the traumatized incised capsule. The objectives of the surgery itself can contribute to hypomobility. If, for instance, alloplastic or autogenous material is placed in the joint, mandibular movement will more than likely be restricted in the initial phases of recovery. If the posterior tissues are shortened surgically, a restriction in mandibular dynamics may result. It is important for the physical therapist to recognize that hypomobility postsurgery may be due to a variety of reasons other than capsular tightness. Treatments, therefore, must be tailored to individual situations. If the physical therapist has any questions about the contraindications of a particular technique/procedure, a discussion with the oral surgeon is in order.

Postarthroscopy.   Trauma to the joint capsule is not as extensive after arthroscopy as it would be for arthrotomy. Most patients postarthroscopy that have restrictions in mandibular dynamics recover their ROM quickly with physical therapy treatments. Physical therapy treatments for rehabilitating the TMJ after arthroscopy will follow procedures discussed in this section as well as in Chapter 10 *(Postarthroscopic Surgery)*. Additional articles discussing physical therapy protocol postarthroscopic can be obtained from the bibliography.[91-93]

Postorthognathic Surgery.   Mandibular hypomobility is sometimes a complication of orthognathic surgery.[94] As discussed with arthrotomy, mandibular restriction may be related to factors other than capsular tightness. Reduced mobility may be related to surgery-induced changes in condyle position,[94] the degree of surgical trauma,[95] duration of maxillomandibular fixation,[95] and non-rigid fixation.[96] The biochemical and biomechanical changes of capsular tissue after hypomobility, more likely postintermaxillary fixation, contribute to a decrease in interincisal opening. Early restoration of mobility postorthognathic surgery is discussed in Chapters 9 and 10 *(Postorthognathic Surgery)*.

Polyarthritides. As mentioned in the section on inflammation, polyarthritides are best treated by the medical/dental profession. The end result of some polyarthritides is an increase in collagen fiber content, contributing to the loss of capsular extensibility.[97] The more destructive the process, the more vigorous is the repair response and collagen production during resolution. Increase in capsular tissue collagen production secondary to the polyarthritides becomes a more difficult situation to resolve. Remodeling of the excess collagen and realignment of the collagen fibers and abnormally placed cross-links among the collagen fibers are all factors that may hamper normalization of capsular extensibility.[85,97] Fortunately, polyarthritides of the TMJ are rare.[1]

Examination. Insight into the history and physical examination of periarticular tightness may increase the awareness of the clinician to a condition that is often overlooked as a contributing cause to restriction of mandibular dynamics. Specifics of the examination are not addressed.

History. Inquire about the occurrence of possible etiologies of capsular tightness previously covered.

Physical Examination. Translation is most often the accessory movement that is restricted. Whenever translation is restricted, rotation of the condyle still permits up to 20 to 25 mm of mandibular opening.[98,99] If unilateral capsular involvement is present, the following **osteokinematic restrictions and aberrant movements** of the mandible will be observed:

1. Less than functional opening with deflection to the side of the involved joint with mandibular depression
2. Less than functional protrusion with deflection to the side of the involved joint
3. Normal lateral excursion to the side of the involved joint; less than functional lateral excursion to the opposite side of the involved joint

Inflammation and masticatory muscle hyperactivity associated with periarticular tightness will influence the overall amount of active movement and degree of mandibular deflection. The previous restrictions in osteokinematic movements associated with periarticular tightness are similar to those associated with an acute disc displacement that does not reduce. Depending on treatment goals (i.e., restore mandibular dynamics regardless of cause or to attempt to reduce a nonreducing disc), a differential diagnostic evaluation will need to be performed to know which condition the patient may have.

As part of a differential diagnosis, especially if inflammation and/or masticatory muscle hyperactivity is present, the clinician may need to examine for capsular tightness by assessing the amount of **passive accessory movements** with intraoral passive mobility examination techniques. Hand placement, direction of force, and stabilization of the patient for the application of these joint play examination techniques will be covered under the treatment section. The main differences between examination and treatment using intraoral techniques are the force and duration used.

When evaluating for joint play, the force is a slow, steady, deliberate pressure to feel a "yield" at the end of the expected range. The amount of time applying the force to determine the "yield" is very short (i.e., 1 to 2 seconds). If the force is applied for a longer period of time, the examination becomes a treatment. The stabilizing hand should be positioned so that an index or middle finger can be placed over the lateral pole to assess movement (Fig. 7-8). A capsular restriction is determined by the clinician's conceptualization of "normal" for the movement tested. A "gummy" end feel describes what the end range of a pathologic tight capsule feels like. If possible, the state of the dysfunctional joint can be compared with the noninvolved contralateral joint. The patient's report of irritability is to be considered. Clinician knowledge of anat-

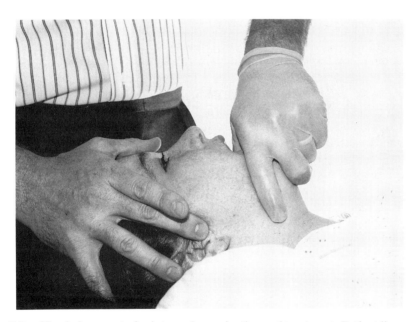

Fig. 7-8. Hand placements for intraoral examination and treatment. Patient lies supine with the cervical spine supported. At the same time that the right hand stabilizes the patient's head, the middle or index finger palpates the lateral pole to assess movement. The thumb of the other hand is placed in the patient's mouth. Thumb position will be better appreciated in Figures 7-11, 7-12, and 7-13. Hand placements are the same for both the examination and treatment of passive accessory movements and for the treatment of an acute disc displacement without reduction (ADDWoR).

omy and kinematics and clinician expertise with respect to application of force and patient stabilization will aid assessment of passive accessory movements.

As a general rule, this author would like at least 20 to 25 mm of active mandibular opening before initiating the treatment procedures that follow. In the absence of translation, rotation will allow 20 to 25 mm of opening. Anything less than 20 to 25 mm typically indicates either inflammation and/or masticatory muscle hyperactivity. Inflammation and masticatory muscle hyperactivity should be addressed before implementing techniques to treat capsular tightness.

Treatment. Techniques that follow are applied clinically in the same order as they are introduced here. A technique is continued as long as improvement is noted by assessing the patient's signs and symptoms. It is difficult to give guidance as to how much force, how long, and how often the technique should be repeated. The subjective and objective presentation of the patient will help to identify individual therapeutic parameters. Clearly, if hypomobility is caused by surgical intervention to the TMJ, the surgeon needs to understand what treatments the physical therapist will be offering, and the physical therapist needs to have a clear understanding of what surgical procedures were performed and to what tissue. Communication between health professionals will deter any complications that could arise during the rehabilitation process. It is important to emphasize that the following treatments are not to be offered in a cookbook fashion, but instead such treatment must be rendered by a physical therapist using sound clinical judgment.

Tongue Up and Open and Close With Speed. The instructions given to the patient for this exercise were covered in the section on Inflammation (Fig. 7-5). The therapeutic value of this exercise is to get the patient's jaw moving in a controlled manner. Tongue up as discussed earlier will control translation. Movement is then performed to counter the effects of immobility. Increase in pain will seldom occur with this exercise. If pain is a factor, modalities to control pain can be administered.

The opening and closing movement regardless of movement velocity is postulated to have an effect of "pumping" similar to continuous passive motion (CPM).[100] Intra-articular pressure alternately raised and lowered through movement presumably facilitates the clearance of fluid and diffusable particles from the joint space into the interstitial tissues.[101] Postarthrotomy, this exercise is postulated to permit therapeutic stress on repaired tissues without inciting inflammatory reactions in these same tissues.[86] When performed in the upright position, gravity offers active assistance in enhancing ROM. Opening and closing can be performed continuously based on the patient's motivation.

Finger Spread Exercise. The patient rests supine, with the clinician standing at the head of the patient. Using the hand opposite the involved joint, the clinician places his or her thumb on the tip of the patient's lower central incisors and index finger on the tip of the top central incisors (Fig. 7-9). The patient is

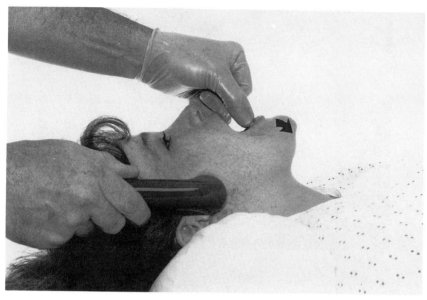

Fig. 7-9. Finger spread exercise. This exercise is performed for the diagnosis of periarticular tissue tightness or ADDWoR. The clinician's free hand is performing an ultrasound treatment during the finger spread exercise.

asked to open actively as the clinician follows with his or her fingertips on the patient's incisors. At the end of the available range, overpressure is applied with the clinician's fingertips.

An important modification to this manual exercise is performed at the time the patient can actively achieve 20 to 25 mm. The patient is instructed to first protrude the mandible forward (1 to 2 mm) and then open the mouth. This will encourage the condyle to enter into the translation phase to avoid possibly forcing rotation beyond 20 to 25 mm. Ultrasound can simultaneously be applied to the involved joint while performing this exercise. Also, this same exercise can be shown to the patient to do at home.

Touch and Bite Exercise.   Capsular tightness affecting the mechanoreceptor activity will alter afferent input to the central nervous system (CNS) about jaw position and movement. What appears to be a limitation in active mandibular movement may be related to a problem in coordination and proprioceptive feedback. The touch and bite exercise aids in the retraining of mandibular protrusion and lateral excursion.

The patient is lying supine, with the clinician standing at the patient's head. Using the hand opposite the involved joint, the clinician places his or her index finger on the outside of the patient's maxillary canine, opposite to the involved joint (Fig. 7-10A). The clinician asks the patient to "reach over and bite my finger." Mandibular movement toward the canine encourages active lateral excursion to that side and condylar translation on the opposite side. Touching

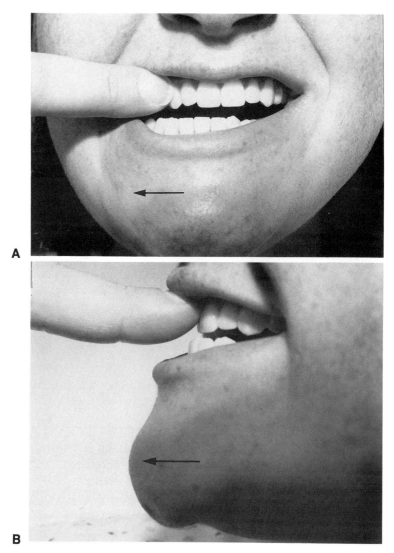

Fig. 7-10.   Touch and bite exercise. **(A)** This exercise is used to coordinate movement of lateral excursion through proprioceptive feedback as well as to treat restricted translation secondary to periarticular tissue tightness and an ADDWoR. In this photograph, the movement is right lateral excursion. The joint that would be restricted in translation would be the left. This exercise can be performed with the patient in the supine position with the clinician standing at the top of the patient's head, touching the patient's right maxillary canine. The clinician's other hand could be performing an ultrasound to the involved joint. **(B)** This exercise is for coordinating movement of protrusion through proprioceptive feedback as well as to treat restricted translation secondary to periarticular tissue tightness and an ADDWoR. This exercise can be performed by the clinician as described in Figure A. The clinician, however, touches the patient's maxillary central incisors with one hand as the other hand could be performing an ultrasound to the involved joint.

the canine gives proprioceptive feedback to the patient as to the required direction of movement. This exercise can also be performed for protrusion (Fig. 7-10B). The clinician would instead touch the front of the patient's central incisors.

While doing this exercise, ultrasound can be applied to the involved joint. This exercise can also be shown to the patient to do at home.

Joint Mobilization Techniques. *Joint mobilization* is a very general term that might be applied to any active or passive attempt to increase movement of a joint. Passive joint mobilization has been a popular treatment for the restoration of joint motion for many years. Passive intraoral joint mobilization techniques will be those techniques applied to the TMJ to address more specifically the restoration of the passive accessory movements of distraction, translation, and lateral glide. Identifying restrictions in passive accessory movements will be determined by performing the intraoral passive accessory movement examination techniques as covered in the previous section, *Physical Examination/Passive Accessory Movement.* Hand placements for examination and treatment will be identical for both. These techniques can be performed with the patient sitting rather than supine, but patient relaxation may be more difficult.

Distraction refers to a force applied parallel to the longitudinal axis of the bone, in this case, the mandible. Distraction is the first choice of the intraoral techniques to use due to the safety, ease, and effectiveness of application.

The clinician will be standing opposite the involved joint with the patient lying supine, with appropriate support given to the cervical spine (Fig. 7-11). The clinician's thumb is placed on the patient's molars on the side of the involved joint. The remaining fingers are wrapped around the chin comfortably. The clinician's other hand stabilizes the patient's cranium; the middle or index finger palpates the lateral pole for movement. If limitation of jaw opening prevents the placement of the thumb on top of the molars, the thumb may be positioned in the premolar area. Premolar contact will tend to encourage the novice clinician to induce osteokinematic depression versus arthrokinematic distraction unless the clinician is careful to generate the forces correctly on the mandible.

There are three stages of distraction[102] that can be applied, depending on patient signs and symptoms:

Stage I: Piccolo: movement is so small that only the compression effect in the joint is released while the joint pressure is neutralized. The joint surfaces are not separated from each other.

Stage II: The slack is taken up moving the joint partner as far as the soft tissues allow using minimal force.

Stage III: This is a continuation and an extension of stage II, but uses more force to progress into the pathologic limits of the restricted tissue.

To enhance the mobilization technique of distraction, active participation

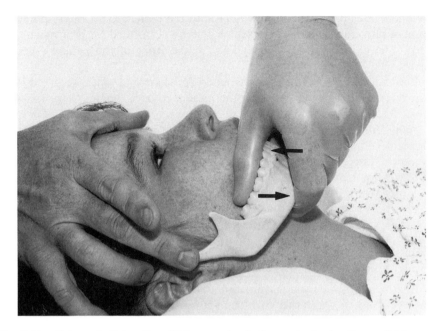

Fig. 7-11. Intraoral distraction. This exercise is for periarticular tissue tightness or ADDWoR. Clinician and patient positions are described in Figure 7-8. The clinician's thumb is positioned to apply a distraction force. *Arrows* demonstrate the direction of force applied with the left thumb and hand.

by the patient is encouraged. For example, while performing the distractional technique, have the patient actively open or close on command using *minimal* muscle contraction. When the patient relaxes, additional distraction forces can be applied. Performing the distractional technique during active participation by the patient allows the patient to experience a less stressful, less painful movement of the joint.

For **translation,** the clinician's body position and stabilizing and mobilizing hand placements are the same as in the distraction technique. The clinician's mobilizing hand will translate the condyle in an anterior direction. *Translation* is not just performed in the sagittal plane but also in an oblique plane slightly across midline (Fig. 7-12). Translation should be performed in the presence of either stage I, II, or III distraction, which will aid in patient comfort.

For **lateral glide,** the clinician's body position and stabilizing hand are the same as in the distraction technique. The thumb contact of the mobilizing hand, however, is different. Thumb contact for lateral glide technique is on the top/ inside of the molars. The rest of the fingers wrap around the mandible comfortably. Lateral glide is performed by pressing laterally with the thumb, at the same time force is directed toward the table and patient's feet (Fig. 7-13). These multiple directions of force avoid discomfort on the contralateral side that would be likely if a lateral force alone is used.

Graded rhythmic oscillatory movements may be applied simultaneously

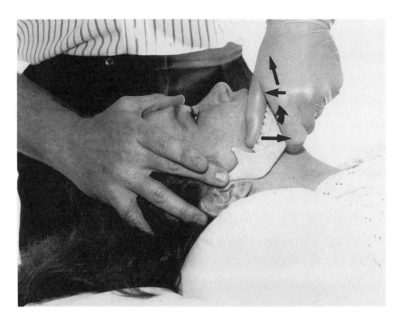

Fig. 7-12. Intraoral translation. This exercise is for periarticular tissue tightness or ADDWoR. Clinician and patient positions are described in Figure 7-8. The clinician's thumb is positioned to apply a translation force. The clinician will also be applying either a stage 1, 2, or 3 distraction. *Arrows* demonstrate the direction of force applied with the left thumb and hand.

while applying distraction, translation, and lateral glide joint play techniques. Rhythmic oscillatory movements are graded 1 to 4, whereas a grade 5 involves a thrust.[104] Grades of oscillations distinguish range and amplitude of oscillations (Fig. 7-14A). The range is based on the pathologic limits of range and not the limits of passive accessory movements for the joint under normal conditions (Fig. 7-14B).

Grade I: Small amplitude motion performed at the beginning of the available range
Grade II: Large amplitude motion performed within the available range
Grade III: Large amplitude motion performed up to the limit of range available
Grade IV: Small amplitude motion performed at the limit of range
Grade V: Manipulation, a high-velocity, low-amplitude thrust, performed at the limits of the available range. Clinically, I have never found the need to apply a thrust to the TMJ and would not advise to do so.

The rationale for applying oscillatory techniques during distraction, translation, and lateral glide movements is either neurophysiologic and/or mechanical.[103]

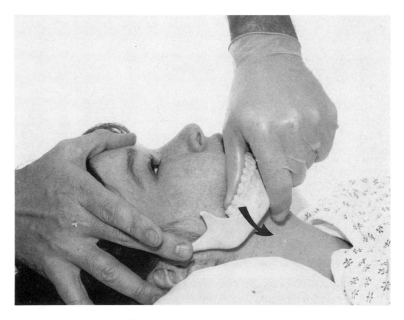

Fig. 7-13.   Intraoral lateral glide. This exercise is for periarticular tissue tightness. Clinician and patient positions are described in Figure 7-8. The clinician's thumb is positioned to apply a lateral glide force. *Arrows* demonstrate the direction of force applied with the left thumb and hand.

Stages I and II distraction and oscillatory techniques of grades I and II are primarily influencing the mechanoreceptors because these techniques are performed well within the available pathologic range. Increased ROM after these maneuvers derives from the **neurophysiologic effects** of a decrease in pain (gaiting) or decrease in masticatory muscle tone via joint mechanoreceptor influences.[104,105]

The **mechanical effects** of joint mobilization are achieved with stage III distraction and grades III and IV oscillatory techniques and the grade V thrust technique. Neurophysiologic effects will no doubt accompany any mechanical forces applied to a joint.

Connective tissue responds to mechanical stress in a time-dependent or viscoelastic manner (Fig. 7-15). The force/load applied needs to exceed the elastic range of a tissue, otherwise, the tissue will return to its original shape and no permanent elongation of the tissue will have occurred.[106,107] Beyond the elastic range or yield point is the plastic range of the tissue.[106,107] Long-lasting or plastic elongation is dependent on the intensity and duration of force applied.[108,109] If loading is continued too far into the plastic range (fatigue point), tissue damage may result.

The clinician may not be able to maintain either the necessary force or duration of force required to achieve plastic elongation of the tissue with intraoral techniques. If patient tolerance of intraoral techniques is good but ROM

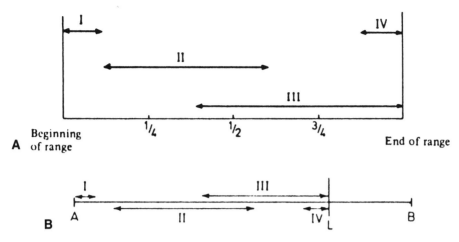

Fig. 7-14. (A) Grades of passive movement: I, small amplitude in beginning of range; II, large amplitude within the range; III, large amplitude up to the end of range; and IV, small amplitude up to the end of range. (B) Normal range of joint movement is limited. *A,* beginning of range of movement; *B,* average anatomic limit; *L,* pathologic limit of range. Grades III and IV are restricted to the new limit of the range. Grade II movements are restricted to smaller amplitudes. (From Maitland,[103] with permission.)

between treatments is not maintained, progression to the static tongue blade technique (Fig. 7-16) may be necessary.

General rules to follow when applying joint play intraoral techniques to the TMJ are

1. Patient and clinician must be properly positioned and relaxed.
2. Patient should be stabilized firmly.

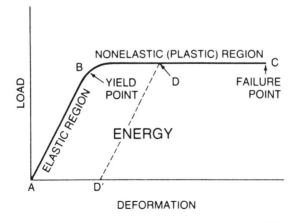

Fig. 7-15. Load–deformation curve. (From Frankel and Nordin,[164] with permission.)

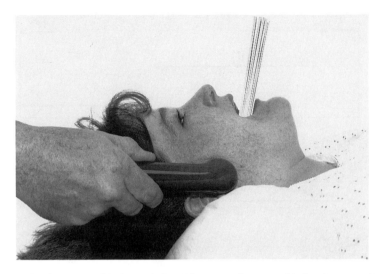

Fig. 7-16. Static tongue blade exercise. The use of tongue blades is to apply a low-load prolonged stretch. This exercise can be performed for periarticular tightness, ADDWoR, or tight elevator muscles of the mandible that have gone through length-associated changes. The clinician can apply heat and/or ultrasound during the duration of the stretch.

3. Clinician must be willing to modify the technique based on the tissue's response and needs. The clinician must be able to "think" through his or her fingers. This is known as "tissue tension sense."

4. Clinician should use the minimum of force consistent with achieving the objective of restoring capsular extensibility.

Mobilization techniques when performed incorrectly or not indicated may result in the following:

1. Increase in pain
2. Increase in swelling and/or muscle guarding
3. Decrease in mobility

Cotton Roll Distraction. Cotton roll distraction is a home exercise that permits self-distraction to the involved joint (Fig. 7-17). This is a *passive* exercise and not active. The patient will be sitting in a comfortable supported position. The patient places a dental roll $\frac{1}{4}$ inch in diameter between the back molars on the side that is to be distracted. The patient places one hand (palm area) under the chin. The other hand is placed on the top of the head toward the front. Both hands are therefore in front of the dental roll. With the patient's jaw as relaxed as possible, the chin hand applies a slight pressure superiorly as the other hand stabilizes the head. Hand pressure in the presence of relaxed

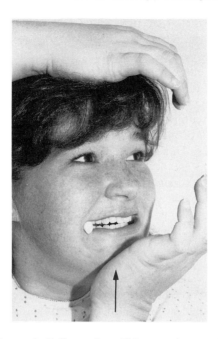

Fig. 7-17. Cotton ball distraction. This exercise can be used when joint unloading is required for such conditions as inflammation, masticatory muscle hyperactivity, periarticular tightness, or attempting to reduce an ADDWoR. A stage I, II, or III can be performed by the patient with proper instructions. If this technique is performed to progress an AADWoR to a chronic disc displacement without reduction (CDDWoR), a stage I distraction is performed as the patient protrudes their jaw to address translation more aggressively.

jaw muscles creates a pivot over the dental roll with the end result being distraction of the condyle.

Static Tongue Blade Exercise. The use of tongue blades is for applying a low-load prolonged stretch (LLPS) to promote long-lasting elongation of the periarticular tissue. The effectiveness of LLPS has been well documented by laboratory studies.[109–111] The patient should be positioned supine for this procedure. The patient is instructed to place tongue blades on the side of the involved joint in the area of the molars. (Fig. 7-16). As a general guideline, one tongue blade positioned on the molars is equal to approximately 3 mm of opening. The patient is told to "take up the slack and then some" with the tongue blades. If more than five tongue blades are used, try taping or gluing all but three of them together. The last tongue blade can be slid in or out between the remaining tongue blades. Working up to a 10- to 20-minute LLPS using tongue blades seems to be satisfactory. Actual duration of the LLPS will usually be dependent on patient tolerance.

Studies have shown that by raising the temperature of the tissue being stretched and allowing the tissue to cool in a loaded position, a greater elongation of the treated tissue(s) is produced.[111-113] Before the patient is placed on a LLPS, moist heat can be applied over the involved joint. The moist heat can be continued while the tongue blades are in place for 10 minutes. A 6- to 8-minute ultrasound can be applied with tongue blades still in place to complete the LLPS session. On completion of the session, moist heat can be applied again while the clinician or patient performs the finger spread exercise for an additional 2 to 4 minutes. This exercise can be performed as a home exercise. The patient is advised to use heat, applied as directed above.

Although not always recommended, some patients may need to grasp the end of the tongue blades and pry down. This will encourage osteokinematic opening rather than arthrokinematic distraction. Those patients with painless restriction who are responding slowly may require this technique to encourage increased mandibular opening.

Horizontal Tongue Blade Exercise.   This exercise directly addresses limitation in translation. This is a home exercise for the patient. The patient places seven tongue blades, taped or glued together horizontally, between the upper and lower anterior teeth (Fig. 7-18). The patient does not bite on the tongue blades, but instead the tongue blades are held in position by the patient's hands.

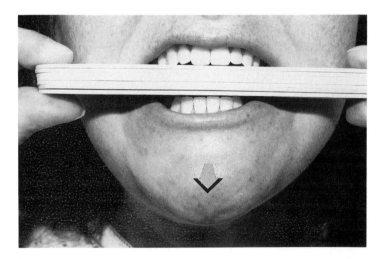

Fig. 7-18.   Horizontal tongue blade stretch. This exercise addresses limitation in translation secondary to periarticular tightness or an ADDWoR. When treating periarticular tissue tightness, the patient holds seven tongue blades horizontally between the central incisors. Patients can actively move their jaw forward or forward and slightly toward the opposite side of the involved joint. If trying to progress an ADDWoR to a CDDWoR, the tongue blades are reduced to three or four.

Seven tongue blades equal approximately 11 mm. At approximately 11 mm, translation normally begins.[98,99] With tongue blades in place, the patient will move the mandible forward and then back repetitively. The forward and back motion of the mandible will specifically address limitation in condylar translation. Should repetitive translation be performed with less than 11 mm of jaw opening, discomfort/pain will usually occur.

Continuous Passive Motion. The importance of initiating early motion during the inflammatory phase, especially after surgical intervention, is becoming widely accepted in the rehabilitation of other joints such as the knee.[114] Use of passive motion on a continuous basis as was introduced by Salter et al in 1970 has become an important area of study.[115] Salter[115] has shown that CPM applied in experimental animal studies is beneficial to soft tissue healing, bone and cartilage healing, swelling, hemarthrosis, and joint function. It is reported that CPM in humans has resulted in positive effects on joint effusions, wound edema, pain, and reduction of capsular contractures and joint stiffness.[100,114] Even though CPM has been used in a variety of orthopaedic conditions, present indications and clinical studies for the use of CPM have largely focused on the rehabilitation of various knee disorders.

Although the potential benefit of CPM is known, there is insufficient clinical research to define the most appropriate device and protocol for CPM use after postarthroscopy or arthrotomy to the TMJ. Measurable outcomes of the therapeutic value and cost-effectiveness of CPM for TMD have not been fully researched. CPM is more likely to be indicated after surgical interventions for ankylosed conditions or after total joint replacements secondary to polyarthritides. In the vast majority of post-TMJ surgical cases, timely physical therapy produces therapeutic outcomes acceptable to both the patient and surgeon, and the inconvenience of CPM may be avoided.

Secondary Benefits of Treatment. In the presence of hypomobility, the temporalis, masseter, and internal pterygoid muscles are unable to lengthen. Treatment for joint hypomobility will also thus influence the elevator muscles of the mandible.

Animal studies have shown when a muscle is subjected to changes in length, it undergoes anatomic, biochemical, and physiologic changes that are not immediately obvious nor readily considered by the clinician.[116] These length-associated changes occur within a few hours, days, or weeks of being immobilized. Animal studies indicate muscles that cannot lengthen will undergo decrease in numbers of sarcomeres in both the young and adult. In the young, there will be a decrease in the rate of additional new sarcomeres, whereas in the adult, there is an absolute loss of sarcomeres.[117] Biochemical changes that occur to a muscle that cannot lengthen demonstrate an increase catabolism and a concomitant loss of weight.[118] Physiologically, the amount of passive and active tension developed by a shortened muscle is less than normal muscles.[119] Studies indicate that when immobilization has been terminated, full recovery from anatomic, biochemical, and physiologic changes occurs.[116] Recovery is time-dependent and may require from a few days to as long as 60 days after termination of immobilization of the muscle.

Length-associated changes in muscle emphasize the need to regain normal mandibular dynamics as soon as possible. The reader is cautioned not to confuse a tight muscle undergoing length-associated changes with a muscle demonstrating heightened tone secondary to an increase in γ motor neuron activity. If altered afferent input affects the cranial V motor neuron activity, an increase in muscle tone/tightness will exist with those muscles innervated by cranial V. Pertinent to this discussion are the elevator muscles of the mandible (i.e., temporalis, masseter, and internal pterygoid muscles). The clinician risks actually facilitating an increase in muscle tone (secondary to altered γ motor neuron activity) by placing the muscle and the associated shortened muscle spindles on stretch. This procedure could facilitate an increase in muscle tone, especially if performed too rapidly.[120] A muscle having a length-associated increase in tone is hypothesized to have less facilitation to stretch than a muscle that has an increase in tone secondary to altered γ motor neuron activity. Understanding why a muscle is tight (length-associated changes versus altered γ motor neuron activity) bears important implications when placing a tight/ tense muscle on stretch. The following areas may contribute to altered γ motor neuron activity of the elevator muscles, resulting in a decrease in mandibular opening, and should therefore be managed first before placing the elevator muscles on stretch.

Occlusion: If a malocclusion is suspected, treat using an occlusal appliance.

TMD: If inflammation is present, follow guidelines discussed for treating inflammation.

Cervical spine disorder: If a symptomatic cervical spine disorder is present, treat with guidelines covered in Chapter 11.

Emotions: Treat with biofeedback using concepts discussed in the TTBS section and patient education. If necessary, professional counseling may be required.

Hypomobility Caused by Disc Displacement

Disc displacement is the most common TMJ arthropathy.[1] Several controversies are associated with treatment of disc displacement that center on the following questions:

1. Is the position of the disc important?
2. Should treatment be reversible or irreversible to be "successful" in treating a disc displacement?

An attempt to answer these two questions is not the intention or objective of this section. However, to introduce the role of physical therapy in management of disc displacements, a general response is necessary.

Disc displacement is commonly defined as an abnormal relation or misalignment of the articular disc and condyle.[1] By using the term *displacement,* it is implied "that the disc of internally deranged articulations had been in a normal position at an earlier time and was then displaced through some kind of precipitating event."[121] Although the cause of disc displacement is not totally agreed on, it is believed that for the disc to displace, stretched or torn ligaments must precede displacement.[122] The general consensus is that the direction of disc displacement is anterior or anteromedial to the condyle.[123] The end result is the posterior band of the disc lies in front of the condyle, with the condyle functioning on the posterior attachment. Once displaced, the disc can be subcategorized into[1]

1. Disc displacement with reduction
2. Disc displacement without reduction: acute or chronic

The morbidity of the disc functioning off the condyle has not been demonstrated to be entirely pathologic.[124–127] Imaging studies have documented the presence of disc displacements in many patients and nonpatients having no signs and symptoms of a disc displacement.[128,131] So common are disc displacements with otherwise asymptomatic healthy joints that several authors suggest that disc displacements should be considered within the normal range of anatomic variability.[128,132–134]

Treatments for disc displacements have focused in past years on occlusal appliances.[135,136] In a review of the literature, Zamburlini and Austin[135] concluded that "the recapture of the disc is permanent in only a small percentage of patients suggesting that the use of irreversible procedures must be carefully evaluated." Improvement of mandibular opening and decrease in pain that frequently occurs after arthroscopy for disc displacements does not occur from altering the position of the displaced disc.[88,137–139] Success from arthrotomy is not always based on a normal disc–condyle relationship despite improved condylar translation and positive patient response.[140,141] In summary, success of treatment is not dependent on the positioning of the disc or the absence of joint noises, but instead success is defined as freedom from pain and functional limitations of the TMJ.[142,143] Conservative treatment should be initiated first irrespective of the position of the disc.[142]

Studies that investigate disc displacements in nonpatient and patient populations can be used for general guidance in the understanding and management of most patients experiencing TMD. However, each patient must be dealt with as an individual with clinical decisions based on the *individual's* signs and symptoms and goals of treatment. A decision to treat with a particular modality or procedure should be supported when possible by the literature, especially if the treatment is irreversible. Otherwise, treatment offered to an individual patient is based on clinical experience and expertise of the clinician, which is influenced by any one or combination of the following nine factors:

1. Age of the patient

2. Chronicity of the disc displacement complaint
3. Severity of the disc displacement's interference with the patient's function and life style
4. Past treatment that failed in which the clinician believes that past treatment did not meet his or her standards of excellence
5. Past treatments that the clinician believes have been properly executed but have failed for unknown reasons
6. Refusal by the patient to consider surgery under any circumstances
7. Criteria for success of treatment differ between clinician and patient
8. Compliance by the patient seriously doubted by the clinician
9. Clinician bias and treatment philosophy

This list is not meant to be all-inclusive. This list can also be applied to other disorders of the TMJ as well as other musculoskeletal problems in which similar dilemmas surrounding treatment choices exist.

Physical therapist and dentist are often confronted with patients who have a disc displacement. I would suggest that if the physical therapist or dentist is not "specialized" in the management of TMD, a consultation with such specialists to review/oversee the treatment program is advised. It is not uncommon for the working diagnosis to change as treatments are rendered. Having a team approach among health professionals will allow for a quicker and smoother change in treatment plan to occur if necessary.

Treatment. As stated earlier, disc displacements are not always painful. If pain/inflammation is present along with a confirmed disc displacement, the clinician should first try to reduce inflammation regardless of the disc displacement[144] (refer to Inflammation). If inflammation continues after 4 to 6 weeks of physical therapy, an appropriate occlusal appliance along with anti-inflammatory medication is then suggested to help control inflammation and masticatory muscle hyperactivity.[145]

If inflammation continues for more than 1 to 3 months with continued physical therapy, an occlusal appliance, and medication, then the confirmed disc displacement may be the perpetuating cause of the inflammation and needs to be addressed. Treatment for a disc displacement without reduction may need to be started within the first 3 months because decrease in mandibular function is frequently present. However, it is not unusual for a nonreducing disc to reduce once inflammation and masticatory muscle hyperactivity is controlled.

General Comments on Treatment for an Acute Disc Displacement Without Reduction. Of the two categories of disc displacements (i.e., reducing and nonreducing), emphasis will be on the acute nonreducing disc because it contributes to hypomobility. The cardinal clinical sign for an acute disc displacement without reduction (ADDWoR) is locking.[146] Locking implies the inability to open the mouth beyond 20 to 25 mm.[147] However, an opening of 20 to 25 mm can also be caused by other nondiseased disorders such as inflammation, periarticular tightness, and masticatory muscle hyperactivity. The history and physical examination will aid in a differential diagnosis.

Physical therapy objectives in the treatment of an ADDWoR can be one of the following:

1. To return an ADDWoR to its normal position
2. To make an ADDWoR become a disc displacement with reduction (DDWR)
3. To allow an ADDWoR to become a chronic disc displacement without reduction (CDDWoR)

To Return an ADDWoR to Its Normal Position: The reality of the disc returning to its normal position with physical therapy treatment is not likely. The only time this author may anticipate the disc to stay in place once it is reduced with intraoral techniques is with a very young patient. Disc position may be maintained after treatment in a young patient provided the lock is recent (within 72 hours) and trauma to the mandible is not an immediate precipitating event. Isometric exercises (see Hypermobility) may assist in this case. An occlusal appliance is often used in conjunction to the intraoral techniques and isometric exercises. The clinician should not offer false hope to the older patient that the disc position will be stable if it is reduced. Reoccurrence of disc displacement is high even with the use of an occlusal appliance.[135,136]

To Make an ADDWoR Become a Disc Displacement With Reduction: Physical therapy treatments may allow an ADDWoR to become a DDWR. The clinical sign of a DDWR is usually the reciprocal click.[148] The primary benefit of an ADDWoR becoming a DDWR is a return of functional mandibular dynamics. If physical therapy is beneficial at allowing an ADDWoR to become a DDWR, several situations may follow:

1. The disc displacement stays as a DDWR without pain. No other treatment may be necessary.
2. The disc displacement stays as a DDWR but is painful. All efforts to control inflammation and masticatory muscle hyperactivity are unsuccessful. Treatments may need to progress with the application of an occlusal appliance as covered in Chapter 6. Other options with or without attempting an occlusal appliance can be surgery involving arthroscopy (see Ch. 8) or arthrotomy (see Ch. 9).
3. The disc displacement becomes a DDWR but returns quickly back to the state of an ADDWoR as soon as the patient brings the teeth into occlusion. One has several options in this situation:
    a. Immediately after the physical therapist reduces the disc, the therapist places dental roles on the patient's back molars. The patient, who has already had a consultation with a dentist, goes to the dentist to receive an occlusal appliance (i.e., a nonrepositioning or an anterior repositioning appliance).

b. "a" option is unsatisfactory, and the patient is referred on to have surgery, either arthroscopy or arthrotomy.

c. The physical therapist, dentist, and patient are determined that surgery is not an option. The choice is made to progress the patient to a CDDWoR.

To Allow an ADDWoR to Become a Chronic Disc Displacement Without Reduction: When the disc is displaced, the condyle functions on the posterior attachment of the disc. The condyle exerts compressive forces onto the posterior attachments and can do so without the patient experiencing pain.[149] It appears that the tissues posterior to the disc are capable of remolding and fibrosing when loaded in the presence of a disc displacement. Thus, a pseudo disc may be said to have developed.[149] In some patients, remolding of the posterior attachment does not occur, occurs but is inadequate, or occurs and is adequate for a time and then fails.[150] In cases in which the posterior attachment fails to withstand compressive forces and pain results, surgical options can be investigated.

Treatment for an Acute Disc Displacement Without Reduction.   Several studies have shown that intraoral mobilization techniques and exercises are successful as a conservative choice in the treatment of an ADDWoR.[151,155]

Joint Mobilization Techniques.   An increase in translation in the upper joint space is the primary objective of intraoral techniques. Increasing translation in the upper joint space allows for a return of functional mandibular dynamics. An increase in opening is probably achieved by elongation of the posterior attachment, with further displacement and advanced deformation of the disc.[148,56] Nitzan and Dolwick[157] attribute an increase in translation to a release of adherence of the disc to the fossa, caused by a reversible effect such as a vacuum or viscous synovial fluid. Even though Nitzan and Dolwick's comments were made on the effects of a lavage in the superior joint space, one can hypothesize that intraoral techniques and exercises have similar effects. Several studies have shown that manual manipulation applied to an ADDWoR can restore mandibular ROM regardless of the duration the patient has been in an acute nonreducing disc state.[153] Instead of an ADDWoR taking its natural course at becoming a CDDWoR, the entire process is sped up by manual techniques because of the importance of regaining functional mandibular dynamics.[131,158,159]

Hand placement for the treatment of an ADDWoR is the same as described in Joint Mobilization Techniques: Treatment For Periarticular Tightness. Intraoral techniques will include only distraction and translation. Lateral glide does not seem to be that beneficial for the treatment of an ADDWoR.

If the objective is to get the disc to reduce, then a stage III distraction followed by translation is performed. If instead the objective is simply to restore translation in the upper joint space, then a stage I or II distraction is applied for patient comfort, followed by translation. The amount of force used depends entirely on joint irritability and the amount of masticatory muscle hyperactivity. In general, intraoral mobilization forces used in treating an ADDWoR are much greater than those used to treat for periarticular tightness, especially if periarticular tightness is secondary to arthrotomy.

I would suggest a frequency of three times a week for 4 to 6 weeks of treatments before determining if a return to functional mandibular dynamics can be achieved. During this 4- to 6-week period, a home exercise program to increase translation in the upper joint space will involve most exercises covered in Treatment for Periarticular Tightness. These exercises are

Finger spread exercise: Throughout the opening phase of this exercise, protrusion of the mandible is performed simultaneously with opening to place emphasis on translation.

Touch and bite exercise: Benefits protrusion as well as lateral excursion to the opposite side of the ADDWoR

Cotton roll distraction: Cotton ball is placed on the same side of the ADDWoR; less distraction is applied while the patient actively protrudes the mandible.

Static tongue blade exercise: Tongue blades are placed on the same side of the ADDWoR; A prying motion on the tongue blades may be helpful here.

Horizontal tongue blade exercise: The number of tongue blades is reduced to three or four, depending on the patient's comfort, to engage translation more.

If joint noises occur during treatment, the clinician will place little emphasis on them. Of the publications reviewed by Wabeke[160] and Spruijt,[161] they found that little attention should be given to joint noises and that treatment should not be performed for noises alone. Clicking can also be related to factors other than a disc displacement with reduction.[160] Treatment for clicking should only be considered when the clicking is associated with pain or troublesome symptoms (e.g., restricted movement).[160,161] In most cases involving disc displacements, the primary objective is to achieve functional mandibular dynamics regardless of disc position.

CONCLUSION

Physical therapy plays an important role in the management of the common disorders that affect the TMJ. A physical therapist can offer significant input into the evaluation and management of inflammation, hypermobility, and hypomobility conditions of the TMJ. Treatments should not be applied in a cookbook way. Sound clinical reasoning by a physical therapist aids in the choice, sequence, and duration of treatments. Therapist's knowledge of the physiologic rationale for treatment is essential for effective physical therapy management of patients with unusual and complex TMD presentations. In combination with other health professionals (dental, medical, and psychological), physical therapists may facilitate improved scope and quality of care in the symptomatic TMD patient.

ACKNOWLEDGMENT

I would like to thank Carolyn Law, M.P.T., for her invaluable assistance with manuscript preparation.

REFERENCES

1. McNeill C (ed): Temporomandibular Disorders; Guidelines for Classification, Assessment, and Management. The American Academy of Orofacial Pain. Quintessence Publishing Co., Chicago, 1993
2. White LW: The temporomandibular joint and craniomandibular disorders. J Clin Orthod 26:607, 1992
3. Danzig W, May S, McNeill C et al: Effect of an anesthetic injected into the temporomandibular joint space in patients with TMD. J Craniomandib Disord Facial Oral Pain 6:288, 1992
4. McCreary C, Clark G, Oakley M et al: Predicting response to treatment for temporomandibular disorders. J Craniomandib Disord Facial Oral Pain 6:161, 1992
5. Dworkin S: Approach to the problem. J Craniomandib Disord Facial Oral Pain 6:302, 1992
6. Ohrbach R: Review of the literature: part I—a current diagnostic system. J Craniomandib Disord Facial Oral Pain 6:307, 1992
7. American Academy of Craniomandibular Disorders: Craniomandibular Disorders. Guidelines for Evaluation, Diagnosis & Management. Quintessence Publishing Co., Lombard, Illinois, 1990
8. Kraus SL: Evaluation and Management of Temporomandibular Disorders. In Saunders HD, Saunders R (eds): Evaluation, Treatment and Prevention of Musculoskeletal Disorders. The Saunders Group, Minneapolis, 1993
9. Spierings ELH, Miree LF: Non-compliance with follow-up and improvement after treatment at a headache center. Headache 33:205, 1993
10. Sluijs EM: Patient Education in Physical Therapy. NIVEL, Utrecht, Netherlands, 1991
11. Boyd RL, Gibbs CH, Mahan PE et al: Temporomandibular joint forces measured at the condyle of macaca arctoides. Am J Orthod Dentofac Orthop 97:472, 1990
12. Kaplan AS, Leon A: Temporomandibular Disorders: Diagnosis & Treatment. WB Saunders, Philadelphia, 1991
13. Schnurr RF, Rollman GB, Brooke RI: Are there psychologic predictors of treatment in temporomandibular joint pain and dysfunction? Oral Surg Oral Med Oral Pathol 72:550, 1991
14. Schiffman EL, Fricton JR, Haley DP et al: The prevalence and treatment needs of subjects with temporomandibular disorders. J Am Dent Assoc 120:295, 1990
15. Ehrlich J, Hochman N, Yaffe A: Contribution of oral habits to dental disorders. J Craniomandib Pract 10:144, 1992
16. Rugh JD, Drago CJ: Vertical dimension: a study of clinical rest position and jaw muscle activity. J Prosthet Dent 45:670, 1981

17. Schoen R, et al: Der Kieferzungenreflex und andre proriozeptive reflexe der zunge und der Kiefermuskulatur. Arch Exp Pathol Pharmacol 160:29, 1931
18. Morimoto T, Kawamura Y: Properties of tongue and jaw movements elicited by stimulation of the orbital gyrus of cat. Arch Oral Biol 18:361, 1973
19. Sauerland EK, Mitchell SP: Electromyographic activity of intrinsic and extrinsic muscles of the human tongue. Tex Rep Biol Med 33:258, 1975
20. Proffit W: Equilibrium theory revisited: factors influencing position of the teeth. Angle Orthod 48:172, 1978
21. Fish F: The functional anatomy of the rest position of the mandible. Dent Practioner 11:178, 1961
22. Atwood DA: A critique of research of the rest position of the mandible. J Prosthet Dent 16:848, 1966
23. Emslie RD, Massler M, Zwemer JO: Mouthbreathing: I etiology and effects. J Am Dent Assoc 44:506, 1952
24. Sharp J, Druz W, Danon J et al: Respiratory muscle function and the use of respiratory muscle electromyography in the evaluation of respiratory regulation. Chest, suppl. 70:150, 1976
25. Weinberg B: Deglutition: a review of selected topics. In Proceedings of the Workshop, Speech and the Dentofacial Complex: The State of the Art: ASHA Reports 5. American Speech and Hearing Association, Washington, DC, 1970
26. Kelly J, Sanchez M, Van Kirk L: An assessment of the occlusion of teeth of children. National Center for Health Statistics, US Public Health Service, 1973
27. Lawerence ES, Samson GS: Growth development influences on the craniomandibular region. In Kraus SL (ed): TMJ Disorders: Management of the Craniomandibular Complex. 1st Ed. Churchill Livingstone, New York, 1988
28. Kraus SL: Influences of the cervical spine on the stomatognathic system. In Donatelli R, Wooden M (eds): Orthopaedic Physical Therapy. 2nd Ed. Churchill Livingstone, New York, 1993
29. Milidonis MK, Kraus SL, Segal RL, Widmer CG: Genioglossi muscle activity in response to changes in anterior/neutral head posture. Am J Orthod Dentofac Orthop 103:39, 1993
30. Yamashita S, Ai M, Mizutani H: Tooth contact patterns in patients with temporomandibular dysfunction. J Oral Rehabil 18:431, 1991
31. Barrett R, Hanson M: Oral Myofunctional Disorders. CV Mosby, St. Louis, 1978
32. Mannheimer JS: Physical therapy concepts in the evaluation and treatment of the upper quarter, therapeutic modalities. In Kraus SL (ed): TMJ Disorders: Management of the Craniomandibular Complex. 1st Ed. 1988
33. Keith DA: Surgery of the Temporomandibular Joint. Blackwell Scientific Publications, Boston, 1988
34. Buckingham RB, Braun T, Harenstein DA et al: Temporomandibular joint dysfunction syndrome: a close association with systemic joint laxity (the hypermobile joint syndrome). Oral Surg Oral Med Oral Pathol 72:514, 1991
35. Westling L, Mattiasson A: General joint hypermobility and temporomandibular joint derangement in adolescents. Ann Rheum Dis 51:87, 1992
36. Dijkstra PU, Lambert de Bont GM, Stegenga B et al: Temporomandibular joint osteoarthrosis and generalized joint hypermobility. J Craniomandib Pract 10:221, 1992
37. Westling L: Craniomandibular disorders & general joint mobility. Acta Odontol Scand 47:293, 1989
38. Esposito C, Clear M, Veal S: Arthroscopic surgical treatment of temporoman-

dibular joint hypermobility with recurrent anterior dislocation: an alternative to open surgery. J Craniomandib Pract 9:286, 1991

39. Whear NM, Langdon JD, Macpherson DW: Temporomandibular joint eminence augmentation by down-fracture & inter-positional cartilage graft: a new surgical technique. Int J Oral Maxillofac Surg 20:357, 1991

40. Goss CM (ed): Gray's Anatomy. 29th Am. Ed. Lea & Febiger, Philadelphia 1973

41. Schwartz L: Therapeutic exercises. p. 223. In Schwartz L (ed): Disorders of the Temporomandibular Joint. WB Saunders, Philadelphia, 1959

42. Zarb G, Speck J: The treatment of mandibular dysfunction p. 382. In Zarb G, Carlsson G (eds): Temporomandibular Joint, Function and Dysfunction. CV Mosby, St. Louis, 1979

43. Guyton AC: Textbook of Medical Physiology. WB Saunders, Philadelphia, 1971

44. Au AR, Klineberg IV: Isokinetic exercise management of temporomandibular joint clicking in young adults. J Prosthet Dent 70:33, 1993

45. Muir CB, Goss AN: The radiologic morphology of asymptomatic temporomandibular joints. Oral Surg Oral Med Oral Pathol 70:349, 1990

46. Stockstill JW, Harn SD, Underhill TE: Clinical implications of anomalous muscle insertion relative to jaw movement and mandibular dysfunction: the anterior belly of the diagastric muscle in a cadaver. J Craniomandib Disord Facial Oral Pain 5: 64, 1991

47. DeAndrade J, Grant C, Dixon A: Joint distention and reflex muscle inhibition in the knee. J Bone Joint Surg 47(A):313, 1965

48. Larsson L, Thilander B: Mandibular positioning, the effect of pressure on joint capsule. Acta Neurol Scand 40:131, 1964

49. Smith AM: The coactivation of antagonist muscles. Can J Physiol Pharmacol 59: 733, 1981

50. Burke D: Critical examination of the case for or against fusimotor involvement in disorders of muscle tone. p. 133. In Desmedt JE (ed): Motor Control Mechanisms in Health and Disease. Raven Press, New York, 1983

51. Tanigawa MC: Comparison of the hold–relax procedure and passive mobilization on increasing muscle length. Phys Ther 52:725, 1972

52. Peacock E Jr: Some biochemical and biophysical aspects of joint stiffness. Ann Surg 164:1, 1968

53. Salter R, Simmonds D, Malcolm BW et al: The biological effect of continuous passive motion on the healing of full-thickness defects in articular cartilage. Clin Orthop 176:305, 1983

54. Salter RB, Hamilton WH, Wedge JH et al: Clinical applications of basic research on continuous passive motion for disorders and injuries of synovial joints, a preliminary report of a feasibility study. J Orthop Res 3:325, 1983

55. Ilyinsky OB, Krasnikova TL, Akoev GN et al: Functional organization of mechanoreceptors. Prog Brain Res 43:195, 1976

56. McCloskey DI: Kinesthetic sensibility. Physiol Rev 58:763, 1978

57. Wyke B: The neurology of joints. Ann R Coll Surg Engl 41:25, 1967

58. Griffin CJ, Hawthorn R, Harris R: Anatomy and histology of the human temporomandibular joint. Monogr Oral Sci 4:1, 1975

59. Gray's Anatomy. 35th Br. Ed. WB Saunders, Philadelphia, 1973

60. MacConaill MA: Studies in the mechanics of synovial joints II. I J Med Sci 6:223, 1946

61. MacConaill MA, Basmajian JV: Muscles and movements: a basis for human kinesiology. Williams & Wilkins, Baltimore, 1969

62. Moss M: The functional matrix concept and its relationship to temporomandibular joint dysfunction and treatment. Dent Clin North Am 27:445, 1983

63. MacConaill MA: The movements of bones and joints. J Bone Joint Surg 35(B): 290, 1953

64. MacConaill MA: The geometry and algebra of articular kinematics. Biomed Eng 1:205, 1966

65. MacConaill MA: Joint movement. Physiotherapy Nov:359, 1964

66. Mennell J: Joint Pain; Diagnosis and Treatment Using Manipulative Techniques. Little, Brown and Co., Boston, 1964

67. Zohn DA, Mennell JM: Musculoskeletal Pain: Diagnosis and Physical Treatment. Little, Brown and Co., Boston, 1976

68. Cotta H, Puhl W: The pathophysiology of damage to articular cartilage. Prog Orthop Surg 3:20,1978

69. Burkhart S: The rationale for joint mobilization. p. 155. In Kent B (ed): Proceedings of the International Federation of Orthopaedic Manipulative Therapists. Third International Seminar, Hayward, California, 1977

70. Radin EL, Paul IL: Response of joints to impact loading. Arthritis Rheum 14:356, 1971

71. Radin EL, Paul IL: Does cartilage compliance reduce skeletal impact loads? Arthritis Rheum 13:139, 1970

72. Glineburg RW, Laskin DM, Blaustein DI: The effects of immobilization on the primate temporomandibular joint: a histologic and histochemical study. J Oral Maxillofac Surg 40:3, 1982

73. Thilander B: Innervation of the temporomandibular joint capsule in man. Trans R Sch Dent Stockholm 7:1, 1961

74. Clark RKF, Wyke BD: Contributions of temporomandibular articular mechanoreceptors to the control of mandibular posture: an experimental study. J Dent 2: 121, 1974

75. Harris R, Griffin CJ: Neuromuscular mechanisms and the masticatory apparatus. Monogr Oral Sci 4:45, 1975

76. Klineberg IJ, Greenfield BE, Wyke BD: Contributions to the reflex control of mastication from mechanoreceptors in the temporomandibular joint capsule. Dent Practioner Dent Rec 21:73, 1970

77. Wyke BD: Articular neurology—a review. Physiotherapy 58:94, 1972

78. Wyke BD: Neurology of the cervical spinal joints. Physiotherapy 65:72, 1979

79. Clark R: Neurology of the temporomandibular joints: an experimental study. Ann R Coll Surg Engl 58:43, 1976

80. Pagonis E: Where is the optimum position of the temporomandibular joint condyle? Ohio Dent J 64:20, 1990

81. Ogus HD, Toller PA: Common Disorders of the Temporomandibular Joint. 2nd Ed. Wright and Bristol, England, 1986

82. Dorland's Illustrated Medical Dictionary. 24th Ed. WB Saunders, Philadelphia, London, 1965

83. Akeson WH: An experimental study of joint stiffness. J Bone Joint Surg 43(A): 1022, 1961

84. Akeson WH, Amiel D, LaViolette D et al: The connective tissue response to immobility: an accelerated aging response. Exp Gerontol 3:289, 1968

85. Akeson WH, Amiel D, Woo S: Immobility effects of synovial joints: the pathomechanics of joint contracture. Biorheology 17:95, 1980

86. Hardy M: The biology of scar formation. Phys Ther 69:1014, 1990

87. Sanders B: Arthroscopic surgery of the temporomandibular joint: treatment of internal derangement with persistent closed lock. Oral Surg Oral Med Oral Pathol 62:361, 1986

88. Nitzan DW, Dolwick MF, Heft MW: Arthroscopic lavage and lysis of the temporomandibular joint. J Oral Maxillofac Surg 48:798, 1990

89. Clark RKF, Wyke BD: Temporomandibular arthrokinetic reflex control of the mandibular musculature. Br J Oral Surg 13:196, 1975

90. Bertolucci LE: Postoperative physical therapy in temporomandibular joint arthroplasty. J Craniomandib Pract 10:211, 1992

91. Wilk BR, McCain JP: Rehabilitation of the temporomandibular joint after arthroscopic surgery. Oral Surg Oral Med Oral Pathol 73:531, 1992

92. Zislis MW, Wank HA, Gottehrer NR: TMJ arthroscopy—a preoperative & postoperative rehabilitation protocol. J Craniomandib Disord Facial Oral Pain 3:218, 1989

93. Wilk BR, Stenback JT, McCain JP: Postarthroscopy physical therapy management of a patient with temporomandibular joint dysfunction. JOSPT 18:473, 1993

94. Zimmer B, Schwestka R, Kubein-Meesenburg D: Changes in mandibular mobility after different procedures of orthognathic surgery. Eur J Orthod 14:188, 1992

95. Athanasiou AE, Melsen B: Craniomandibular dysfunction following surgical correction of mandibular prognathism. Angle Orthod 6:9, 1992

96. Magnusson T, Ahlborg G, Svartz K: Function of the masticatory system in 20 patients with mandibular hypo- or hyperplasia after correction by a sagittal split osteotomy. Int J Oral Maxillofac Surg 19:289, 1990

97. Hussey HH (ed): Rheumatoid arthritis, section 7 (supplement). AMA 224:687, 1973

98. Posselt U: Hinge opening axis of the mandible. Acta Odontol Scand 14:61, 1956

99. Osborn JW: The disc of the human temporomandibular joint: design, function and failure. J Oral Rehabil 12:279, 1985

100. McCarthy MR, O'Donoghue PC, Yates CK et al: The clinical use of continuous passive motion in physical therapy. JOSPT 15:132, 1992

101. O'Driscoll SW, Kumar A, Salter RB: The effect of the volume of effusion, joint position and continuous passive motion on intraarticular pressure in the rabbit knee. J Rheumatol 10:360, 1983

102. Kaltenborn FM: Manual Therapy for the Extremity Joints. 2nd Ed. Olaf Norlis Bokhandel, Oslo, 1976

103. Maitland GD: Vertebral Manipulation. Butterworths, London, 1981

104. Newton R: Joint recepter contributions to reflexive and kinesthetic responses. Phys Ther 62:22, 1982

105. Freeman M, Wyke B: The innervation of the knee joint: an anatomical and histological study in the cat. J Anat 101:505, 1967

106. Wright V, Dowson D, Longfield M: Joint stiffness—its characterization & significance. Biomed Eng 4:8, 1969

107. Randall T, Portney L, Harris BA: Effects of joint mobilization on joint stiffness and active motion of the metacarpal-phalangeal joint. JOSPT 16:30, 1992

108. Stromberg D, Wiederhielm CA: Viscoelastic description of a collagenous tissue in simple elongation. J Appl Physiol 26:857, 1969

109. LaBan MM: Collagen tissue: implications of its response to stress in vitro. Arch Phys Med Rehabil 43:461, 1962

110. Lehmann J, Masock A, Warren C et al: Effect of therapeutic temperature on tendon extensibility. Arch Phys Med Rehabil 51:481, 1970

111. Warren C, Lehman J, Koblanski J: Heat and stretch procedures: an evaluation using rat tail tendon. Arch Phys Med Rehabil 57:122, 1976

112. Lentell G, Hetherington T, Eagan J et al: The use of thermal agents to influence the effectiveness of a low-load prolonged stretch. JOSPT 16:200, 1992

113. Warren C, Lehmann J, Koblanski J: Elongation of rat tail tendon; effect of load and temperature. Arch Phys Med Rehabil 52:465, 1971

114. McCarthy MR, Yates CK, Anderson MA et al: The effects of immediate continuous passive motion on pain during the inflammatory phase of soft tissue healing following anterior cruciate reconstruction. JOSPT 17:96, 1993

115. Salter RB: The biological concept of continuous passive motion of synovial joints. The first 18 years of basic research and its clinical application. Clin Orthop 242: 12, 1989

116. Gossman MR, Sharmann SA, Rose SJ: Review of length-associated changes in muscle. Phys Ther 62:1799, 1979

117. Tabary JC, Tabary C, Tardieu G et al: Physiological and structural changes in the cat's soleus muscle due to immobilization at different lengths by plaster casts. J Physiol (Lond) 224:231, 1972

118. Schar I, Takacs O, Guba F: The influence of immobilization on soluble proteins in muscle. Acta Biol Med Germanica 36:1621, 1977

119. Goldspink G, Williams PE: The nature of the increased passive resistance in muscle following immobilization of the mouse soleus muscle. Physiol Soc Dec:55, 1978

120. Jacobs M: Neurophysiological implications of slow active stretching. Am Corr Ther J 30:151, 1976

121. Luder HU, Bobst P, Schroeder HE: Histometric study of synovial cavity dimensions of human temporomandibular joints with normal & anterior disc position. J Orofac Pain 7:263, 1993

122. Stegenga B: Temporomandibular joint osteoarthrosis and internal derangement: diagnostic and therapeutic outcome assessment. Thesis. Groningen, Netherlands, 1991

123. Hansson TL: Pathological aspects of arthritides and derangements. p. 165. In: Sarnat BG, Laskin DM (eds): The Temporomandibular Joint: A Biological Basis for Clinical Practice. 4th Ed. WB Saunders, Philadelphia, 1992

124. Toller P: Non-surgical treatment of the temporomandibular joint. Oral Sci Rev 7: 70, 1976

125. Rasmussen OC: Description of population and progress of symptoms in a longitudinal study of temporomandibular arthropathy. Scand J Dent Res 89:196, 1981

126. Clark GT, Mulligan RA: A review of the prevalence of temporomandibular dysfunction. J Gerodontol 3:231, 1986

127. Greene CS, Turner C, Laskin DM: Long-term outcome of TMJ clicking in 100 MPD patients. J Dent Res 61:218, 1982

128. Kircos LT, Ortendahl DA, Mark AS et al: Magnetic resonance imaging of the TMJ disc in asymptomatic volunteers. J Oral Maxillofac Surg 45:852, 1987

129. Hatala MP, Westesson P-L, Tallents RH: TMJ disc displacement in asymptomatic volunteers detected by MR imaging. J Dent Res April 1991

130. Pothitaskis MC, Zeitler DL, Moore TE: Bilateral TMJ MRI studies in patients with unilateral symptoms. J Dent Res April 1991

131. Eriksson L, Westesson PL: Clinical & radiological study of patients with anterior disc displacement of the temporomandibular joint. Swed Dent J 7:55, 1983

132. Turell J, Ruiz HG: Normal and abnormal findings in temporomandibular joints in autopsy specimens. J Craniomandib Disord Facial Oral Pain 1:257, 1987

133. Hellsing G, Holmlund A: Development of anterior disk displacement in the temporomandibular joint: an autopsy study. J Prosthet Dent 53:397, 1985.

134. Westesson PL, Eriksson L, Kurita K: Reliability of a negative clinical temporo-

mandibular joint examination: prevalence of disk displacement in asymptomatic temporomandibular joints. Oral Surg Oral Med Oral Pathol 68:551, 1989.

135. Zamburlini I, Austin D: Long-term results of appliance therapies in anterior disk displacement with reduction: a review of the literature. J Craniomandib Pract 9: 361, 1991

136. Orenstein ES: Anterior repositioning appliances when used for anterior disk displacement with reduction—a critical review. J Craniomandib Pract 11:141, 1993

137. Montgomery MT, Van Sickels JE, Harms SE et al: Arthroscopic TMJ surgery: effects on signs, symptoms, and disk position. J Oral Maxillofac Surg 47:1263, 1989

138. Perott DH, Alborzi A, Kaban LB et al: A prospective evaluation of the effectiveness of temporomandibular joint arthroscopy. J Oral Maxillofac Surg 48:1029, 1990

139. Gabler MJ, Greene C, Palacios E et al: Effect of arthroscopic temporomandibular joint surgery on articular disk position. J Craniomandib Disord Facial Oral Pain 191, 1989

140. Farole A: Correlation of postoperative TMJ MRI and patients clinical symptoms. J Oral Maxillofac Surg 48:132, 1990

141. Montgomery M et al: Meniscal repositioning and arthroscopic TMJ surgeries: outcome comparisons. J Dent Res 1004, 1990

142. Vichaichalermvong S, Nilner M, Panmekiate S et al: Clinical follow-up patients with different disc positions. J Orofac Pain 7:61, 1993

143. Moloney F, Howard JA: Internal derangements of the temporomandibular joint: anterior repositioning splint therapy. Aust Dent J 31:30, 1986

144. Murakami K-I, Segami N, Fujimura K et al: Correlation between pain and synovitis in patients with internal derangement of the temporomandibular joint. J Oral Maxillofac Surg 49:1159, 1991

145. Chung S-C, Kim H-S: The effects of the stabilization splint on the TMJ closed locked. J Craniomandib Pract 11:95, 1993

146. Farrar WB: Characteristics of the condylar path in internal derangements of the TMJ. J Prosthet Dent 39:319, 1978

147. Murakami K-I, Segami N, Moriya Y et al: Correlation between pain and dysfunction and intra-articular adhesions in patients with internal derangement of the temporomandibular joint. J Oral Maxillofac Surg 50:705, 1992

148. Dolwick MF, Katzberg RW, Helms CA: Internal derangements of the temporomandibular joint: fact or fiction: J Prosthet Dent 49:415, 1983

149. Scapino RP: The posterior attachments: its structure, function, and appearance in TMJ imaging studies: part 1. J Craniomandib Disord Facial Oral Pain 5:83, 1991

150. Scapino RP: Histopathology of the disc and posterior attachment. In: Disc Displacement Internal Derangements of the TMJ. In Palacios E (ed): Magnetic Resonance Imaging of the temporomandibular joint. Georg Thieme Verlag, Stuttgart, 1990

151. Van Dyke AR, Goldman SM: Manual reduction of displaced disk. J Craniomandib Pract 8:350, 1990

152. Minagi S, Nozaki S, Sato T et al: Manipulation techniques for treatment of anterior disk displacement without reduction. J Prosthet Dent 65:686, 1991

153. Segami N, Murakami K-I, Iizuka T et al: Arthrographic evaluation of disk position following mandibular manipulation technique for internal derangement with close lock of the temporomandibular joint. J Craniomandib Disord Oral Facial Pain 4: 99, 1990

154. Jagger RG: Mandibular manipulation of anterior disc displacement without reduction. J Oral Rehabil 18:497, 1991
155. Friedman MH: Closed lock. A survey of 400 cases. Oral Surg Oral Med Oral Pathol 75:422, 1993
156. Westesson P-L, Bronstein SL, Liedberg J: Internal derangement of the temporomandibular joint: morphologic description with correlation to joint function. Oral Surg Oral Med Oral Pathol 59:323, 1985
157. Nitzan DW, Dolwick FM: An alternative explanation for the gensis of close-lock symptoms in the internal derangement process. J Oral Maxillofac Surg 49:810, 1991
158. Farrar WB, McCarty WL: Inferior joint space arthrography & characteristics of condylar paths in internal derangements of the TMJ. J Prosthet Dent 41:548, 1979
159. Westesson P-L, Lundh H: Arthrographic & clinical characteristics of patients with disk displacement who progressed to closed lock during a 6 month period. Oral Surg Oral Med Oral Pathol 67:654, 1989
160. Wabeke KB, Hansson TL, Hoogstraten J et al: Temporomandibular joint clicking: a literature overview. J Craniomandib Disord Facial Oral Pain 3:163, 1989
161. Spruijt RJ, Hoogstraten J: The research on temporomandibular joint clicking: a methodological review. J Craniomandib Disord Facial Oral Pain 5:45, 1991
162. Donatelli R, Wooden MJ: Orthopaedic Physical Therapy. Churchill Livingstone, New York, 1989
163. Kraus S: Tongue-Teeth-Breathing-Swallowing: Exercise Pad. Stretching Charts, Inc., Tacoma, Washington, 1987
164. Frankel VH, Nordin M: Basic Biomechanics of the Skeletal System. Lea & Febiger, Philadelphia, 1980

8 | Arthroscopy in the Conservative Management of TMD

Robert E. Going, Jr.

TMDs are a significant cause of facial pain and dysfunction. Surgical modalities may be indicated in the conservative management of TMD if certain specific criteria are satisfied. Continually, new advances in small joint arthroscopic instrumentation have established an important option in the treatment of TMDs. Potentially less invasive than open arthrotomy, TMJ arthroscopy offers both diagnostic and therapeutic capabilities in the management of internal derangements and degenerative joint diseases (DJD). An internal derangement or articular disc displacement has been defined by the American Association of Oral & Maxillofacial Surgeons as a "disruption within the internal aspects of the TMJ, in which there is displacement of the disc from its normal functional relationship with the mandibular condyle and the articular posterior of the temporal bone (glenoid fossa and eminence), or alterations in the normal dynamic motion of intracapsular elements leading to joint dysfunction."[1] DJD (osteoarthritis, arthrosis) also has been defined as a noninflammatory focal disorder, characterized by progressive deterioration of the articular surfaces within the joint, usually associated with pain and impaired function.

Arthroscopy is a surgical procedure used to visualize, diagnose, and treat intracapsular TMDs. In an arthroscopic examination, the surgeon makes a small incision to insert a small-diameter arthroscope into the TMJ. The system magnifies the structure inside the joint for projection onto a television monitor. This enables inspection of the TMJ to determine the extent of pathology and allows the performance of a surgical procedure if necessary. Specially designed instruments can be inserted through additional puncture sites to allow for various therapeutic procedures to be accomplished under direct visualization.

Arthroscopy gives the surgeon a precise direct view of the superior joint space and occasionally the inferior joint space and condyle. Recent reports of inferior joint space arthroscopy with a 0.69-mm-diameter ultra-thin arthroscope were noted by Kondoh and Westesson in 1991[2] with limited value. A more detailed and magnified examination of the TMJ can be accomplished with the arthroscope (Fig. 8-1A and B) without disturbance of the component relationships of the joint than with traditional "open joint" TMJ surgical procedures. Areas sometimes difficult to see on a variety of radiographic imaging techniques can be seen during TMJ arthroscopy.

Patients and surgeons have chosen this type of surgical modality over conventional open joint methods because of the small nature of the incision and arthroscopic techniques that do not disrupt muscles or tissues, allowing for less time in the operating room, less requirement for surgical anesthesia, less time in the hospital, few pain-relieving medications postoperatively, incisions that are barely noticeable and faster recovery.

One of the significant advantages in surgically addressing the TMJ with arthroscopic techniques is the ability to diagnose and treat TMJ intracapsular pathology at an earlier stage, so that early return to normal function is possible. This is preventive in nature, as less debilitating future surgeries, such as open joint surgery and total joint reconstruction (and their inherent morbidities), can be avoided. If good diagnosis and treatment planning of TMD are performed at an early stage, then conservative nonsurgical modalities and surgical modalities such as TMJ arthroscopy can virtually "cure" patients and allow return to normal function with minimal to no symptomatology.

The treatment plan should always be based on a thorough and complete diagnosis of the TMJ. This should encompass the extracapsular as well as the intracapsular disorders, as successful TMJ management is dependent on the recognition of the multiple etiologies of TMJ and facial pain. The most common symptom in patients with articular disc displacement is joint pain associated with function (i.e., does it hurt to chew?). Headaches, ear pain, tinnitis, clicking and popping sounds (with or without pain), crepitance, and hypermobility or displacement are other signs and symptoms consistent with TMJ disorders.

The efficacy of TMJ arthroscopy has been reported in many scientific articles. McCain et al[3] in 1992 reported on a 6-year multicenter retrospective study of 4,831 TMJs, showing four outcomes: (1) range of motion (ROM), (2) pain, (3) diet, and (4) disability. Six diagnostic categories were evaluated: (1) acute disc displacement without reduction, (2) a painful disc displacement with reduction, (3) osteoarthritis, (4) hypermobility, (5) fibrous ankylosis, and (6) arthralgia. After arthroscopic surgery, 91.6 percent had good or excellent motion; 91.3 percent had good or excellent pain reduction; 90.6 percent had good or excellent reduction in disability. Mosby[4] in 1993 studied 150 TMJs that underwent arthroscopic surgery with lysis, lavage, and débridement. The patients were evaluated for interincisal opening, lateral and protrusive excursions,

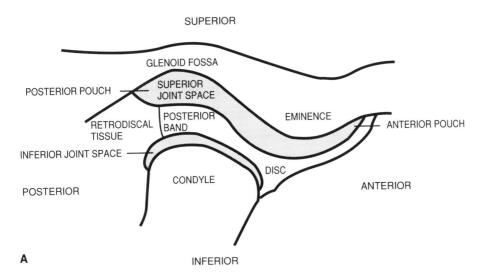

A

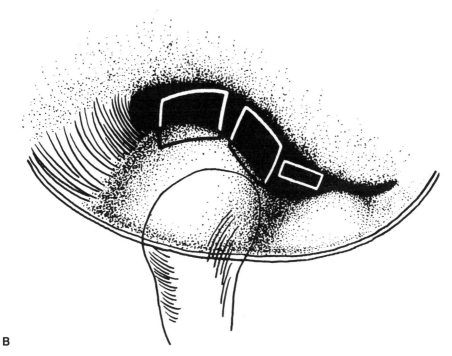

B

Fig. 8-1. (A) Osseous landmarks for anatomic classification. **(B)** Right TMJ superior joint space, posterior band area, and immediate zone area. (From Blaustein and Heffez,[5] with permission.)

and pain. There was a general improvement in all categories of mandibular movement, with a reduction of pain in 93 percent of the patients.[4]

Arthroscopic TMJ surgery has also stimulated changes in theoretic and clinical applications regarding management of disc displacement in the TMJ. The literature supports many patients with documented intra-articular pathology refractory to nonsurgical therapies who underwent TMJ arthroscopy involving lysis and lavage in the superior (upper) joint space. Significant improvement was noted in pain, ROM, and diet, yet no improvement was noted in the incidence of joint sounds, and disc position remained unchanged (anteriorly displaced) in most TMJs. Academic and clinical surgeons now agree that disc positioning may not be needed to achieve clinical success. Disc "recapturing" is not as significant as once thought in the reduction of painful symptomatology in the TMJ. The significance of TMJ noise remains obscure from a prognostic standpoint.

Other reasons for success with TMJ arthroscopy besides lysis, lavage, and débridement should include

1. Dilatation of the lateral capsule (i.e., capsular fibrosis)
2. Decreased potential for fibrous scar formation postsurgically
3. Quicker recovery time in returning to normal mastication and TMJ function

HISTORY OF ARTHROSCOPY

Arthroscopy has been used for various diagnostic and therapeutic procedures since its primitive inception in 1918, when Professor Kengi Takagi, the father of arthroscopy, modified a cystoscope to study the knee joint, using the principles of endoscopy. He invented the "number one" arthroscope and, in 1931, the panendoscope. The nasoscope had been previously reported in 1806 by Bozzini, and the genitourinary cystoscope in 1877 by Nitze. In 1921, Bircher reported knee arthroscopy using a modified cystoscope. In 1925, Kreuscher published an arthroscopic diagnosis of knew menicus disorders. In 1931 in New York, Burman used a 3-mm scope for shoulder, elbow, and hip surgery and performed in vivo cartilage staining with eosin.[5]

Between 1949 and 1969, knee arthroscopy made significant improvements, primarily with the developments of Watanabe and Takeda. They introduced fiberoptics as well as publishing an atlas of knee arthroscopy. In 1959, Dr. Masaki Watanabe was instrumental in the development and design of the first direct and forward oblique viewing #21 arthroscope, which was the single most important development in arthroscopic instrumentation. In 1972, Watanabe developed a small joint arthroscope. During the period between 1959 and 1972, advancement of fiberoptic lens sources and the use of television cameras and video monitors were also introduced.[5]

The first published report of human TMJ arthroscopy was by Ohnishi in 1975[6]; and in 1980, he published on (1) the diagnostic direct observation of the

TMJ, (2) observation of movement, (3) blind biopsy of the TMJ, (4) photographic documentation, and (5) diagnosis and selection of appropriate therapy guided by the arthroscopic examination.[7]

In 1978[8] and 1980,[9] Laskin researched rabbit TMJ arthroscopy and pathology using the arthroscope. Since then, pioneers such as Kino, Murakami, Hellsing, Holmlund, Sanders, Hoshino, Merrill, McCain, Heffez, and Blaustein have contributed to the acceptance of TMJ arthroscopy as a standard of surgical TMJ therapy. They not only demonstrated its ability to be an additional diagnostic tool but also presented its therapeutic future with the lysis of adhesions and treatment of disc displacements without reduction.

INSTRUMENTATION

The arthroscope is a relatively simple device. Its terminal end contains a magnifying lens that can be angled to allow expanded viewing (i.e., 0°, 5°, 15°, 30°). The proximal end of the arthroscope conforms the ocular apparatus, which is coupled to the television camera. Also at this end is the attachment for the fiberoptic light source. This all connects to the arthroscope, which is made up of a rod lens system, also known as the Hopkins rod. This is passed through a slightly larger cannula (the outer sheath), which allows for the ingress and egris of suction and irrigant to insufflate and evacuate the joint of debris. Irrigant can be normal saline or usually lactated Ringer's solution, which has a less variable physiologic pH. An exit port and various surgical ports can be established with a small-gauge needle and/or trochars (Fig. 8-2) to introduce additional cannulas through which specially designed arthroscopic surgical instruments are placed. These can include various laser probes, motorized shavers, forceps, probes, cutting instruments, rasps, files, and biopsy punches and needles.

INDICATIONS FOR ARTHROSCOPY

There are many specific indications for arthroscopy of the TMJ. Indications for diagnostic arthroscopy include those joint conditions that warrant direct examinations to confirm the presence of clinically suspected disease states that cannot be confirmed by other means of evaluation and imaging. Also, when confirmation of the disease will affect the patients' care and direct examination of the joint will enhance an established diagnosis for making treatment decisions, then arthroscopy is indicated. This can include synovial fluid assays with biochemical analysis, visualization, and histopathologic sampling of suspected lesions or disease states. Unexplained persistent TMJ pain unresponsive to nonsurgical modalities including physical therapy, anti-inflammatory and muscle relaxant therapy, and splint therapy is a good indication for diagnostic TMJ arthroscopy. In addition, arthroscopy is indicated if the patient has a suspected perforation but is allergic to radiopaque dye with an arthrogram.

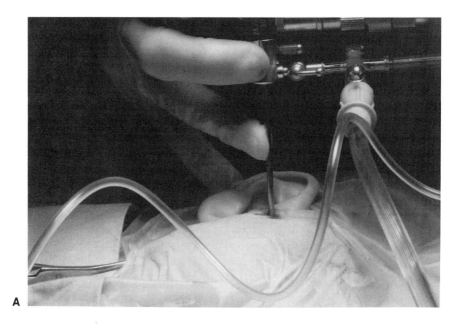

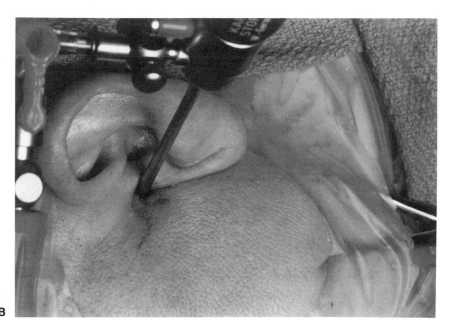

Fig. 8-2. (A)   Right TMJ arthroscopic puncture site. **(B)** Left TMJ arthroscopic puncture site (one port). Towel clamp at angle of mandible.

Specific indications for operative arthroscopy include

1. Acute disc displacement without reduction or frequent intermittent locking (Fig. 8-3)
2. Hypomobility secondary to adhesions in the superior joint space
3. Disc displacement with small perforation of the retrodiscal tissue or disc, provided that the condyle will not catch in the perforation with normal condylar translation
4. Unexplained pain refractory to nonsurgical modalities such as (Figs. 8-4 and 8-5)
    (a) Disc displacement with reduction
    (b) Capsulitis
    (c) Degenerative joint disease
5. Hypermobility, resulting in painful subluxation or dislocation. This can be treated with electrocautery, laser, and chemical sclerosing techniques, which at this time have very positive short-term results

An operative arthroscopy procedure is indicated for selected joint conditions listed above that constitute a disability for the patient, are refractory to dental/medical treatment, and may require internal structural modification.

Indications for an open joint surgery to the TMJ are large meniscal or retrodiscal perforations that are too severe for arthroscopic correction. Other indications for TMJ arthrotomy include fibrous and bony ankylosis, where space for introduction of an arthroscope is not possible. Removal of large tumor masses or alloplastic materials are other indications for open joint surgery. In my experience, a clicking or popping joint is not an indication for surgical therapy (including arthroscopy or arthrotomy techniques) unless it is painful and unresponsive to nonsurgical modalities.

CONTRAINDICATIONS

Contraindications to arthroscopy include skin infection, possible tumor seeding, septic arthritis, certain physiologic disorders rendering the patient a poor surgical candidate, a medically compromised patient (such as one with bleeding disorders) in whom surgery or anesthesia would be deleterious to the patient's health and welfare, and facial pain without a functional intracapsular component (e.g., myofascial pain).

ADVANTAGES

Clinical success is technique-sensitive and requires clinical experience and optimal operative expertise from adequate training and practice. Given such experience and expertise, the advantages for TMJ arthroscopy are

1. High success rate (93 to 98 percent) reported by multiple specialists nationally

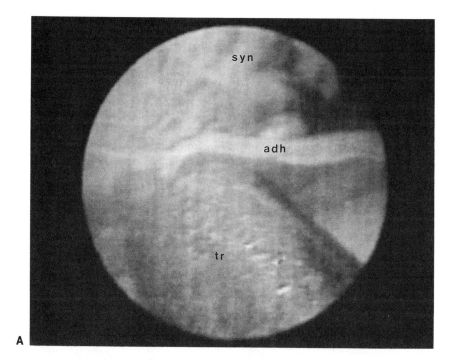

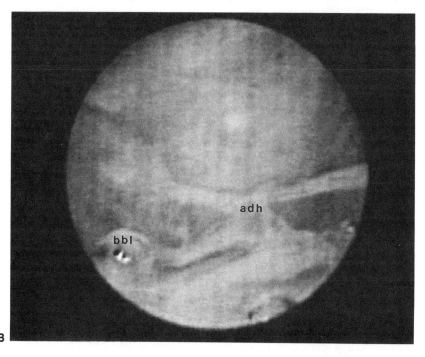

Fig. 8-3. **(A)** Posterior view of right disc displacement with reduction with moderate synovitis and capsulitis, and adhesions. **(B)** Posterior view of right disc displacement without reduction with moderate synovitis and capsulitis, and adhesions (glenoid fossa to retrodiscal tissue and air bubble). adh, adhesion; bbl, air bubble; p, posterior ; syn, synovial ; tr, trocar.

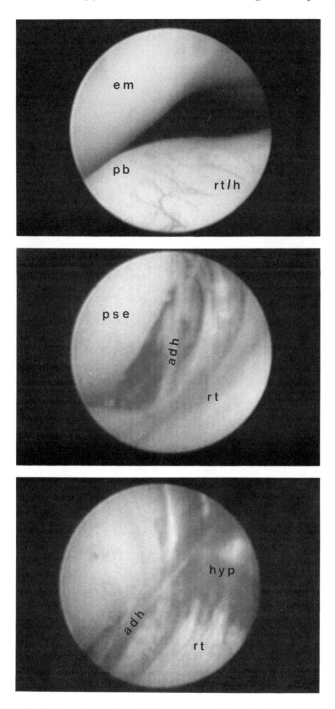

Fig. 8-4. Left TMJ showing a disc displacement with reduction, adhesions, and hyperemia. Views are anterior to posterior going from top to bottom. adh, adhesion; em, eminence; hyp, hyperemia; pb, posterior band; pse, posterior slope eminence; rt, retrodiscal tissue; rt/h, retrodiscal tissue with hyperemia.

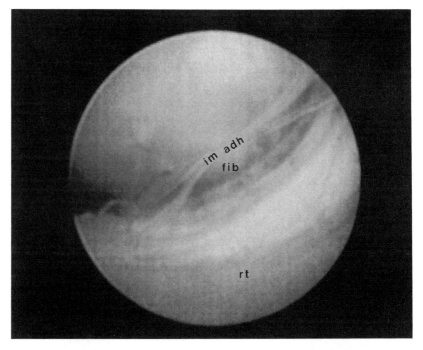

Fig. 8-5. Left disc displacement with reduction, immature adhesions, and fibrillation. im adh, immature adhesion; fib, fibrillation; rt, retrodiscal tissue.

2. Less potential formation of adverse scar tissue (smaller incision)

3. Less repeat TMJ surgery required

4. Less morbidity compared with open joint surgery. TMJ surgical results have been most successful at the first and earliest attempts, as opposed to repeat surgeries on the same TMJ. The success rate is significantly lower (50 percent) for repeat surgery performed with open joint techniques than with arthroscopic techniques

5. Quicker return to normal ROM diet, and mandibular function

6. Less postoperative pain and swelling

7. Less postoperative complications such as temporary and/or permanent hearing changes, sensory and motor nerve deficits of the trigeminal and facial nerves, and occlusal changes such as posterior open bites

8. Various diagnostic procedures may be performed, such as the ability to examine the superior joint space with magnification and to take specific tissue biopsies as necessary

For the reasons stated above, TMJ arthroscopy, in my practice, is the surgical modality of choice for most internal derangements.

PREOPERATIVE EVALUATION AND MANAGEMENT

As noted previously, arthroscopy is a conservative modality for effective surgical treatment of the TMJ. It is specific for treatment of TMJ internal derangement usually manifesting as painful mechanical symptoms. Intracapsular therapy has an indirect effect on myofascial pain resolution by allowing for return to normal functional mechanics of the TMJ (even with a continuation of an internal derangement) and masticatory apparatus (muscle, tendons, fascia, synovium, collagen, etc.) to hasten improvement of myofascial symptoms.

Facial and TMJ pain can commonly be categorized in one or more of the following diagnoses:

1. Masticatory muscle disorders related to
    (a) Stress
    (b) Parafunctional activities
    (c) Internal derangement
    (d) "b" in response to a symptomatic cervical spine disorder
2. Internal derangement of the TMJs
    (a) Disc incoordination
    (b) Disc displacement with reduction
    (c) Disc displacement without reduction
    (d) Disc perforation
3. Degenerative joint disease of the TMJs
4. Hypermobility (subluxation) of the TMJs

The diagnosis can usually be made based on a thorough and complete history and clinical examination supplemented with radiographic or other imaging studies of the TMJ area. The most useful radiograph is a panoramic radiograph, which can serve as a "scout" film to recognize arthritic and sclerotic changes in the condyle, eminence, and fossa. It also allows for observation of the joint space to determine if it is adequate for introduction of the arthroscope and outer cannula into the superior joint. A tomogram can be ordered if severe degenerative changes or tumors are noted on the panorex. Magnetic resonance imaging (MRI) of the TMJ has gained acceptance in the past few years because of the wealth of information obtained for both the hard and soft tissues with a noninvasive technique.

TMJ arthrography is very useful preoperatively with arthroscopy. Dynamic movement, translation, and rotation can be documented as well as hard tissue pathology. By far the most important information obtained with an arthrogram is the disc position in relation to the condylar head and the presence or absence of a perforation in the disc or retrodiscal tissue. This will help organize the surgical treatment plan, allowing definitive patient consent and surgical options to be decided before operating.

The common and most effective forms of nonsurgical therapy, which are almost always used before arthroscopy, include dental occlusal splints, behavior modification (including diet, parafunctional habit identification, and general rest and relaxation), nonsteroidal anti-inflammatory drugs (NSAIDs) and muscle relaxation or nocturnal antianxiety medications, and physical therapy including modalities and procedures such as heat, cold, ultrasound, massage, iontophoresis, phonophoresis, and various forms of electrical stimulation. Active and passive ROM to the jaw and cervical spine and muscle strengthening/ stretching summarize various procedures that can also be used.

Physical therapy is frequently used to increase jaw opening that is less than functional. To simply increase jaw opening without any consideration of disc position usually is deleterious in most cases. However, with proper knowledge of active and passive exercises and a well-informed patient, physical therapy may, in some cases, increase jaw opening with an existing disc displacement (see Ch. 7). Success of physical therapy is often dependent on the degree of masticatory muscle hyperactivity and or capsulitis/synovitis that is present. If pain and limitation of function persists after good compliance with the above nonsurgical modalities, then arthroscopy is indicated.

In summary, accurate and complete diagnosis of the TMJ must be obtained by history and physical examination and radiograph by an oral and maxillofacial surgeon, general dentist, and/or physician. Once that has been completed, then multidisplinary therapy for this multifactorial disorder can be initiated. Evaluation and treatment by a physical therapist experienced in TMJ and facial pain is very important in corroborating the findings of the dentist or surgeon. This preoperative assessment and initiation of physical therapy increases the patient's response to surgical modalities, allowing for postoperative continuity, so important in the first 6 to 8 weeks after TMJ arthroscopy.

SURGICAL TECHNIQUE

TMJ arthroscopic surgery has been reported to have been performed under local anesthetic and intravenous sedation techniques, but by far the most common and effective setting is in the operating room under general anesthesia. Not only are sterile techniques used to reduce the incidence of infections, but general anesthesia enables a more complete surgical procedure. It allows for use of nondeplorizing skeletal muscle relaxation to provide better access to the superior joint space. If the masticatory muscles are relaxed, then focus on the anatomic and mechanical disorders of the TMJ can be much more effective. Manipulation of the mandible under general anesthesia is beneficial to the arthroscopic surgical outcome. Also of importance is the ability to have the patient motionless because of the close proximity of many vital structures such as the inner ear, external auditory meatus and tympanic membrane auxiliary artery, facial nerve, spinal dura, superficial temporal artery, and vein.

A 2-mm vertical skin incision is created over the lateral posterosuperior aspect of the condyle through the skin and subcutaneous tissues after marking the surgical incision with an indelible marker. Next, using straight hemostat and blunt trocar, dissection is performed bluntly down to the lateral capsule.

This is followed with a sharp trocar and arthroscopic sleeve. Once penetration into the superior joint space is accomplished, epinephrine solution 1/200,000 is delivered into the superior joint space for the purpose of providing hemostasis and insufflation. Next, the arthroscope (2.4 mm) is then placed into the TMJ. Warm lactated Ringer's solution is used for insufflation and for irrigation of the joint to allow for examination and arthrocentesis of the superior joint space. Longitudinal, transverse, and dynamic study of the TMJ can be accomplished.

Various surgical techniques using additional ports and the principles of triangulation are sometimes required for definitive surgical correction of the joint disorder. This can include rotary shavers, biopsy forceps, probes and trocars for positioning, tissue sampling, and débridement.

Currently, the holmium: yttrium–aluminum–garnet (YAG) laser is being used for sclerosis, ablation and débridement, tissue "welding," hemostasis, and very specific and controlled surgical dissections. Early reports on the use of the holmium:YAG laser in the TMJ are very favorable. Sclerosing agents for hypermobility have been reported to be effective when injecting into the oblique protuberance using arthroscopic guidance.

Multiple reports using lysis and lavage techniques in the superior joint space confirm the efficiency of this arthroscopic arthrocentesis. At the present time, this is still the standard of care for most TMJ internal derangements requiring arthroscopic surgery. Lysis can be accomplished with a wide variety of arthroscopic techniques, directly or indirectly. Use of probes, lasers, motorized shavers, cutting scissors, and knifes to release (lyse) tissues in the joint has been reported. Lysis usually describes releasing tissues that are pathologic or in a pathologic relationship. Any of the above techniques can be used for lysis but are not always necessary. Instrumentation is dependent on the underlying diagnosis.

Lavage is standardized arthroscopic techniques may use irrigation administered through one or more ports. Reusing of the joint space can be accomplished continuously throughout the procedure under gentle pressure and usually with copious amounts to remove products of inflammation and debris. Once completed, the excess irrigant and debris are removed from the joint space, using suction and pressure. The incision is closed with 6-0 nylon suture in the primary incision and in the secondary incisions. The wound is then dressed with Neosporin ointment, a pressure dressing, and sterile dressing. The pressure dressing is placed for the purposes of preventing excess postoperative edema.

The TMJ encompasses two joint spaces: the lower joint space, also known as the rotational joint space, and the superior joint space, which is the translation joint space responsible for most TMDs. The superior and inferior joint spaces can be entered through the same arthroscopic port in cases with a large disc or retrodiscal perforation. At the present time, diagnostic information can be visualized with inferior joint space arthroscopy, but because of the small size and also rotational function of this space, there is minimal therapeutic benefit to de novo examination of the inferior joint space. Kondoh and Westesson[2] arrived at the same conclusions, as their study reported in 1991.

Currently, smaller instrumentation is being developed to accomplish specific surgical techniques. Yet, the trend today is to use slightly larger (2.7 mm) arthroscopes for greater depth of field and greater panoramic visualization.

Posterior positioning and suturing of the disc is feasible using arthroscopic-guided procedures. Shaving of the synovial lining, glenoid fossa, and meniscal irregularities and removal of fibrillation of the soft tissues, as well as anterior band or lateral pterygoid muscle release, are possible using arthroscopic techniques. Surgical arthroscopic techniques are being reported more frequently. Short-term results appear to be positive and hold promise for more research and data, but at the present time, it's too early to report on long-term stability and significance of these procedures.

COMPLICATIONS

Several reported and potential complications are possible with TMJ arthroscopic surgery. Because of the relatively blind puncture technique before visualization with the arthroscope, complications have been reported. The more experience a surgeon has with the arthroscopic technique, the fewer complications usually occur. Proper location, orientation, and angulation of the instruments must always be the foremost consideration.

Complications of TMJ arthroscopic surgery include the following:

1. Middle ear injury and perforation of the external auditory meatus. Van Sickles et al.[10] reported a case in 1987 of tympanic membrane perforation and ossicle disruption that led to a temporary hearing change
2. Infection and/or persistent drainage
3. Hemorrhage from the superficial temporal vessels, the internal maxillary artery, and the middle meningeal artery
4. Parotid gland injury
5. Perforation of the middle cranial fossa and dura exposure
6. Facial nerve injury, usually transient
7. Trigeminal nerve injury affecting the inferior alveolar, lingual, and/or auriculotemporal nerves
8. Iatrogenic injury to the articular surfaces and meniscal perforation
9. Instrument fracture, because of the small size required for instrumentation of the TMJ
10. Delayed or hypertrophic wound healing
11. Gustatory sweating

NOMENCLATURE OF NORMAL AND PATHOLOGIC ARTHROSCOPIC ANATOMY WITH SUPERIOR JOINT SPACE

Anatomic descriptions are important to both establish reference points when looking through an arthroscopic window and characterize those tissues that are visualized (Fig. 8-1A and B).

Bony landmarks, which are not mobile, are used for orientation. For example, the glenoid fossa can be spatially divided into the pre-eminence, anterior glenoid, and posterior glenoid regions. Also, the eminence serves as a landmark to document disc displacement.

The meniscus and attaching tissues have been described with many terms. These include anterior recess or pouch, disc, intermediate or thin zone, posterior band with a posterior and anterior incline retrodiscal tissue, medial and lateral sulcus, synovial tissue plica (medial), synovial villi (posterior), flexure (V-shaped), or the posterior pouch.

The soft tissue descriptions characterize the disc shape, color, orientation, joint space, and the relationships to topographic landmarks. Also, vascularity can be noted as the superficial surface vessels will fill on closure and empty on opening translation.

Pathologic anatomy is used to describe the location, character, and quantity of abnormal tissues. This can include bony changes such as chondromalacia and eburnation. Osseous remodeling soft tissue changes have also been given many names. Remodeled retrodiscal tissue shows degrees of fibrosis. Adhesions usually are secondary to trauma etiology. Hemorrhage produces lysozyme elucidation leading to fibrosis. Synechiae or immature cobweb-like adhesions are usually pathognomonic for chronic joint immobility. Disc displacement can be based on the posterior band relationship to the condyle and eminence. Synovitis, hyperemia, capsulitis, and vascularity (or vascular markings) anterior to the flexure are pathologic signs of acute or chronic inflammatory changes. Also, fat or loose bodies have been described in the synovial fluid, even though this is rare. Capsular fibrosis is a descriptive term used to quantify the resistance to lateral capsule puncture with the arthroscopic instruments. Iatrogenic trauma can include tearing of the synovial tissue (crabmeat, scuffing) and of the retrodiscal tissue. Perforation of the medial capsule from the puncture sometimes is noted. Perforations of the menicus and retrodiscal tissue demonstrate a severe joint pathology. The character of the perforation edges, whether thickened or inflamed, for example, can give an indication in establishing acute or chronic pathology.

POSTOPERATIVE MANAGEMENT

The first 6 weeks after arthroscopic surgery are critical for the proper healing and return to normal function of the TMJ. Close monitoring of the patient is essential to maximize the surgical goals, resulting in less relapse potential. The patient is encouraged to resume a regular diet beginning the day of surgery. This serves to maintain ROM obtained intraoperatively, which decreases the potential for adhesion formation. Also, gradual strengthening and lengthening of the muscles of mastication is required for a return to normal function. A regular diet (with the exception of gum chewing) is the most important postoperative exercise toward a successful result. The patients have usually been on a soft restricted diet for the preoperative period for months, or possibly, years.

If the dental splint is needed for clenching-bruxing habits, it can be used on an as-needed basis but is not usually required postoperatively.

Cold compresses are beneficial to the sides of the face during the first 3 postoperative days to help reduce postoperative edema. Intravenous steroids are used preoperatively to aid in reduction of postoperative edema. Intracapsular steroids are used by many other practitioners but also are not required during arthroscopic surgery. A return to warm compress is recommended after the third day for resolution of the edema and muscle relaxation. Prophylactic antibiotics and keeping the wound dry during the first week help prevent postoperative infection. Most patients have very minimal discomfort and will take a nonsteroidal analgesic on an as-needed basis.

During the second to fourth postoperative week, if the patient's ROM is not gradually increasing, the reason needs to be aggressively pursued. This complication can be caused by lack of patient motivation or compliance, misunderstanding, discomfort, and/or muscle fibrosis. Physical therapy is very instrumental at this time. This can include supportive measures, such as massage, deep heat or ultrasound, and active stretching exercises. Also benefiting the physical therapist can be the use of tongue blade exercises or Therabite (Therabite Corp., Bryn Mawr, Pennsylvania) use. At the 6 to 8-week postoperative period, most of the wound healing is complete, and the patient's ROM and symptomatology are a guideline for long-term stability.

The patient's expectations after TMJ arthroscopy are dependent on the specific diagnosis. In general, the patient may expect a return to all activities involving the function of the jaw with little or no pain. The disc is rarely "recaptured," and joint noises are sometimes present for a time in the postoperative plan and gradually diminish as remodeling progresses.

FUTURE TRENDS

Future trends in TMJ arthroscopy no doubt will incorporate the basics of lysis, lavage, and débridement. The holmium: YAG laser has some very distinct advantages for small joint arthroscopy. Initial reports show very good results using the laser for specific surgical techniques. In the past decade, research and clinical experience with TMJ arthroscopy has evolutionized the theoretic and practical management of TMDs. Not only has arthroscopic examination of the TMJ proved to be a useful adjunct to history taking, clinical examination and imaging studies in the diagnosis of TMJ pathology, but TMJ arthroscopy is recognized as an acceptable and effective treatment modality for certain types of TMJ pathology.

An example of the impact that arthroscopy and MRI studies have had on the management of TMJ disorders is the concept of disc "recapturing" with surgical plication and anterior repositioning splints. MRI studies before and after open joint surgery demonstrate that the posterior band of the disc remains anterior to the condylar head postsurgically, even though the patient has significant improvement of painful symptoms. Arthroscopic lysis, lavage, débridement product a very significant improvement of function and reduction of pain, even though the disc remains displaced.

Many theories are presently being researched to explain why patients have such a dramatically positive result with arthroscopic surgery, even though the disc position is not posteriorly positioned.

Attempts to reposition the disc posteriorly ("recapture") will continue to be researched and reported, but successful arthroscopic therapy has led to questioning of the need to recapture the anteriorly displaced disc. Normal, pain-free, long-term, stable ROM and function can be accomplished without necessarily surgically "recapturing" the disc. Future techniques that are efficacious and predictable could show that "recapturing" of the disc might be a good alternative, but at the present time, lysis, lavage, and débridement represent the standard of care because of minimal morbidity, long-term stability, and very high success rate.

Lavage of the products of inflammation and mediators of pain in the synovial fluid and lining have been researched by Quinn and Bazan.[11] They have shown with bioassays that prostaglandins, leukotrienes, and bradykinins (LTB_4, PGE_2) are present in the synovial fluid of inflamed TMJs, providing objective data to confirm that the TMJ is a source of the patient's pain.

Arthrocentesis in a clinical setting under sedation has been reported with minimal long-term success. This is usually a "blind" procedure but can be directed with arthrographic techniques. It has been used for palliation of acute, emergency-type arthralgia. Arthrocentesis during arthroscopic surgery has a higher success rate because visualization of the underlying pathology and irrigation of the affected tissues and spaces can be accomplished directly. Also the quantity of lavage irrigant can be copious without patient discomfort and splinting.

Dilation of the lateral capsule is proposed by the author to have an advantageous effect on the lateral capsular fibrosis, much the same as open joint dissection has on the lateral capsule of the TMJ. A dilation or stretching of the lateral capsule, intraoperatively, followed by aggressive postoperative physical therapy techniques to maintain the re-established ROM during the initial soft tissue wound healing, is beneficial to long-term stability and therefore decreased relapse potential of the arthroscopically operated TMJ.

Whatever avenue arthroscopic takes in the future, the most important criteria for the postoperative success is patient screening and selection. Specific intracapsular disorders are managed very effectively with arthroscopic surgery. Extracapsular disorders (masticatory muscle disorders) are only indirectly affected by intracapsular surgery and, therefore, will have a predictable lower success rate.

CONCLUSION

Successful TMJ arthroscopic surgical intervention can be defined as the return to normal, pain-free function. This can be accomplished if accurate diagnostic and proper preoperative management is completed. The postoperative period is critical for optimal results of the surgery. Successful, conservative arthroscopic surgical intervention is dependent on thorough pre- and postoperative management.

ACKNOWLEDGMENTS

I thank Marilyn Barry, Pat Herndon, and Sharon Atkinson, medical librarians at Dekalb Medical Center Library, and Jean Lewis for their kind assistance in preparing this chapter.

REFERENCES

1. American Association of Oral and Maxillofacial Surgeons Position Paper on TMJ, August 1988
2. Kondoh T, Westesson PL: Diagnostic accuracy of temporomandibular joint lower compartment arthroscopy using an ultrathin arthroscope: a postmortem study. J Oral Maxillofac Surg 49:619, 1991
3. McCain JP, Sanders B, Koslin MG et al: Temporomandibular joint arthroscopy: a 6-year multicenter retrospective study of 4,831 joints. J Oral Maxillofac Surg 50: 926, 1992
4. Mosby EL: Efficacy of TMJ arthroscopy: a retrospective study. J Oral Maxillofac Surg 51:17, 1993
5. Blaustein D, Heffez L: Arthroscopic Atlas of the Temporomandibular Joint. Lea & Febiger, Philadelphia, 1990
6. Ohnishi M; Arthroscopy of the temporomandibular joint. J Stomatol Soc Jpn 42: 202, 1975
7. Ohnishi M: Clinical application of arthroscopy in the temporomandibular joint diseases. Bull Tokyo Med Dent Univ 27:141, 1980
8. Hilsabeck R, Laskin D: Arthroscopy of the temporomandibular joint of the rabbit. J Oral Surg 36:938, 1978
9. Williams RA, Laskin DM: Arthroscopic examination of experimentally induced pathologic conditions of the rabbit temporomandibular joint. J Oral Surg 38:652, 1980
10. Van Sickles JE, Nishioka GJ, Hegewald M, Neal G: Middle ear injury resulting from temporomandibular joint arthroscopy. J Oral Maxillofac Surg 45:962, 1987
11. Quinn JH, Bazan NG: Identification of prostaglandin E_2 leukotriene B_4 in the synovial fluid of painful, dysfunctional TMJ. J Oral Maxillofac Surg 48:968, 1990

SUGGESTED READING

AAOMS 1984 Criteria Statement for TMJ Mensicus Surgery
Blaustein D, Heffez L: Diagnostic arthroscopy of the temporomandibular joint, part II: arthroscopic findings of arthrographically diagnosed disk displacements. Oral Surg Oral Med Oral Pathol 65:135, 1988
Buckley MJ, Merrill RG, Braun TW: Surgical management of internal derangement of the temporomandibular joint. J Oral Maxillofac Surg 51:20, 1993

Clark GT, Moody DG, Sanders B: Arthroscopic treatment of temporomandibular joint locking resulting from disc derangement: two year results. J Oral Maxillofac Surg 49:157, 1991

Dolwick M: 1984 Criteria for TMJ Meniscus Surgery. American Association of Oral and Maxillofacial Surgeons, November 1984

Esposito C, Clear M, Veal SJ: Arthroscopic surgical treatment of temporomandibular joint hypermobility with recurrent anterior disclocation: an alternative to open surgery. J Craniomandib Pract 9:286, 1991

Heffez L, Blaustein D: Diagnostic arthroscopy of the temporomandibular joint, part I: normal arthroscopic findings. Oral Surg Oral Med Oral Pathol 64:653, 1987

Hellsing G, Holmlund A, Nordenram A et al: Arthroscopy of the temporomandibular joint. Examination of 2 patients with suspected disk derangement. Int J Oral Surg 13:69, 1984

Holmlund A, Hellsing G, Wredmark T: Arthroscopy of the temporomandibular joint: a clinical study. Int J Oral Maxillofac Surg 15:715, 1986

McCain JP: Arthroscopy of the human temporomandibular joint. J Oral Maxillofac Surg 46:648, 1988

McCain JP, de la Rua H, LeBlanc WG: Correlation of clinical, radiographic and arthroscopic findings in internal derangements of the TMJ. J Oral Maxillofac Surg 47: 913, 1989

Merill RG, Yei WY, Langan MJ: A histologic evaluation of the accuracy of TMJ diagnostic arthroscopy. Oral Surg Oral Med Oral Pathol 70:393, 1990

Montgomery MT, Van Sickels JE, Harms SE, Thrash WJ: Arthroscopic TMJ surgery: effects on signs, symptoms, and disc position. J Oral Maxillofac Surg 47:1263, 1989

Moses JJ, Sartoris D, Glass R et al: The effect of arthroscopic surgical lysis and lavage of the superior joint space on TMJ disc position and mobility. J Oral Maxillofac Surg 47:674, 1989

Moses JJ, Topper DC: A functional approach to the treatment of temporomandibular joint internal derangement. J Craniomandib Disord Facial Oral Pain 5:19, 1991

Murakami K, Hoshini K: Regional anatomical nomenclature and arthroscopic terminology in human temporomandibular joints. Okamimal Folia Anat Jpn 58:745, 1982

Murakami K, Matsuki M, Lizuka T, Ono T: Diagnostic arthroscopy of the TMJ: differential diagnosis in patients with limited jaw opening. J Craniomandib Pract 4:117, 1986

Nitzan DW, Dolwick MF: An alternative explanation for the genesis of closed-lock symptoms in the internal derangement process. J Oral Maxillofac Surg 49:810, 1991

Nitzan DW, Dolwick MF, Heft MW: Arthroscopic lavage and lysis of the temporomandibular joint: a change in perspective. J Oral Maxillofac Surg 48:798, 1990

Nitzan DW, Dolwick MF, Martinez GA: Temporomandibular joint arthrocentesis: a simplified treatment for severe, limited mouth opening. J Oral Maxillofac Surg 49: 1163, 1991

Parrott DH, Alborzi A, Kaban LB, Helms CA: A prospective evaluation of the effectiveness of temporomandibular joint arthroscopy. J Oral Maxillofac Surg 48:1029, 1990

Sanders B: Arthroscopic surgery of the TMJ: treatment of internal derangement with persistent closed lock. Oral Surg Oral Med Oral Pathol 62:361, 1986

Sanders B, Buoncristiani R: Diagnostic and surgical arthroscopy of the temporomandibular joint: clinical experience with 137 procedures over a two year period. J Craniomandib Pract 1:202, 1987

Tarro AW: TMJ arthroscopic diagnosis and surgery: clinical experience with 152 procedures over a $2\frac{1}{2}$ year period. J Craniomandib Pract 9:107, 1991

Westesson PL, Cohen JM, Tallents RH: Magnetic resonance imaging of temporomandibular joint after surgical treatment of internal derangement. Oral Surg Oral Med Oral Pathol 71:407, 1991

Westesson PL, Eriksson L, Liedberg J: The risk of damage to facial nerve, superficial temporal vessels, disk, and articular surfaces during arthroscopic examination of the TMJ. Oral Surg Oral Med Oral Pathol 62:124, 1986

9 | Arthrotomy and Orthognathic Surgery for TMD

Robert A. Bays

ARTHROTOMY

History

Open joint surgery, arthrotomy, of the TMJ has been described for more than a century.[1] The practice of arthrotomy has waxed and waned over this period, even up to the present. In the 1950s, discectomy and condylotomy were popular in Europe and England. Early advocates of discectomy later denounced the procedure as too destructive and fraught with complications.[2-4] The revival of arthrotomy in modern U.S. history was led by Henny,[5] who performed TMJ surgery throughout the 1950s and 1960s. Generally, few surgeons in the United States treated TMD surgically until the late 1970s. McCarty and Farra[6] initiated the most recent interest in the surgical management of TMD by popularizing the concept of internal derangement and its surgical correction by disc plication. Apparently, because many surgeons were unable to achieve success with this procedure or in cases where, in the surgeon's opinion, discs were unrepairable, a plethora of variations began to emerge. Procedures such as eminectomies,[7] condylar shaving,[8] discectomy,[9] condylotomy,[10] and a variety of disc replacements[11-16] have been advocated. Unfortunately, functionally untested alloplastic materials gained popularity.[11,15] Various forms of silicone were used, as well as the very destructive Proplast-Teflon laminate. As a result of many failed surgeries and the growing evidence of the destructiveness of the allo-plasts, autogenous materials were favored. The most common of these include ear cartilage,[14] dermis,[16] and fascia.[12] Techniques for disc repair or replacement

237

with vascularized pedicle flaps have been used.[17,18] As history repeats itself, discectomy without replacement[19] and condylotomy[20] are being recycled. Whether these procedures will prove to be more successful than plication with disc repair is not known, but all are considerably more invasive. Obviously, wide disagreement exists among surgeons regarding the most efficacious method for correcting internal derangement.

Indications

To be considered for surgery, the patient should meet the following criteria:

1. Pain in the TMJ, especially when associated with a function (i.e., chewing, opening, talking, yawning). Absence of pain is almost always a contraindication to surgery except where severe limitation of opening exists.

2. Evidence of a disc displacement such as decreased opening and reciprocal clicking, or the history of either. This is very important because pain in the TMJ can exist even though the disc–condyle relationship is normal. Myofascial pain stemming from the muscles of mastication or referred pain from the cervical spine is a frequent cause of such pain. The exact mechanism is not fully understood, but various joint noises may occur as a result of masticatory muscle disorders (MMD) without the existence of a true disc displacement. Considerable clinical experience and skill are required to determine disc displacement in patients with concomitant MMD.

Even these two indications for arthrotomy are subject to qualification. The pain in the joint must be of a nature that is conducive to surgical management. No strict litmus tests exist to differentiate those TMJ pains that will respond to surgery from those that will not. Because the exact cause for pain in the joint is not understood, treatment schemes are essentially educated guesses. Indications for arthrotomy will vary dramatically among surgeons, as well as the differences in technique once the need for surgery is established.

Alloplastic implant materials previously placed in the joint may represent a new absolute indication for arthrotomy, even in the absence of pain. This topic will be addressed in more detail.

Surgical procedures are performed on the TMJ to relocate and/or repair displaced or perforated discs, to correct bony aberrations in the joints, to overcome bony or fibrous ankylosis, and, occasionally, to reduce fracture displacements of the entire condyle. These various problems are discussed separately.

Internal Derangement of the TMJ Discs

The most common surgical problem of the TMJ is a derangement of the disc. This may take many forms and is often oversimplified. Disc derangement is considered a surgical problem only when stringent criteria are met. Signs and symptoms of disc derangement have been discussed in other chapters and are not reiterated here.

My clinical experience leads me to believe that disc plication surgery is indicated in cases of documented disc displacement with or without reduction when quality nonsurgical therapy has failed and if, in the clinical judgment of the treating team, the primary source of pain is from the joint and not elsewhere. This is a crucial point because pain frequently is elicited from sources other than the joint. Surgery will probably not alleviate pain from these other sources. Physical therapy, splint therapy, and other nonsurgical therapies not only assist in pain management of these patients, but often give diagnostic insight into the value of disc plication surgery.

Controversy exists about whether disc position is important. Clearly, in many people it is not. Many pain-free individuals have a disc displacement for years without any other problems. Also, there are several treatments that do not attempt to reposition discs but often give relief of pain, such as splint therapy, arthroscopy, arthrocentesis (joint lavage), physical therapy, stress management, and a variety of medical regimens. The success of such a variety of therapies simply underscores the multifactorial nature of TMD. Although some would claim that even disc plication surgery does not relocate the disc,[21] others have found a close correlation between postoperative disc position and pain relief.[22] Therefore, clinical experience and operator preference dictate therapy. In my experience, disc plication surgery successfully reduces pain and disc position in patients with a painful disc displacement with or without reduction.

Disc Displacement With Reduction

Probably the most widely agreed on indication for arthrotomy is a painful disc displacement with reduction that has not responded to nonsurgical management such as splint therapy, physical therapy, or medical treatments. These patients typically will give a history of reciprocal clicking with pain. Reciprocal clicking of the TMJ is found in up to 40 percent of the population; only 2 to 3 percent of these displacements are painful.[23] Many of these may reasonably be assumed to represent nonpainful disc displacements. With this is in mind, one must be careful about overtreating painful disc displacement.

Occasional locking (disc displacement without reduction) may occur. If the reciprocal clicking and locking is treated with an anterior repositioning splint the disc often reduces and the pain and clicking will often disappear. Usually, after a few months of anterior repositioning, these patients are returned to a centric position of the mandible by splint therapy. Frequently, they remain comfortable and no further treatment is needed; however, if painful clicking or locking returns, arthrotomy with disc plication will generally ensure a very high probability of success.[24,25] The key here is that the clicking is associated with pain and the pain is localized to the joint. Furthermore, if reducing the disc with splints eliminates the pain, this is additional evidence that disc repositioning surgery will be successful.

If a disc–condyle derangement causes clicking but is not painful, does not limit function, and is not bothersome to the patient, I believe that the physical therapist and physician should make the patient aware of but not alarmed about the condition. If the clinician(s) is treating the patient for cervical or headache pains, it would be most appropriate to monitor the patient and re-evaluate the TMJ. If the clicking becomes painful or changes in nature, referral of the patient to an appropriate dentist/oral surgeon is in order.

Disc Displacement Without Reduction

Typically, these patients have a history of clicking and reciprocal clicking that has proceeded to locking. A significant decrease in range of motion (ROM) accompanies this locking in the early stages, but, with time, maximum inter-incisional opening (MIO) will usually increase almost back to normal. This condition may not include pain, or it may initially involve pain that resolves with or without treatment. Whether to treat a nonpainful displaced disc with or without reduction is always a difficult clinical judgment and must be made on the basis of other procedures contemplated in the patient's overall care. A dilemma emerges because many of these patients will improve without treatment or with nonsurgical treatments such as those mentioned above. However, in those that worsen or fail to improve, disc plication surgery is more likely to be successful the sooner it is performed in the displacement process. It is fairly well agreed that in many cases, if left untreated, disc displacement will lead to degenerative changes in the joint. Some of these will not result in pain or dysfunction, but some will. No one knows the formula to predict the prognosis of an individual case when seen in the early stages. The success rate for total relief of pain in these patients is less than in patients with reducing discs but can be quite good if the diagnosis is accurate. The essential ingredient is always an accurate diagnosis.

Alternatives to disc plication include partial or total discectomy with grafts or without replacement. The degree of disc deformation and health of the intracapsular disc attachments dictate the feasibility of plication (see Disc Perforation and Degeneration). Arthroscopy is also often recommended for displacement without reduction; however, it is not clear whether this offers any advantages over arthrocentesis with lavage.

A physical therapist whose patient has an anteriorly displaced disc that cannot be reduced may be asked to allow the disc to remain anteriorly displaced without any further attempts at relocation. This greatly depends on whether the patient has pain or limitation of function or is in some other way inhibited by the displacement. It is also heavily influenced by any future treatment to the occlusion that may be contemplated by the patient, especially orthodontic, major dental restoration, or orthognathic repositioning of the jaws for esthetic or functional purposes. All these treatments have a profound influence on the occlusion. Even if treatment by such means is anticipated, the therapist and/or patient may decide not to attempt surgical relocation of the discs if patient complaints are minimal. The patient must be made fully aware of the condition, however, and must also be warned that pain or increase in dysfunction may result from major changes in occlusion.

Disc Displacement and MMD

Once the patient has been determined to have a disc displacement that is painful and cannot be corrected without surgery, an assessment is made of the muscles of mastication as a contributing factor. Many patients with disc displacements have a large amount of both MMD and cervical spine muscle disorders either secondary to or preceding disc displacement. The sequence of symptoms is important to ascertain. If MMD is secondary to disc displacement, it is reasonable to assume that correction of the disc position, proper occlusal management of jaw position, and physical therapy to the cervical spine and jaw, as indicated, should lead postoperatively to a great reduction or elimination of MMD. If MMD has preceded disc displacement, however, and has possibly been the cause of it by the constant forces delivered to the TMJ by parafunctional activity, disc repair may have little effect on pain experienced by the patient unless MMD can be decreased postoperatively. A complete history of the patient's pain complaints and skillful clinical analysis are required to make this differentiation.

Important historical facts include the timing of clicking and reciprocal clicking relative to pain and limitation of opening. Often, clicking and reciprocal clicking have occurred for several years during the patient's teenage years, after which clicking ceases and a limitation of opening is noticed. Years later, opening and ROM improve and crepitus ensues. This is typical of a disc displacement with reduction proceeding to an acute disc displacement without reduction and ending with a perforation and degenerative changes in the joint (chronic disc displacement without reduction).

A history of atypical migraines, neck and shoulder pain, or other vague types of facial and neck pain may indicate that myofascial involvement of the jaw and neck preceded internal joint pathology. Known psychosomatic illnesses (gastrointestinal disturbances, such as frequent indigestion, peptic ulcer disease, Crohn's disease, ulcerative colitis, or chronic diarrhea; psoriasis; lower back pain; neurogenic bladder; certain types of asthma associated with stress; palpitations of the heart) that have been ascertained by appropriate medical experts and either left untreated or treated with medicines such as tranquilizers, antidepressants, mood elevators, β-blockers, or hypnotics indicate that considerable emotional input may contribute to a patient's complaints. Emotional and psychosomatic influences play a large role in myofascial pain and should affect internal joint pathology only secondarily.[26]

Finally, the clinician should note the effect of local anesthesia injected into and around the joint capsule either diagnostically or for the purpose of arthrography. In patients with myofascial pain, the preauricular pain usually radiates into the temple or neck and increases in intensity after adequate anesthesia of the joint has been achieved. This is a clear indication that most of the pain does not originate in the capsular or intracapsular structures.

Imaging

The most conclusive evidence of disc displacement is the arthrogram.[27] Arthrography is a dynamic study that is performed to evaluate disc position during function. Computed tomography (CT scan) was advocated as a replacement for arthrography. Several studies, however, have shown that other soft tissue structures can be confused with the disc on CT scans.[28-30] Magnetic resonance imaging (MRI) has become the standard for most cases with a clinical diagnosis of disc displacement.[31]

Arthrography or MRI should be considered if temporomandibular (TM) surgery is contemplated. However, in many cases, the disc displacement may be so clinically obvious that imaging is not necessary to make a decision regarding surgery. Imaging is often performed after conservative TMJ treatment (i.e., splint therapy) has failed. Although imaging identification of a disc displacement might be interesting before any treatment, it is usually not performed because of the satisfactory success rate of conservative therapy when performed by qualified clinicians.

Arthrographic Technique

Arthrography is performed in the fluoroscopy room of a hospital radiology department. The patient is placed on one side so that a transcranial view of the TMJ can be achieved. Local anesthetic is injected over the TMJ to anesthetize the soft tissues and capsule surrounding the joint. In experienced hands, this should be a relatively pain-free procedure. After the achievement of complete local anesthesia, a radiopaque medium is injected into the inferior joint space, using only enough volume so that it can be detected on the fluoroscopy monitors. This procedure is videotaped while the patient is asked to open, close, and go into lateral and protrusive excursions of the mandible. In some cases, the patient may be asked to attempt to cause clicking if it is not readily apparent. It is sometimes helpful to inject the radiopaque medium into the superior joint space, especially for delineation of the disc displacement without reduction.

In my experience with arthrograms, I have seen no complications beyond occasional postarthrogram tenderness. This occurs after a difficult entry into the inferior joint space. Most arthrograms leave the patient with no more soreness than any other soft tissue injection.

Arthrograms may be performed by oral surgeons, radiologists, or any other trained clinician. I believe, however, that the clinician caring for the patient will often be the one who is most gentle in performing arthrography, although most trained clinicians can do this with minimum discomfort and maximum effectiveness.

Clearly, the most common cause for inaccurate arthrography is operator error. Experience has shown that the most common false-positive is the movement of the dye from the inferior to the superior joint space, indicating a possible perforation. Indeed, the dye may escape around the needle because of excessive manipulation at the time of injection, and possibly no perforation will exist. False-negatives occur if the inferior joint space is overfilled with dye and effectively "washes out" the click, causing a normal disc–condyle relationship to appear on an arthrogram when the disc is actually displaced. The details of MRI are described elsewhere (see Ch. 5).

Preoperative Management

In cases of painful internal derangement of the TMJ, nonsurgical therapy should almost always be attempted before consideration of surgery. Physical therapy and splint therapy generally have been successful in maintaining the disc in the proper relationship.[32]

If a painful disc is being treated conservatively with physical therapy, 6 to 8 weeks would probably be an adequate period to use this mode of therapy before proceeding to other techniques. Even if the decision has been made to perform intracapsular surgery to correct a disc displacement, all efforts should be made preoperatively to decrease myofascial pain if it exists. Most of the physical therapy techniques described elsewhere in this book should be considered, depending on the patient's particular complaints.

Many patients with major joint pain, however, may not tolerate preoperative physical therapy. The ability to manage myofascial pain during physical therapy in the face of severe joint pain is decreased.

Splint therapy is somewhat more complex. In some cases, anterior displacement of the disc can be reduced with an anterior repositioning splint. The mandible is generally maintained anterior to the habitual occlusion for 2 to 4 months. If the disc cannot be reduced with the anterior repositioning appliance and if the patient continues to have pain in the forward position, early surgical intervention may be indicated (as early as 1 to 2 months after initiation of anterior repositioning splint therapy). The primary source of pain, however, may not be the joint; if it is not, anterior relocation of the joint with the appliance will not be successful. The overall evaluation of the patient and patient's history together with the signs and symptoms of other causes of pain must be addressed.

After successful reduction of the disc with an anterior repositioning appliance, the splint is changed to a centric relation (CR) splint. Regardless of the name of the splint, the objective is to allow the muscles of mastication to position the mandibular condyles in the most comfortable position without interdigitation or malocclusion of the teeth playing a role.

The subject of condylar positioning is another area of great controversy. I believe that there is no perfect or ideal position for the condyles. Instead, there is a range of positions in which an individual can function in relative comfort. In some persons, the range is very wide, and most any position of the condyle will satisfy them functionally. Other individuals have a very narrow range, and any positioning of the condyles outside that range will precipitate intracapsular or myofascial discomfort and dysfunction. Thus, the practice has been developed of allowing the muscles of mastication to seat the condyles upward and forward against the articular eminence with the disc interposed.[33,34] This appears to be a position that is reproducible and comfortable in most patients. This also obviates the clinician's judgment dictating condylar position and allows the patient's own masticatory musculature to seat the condyles appropriately.

An anteriorly displaced disc may be reduced and maintained pain-free for a period of 2 to 4 months, but on relocation of the condyle–disc complex into the fossa with use of the CR splint, displacement of the disc may recur. The dentist who is treating the patient with splints must use clinical judgment in deciding whether to reattempt an anterior repositioning therapy or to evaluate the patient for surgery. Such patients tend to be excellent surgical candidates because the anterior repositioning appliance and resultant good condyle–disc relationship has provided symptomatic relief short-term. However, the CR splint does not maintain the disc in the appropriate position, long-term and the symptoms return once again. In my clinical experience, such patients have the highest incidence of success from surgical repositioning of the disc.

Patients who have anterior repositioning and CR splint therapy resulting in a satisfactory relocation of the condyle–disc complex but have significant residual muscular pain are not candidates for intracapsular TMJ surgery. Their symptoms of myofascial origin should be treated conservatively as outlined elsewhere in this text.

Finally, in splint management, as in any other mode of therapy, it is extremely important that the individual clinician treating the patient with splints is well versed not only in the technical aspects but also in the theoretic and pathophysiologic considerations underlying the splint therapy. Any dentist or dental specialist can achieve a level of expertise through study and experience. One can, however, place a splint in a patient's mouth without having a full and complete understanding of the basic principles of this therapy. This may lead to failures in conservative therapy that are operator-dependent rather than technique-dependent.

Because the indications for arthrotomy are variable, it is impossible to offer a cookbook regimen of preoperative management. Splint therapy should precede the decision to seek surgical consultation as the success rate is 80 to 90 percent.[34] The type of splint will depend on the diagnosis; however, the patient who is indicated for surgery should be maintained in whatever manner is most comfortable, with or without a splint. Most opt to wear a splint up to the time of surgery.

Conservative TMJ Surgical Technique

Most intracapsular surgery performed today is done to relocate a disc that is displaced. Sometimes the disc may have suffered severe wear and even perforation. Surgical treatment of perforation is described later (see p. 252). Most authors advocate some sort of disc plication when the disc is displaced but not severely damaged.[35] Plication is used to designate a procedure in which a structure, in this case the TMJ disc, is secured or tacked down so that it is either less mobile or is held in place. The dissection I use is as follows.

A modified facelift incision is made in the preauricular area, allowing an esthetic, functional exposure of the TMJ (Fig. 9-1). The dissection is carried under the superficial temporalis fascia down to the level of the zygomatic arch. The TMJ capsule is cleaned off but not divided until it is exposed from the lateral aspect of the glenoid fossa to the neck of the condyle. An incision is made into the superior joint space through the lateral capsule (Fig. 9-2). The lateral collateral ligament of the disc is divided so that the inferior joint is entered and the head of the mandibular condyle is visualized (Fig. 9-3). An assessment is then made of the disc position and its health. If the disc is significantly displaced anteriorly or medially, the surgeon must determine whether excessive tissue exists in the bilaminar zone. If so, a wedge of tissue is removed at the junction of the disc and the bilaminar zone (Fig. 9-4) and is sutured with a long-lasting resorbable suture (Fig. 9-5A). In such cases, one would expect a longer healing period when this wedge of tissue is removed because the support of the posterior attachment, the bilaminar zone, has been weakened

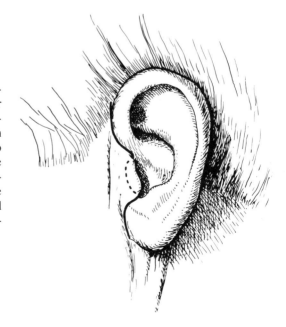

Fig. 9-1. Modified facelift incision is made in the preauricular area. Intrameatal extension to include the skin over the tragus in the anterior flap results in two separated visible portions of the incision that lie in the preauricular fold. Optimal postoperative esthetics and adequate surgical exposure are provided by this approach.

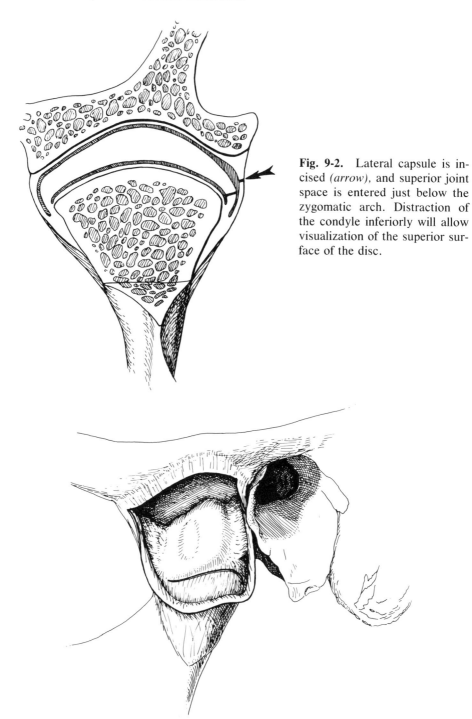

Fig. 9-2. Lateral capsule is incised *(arrow)*, and superior joint space is entered just below the zygomatic arch. Distraction of the condyle inferiorly will allow visualization of the superior surface of the disc.

Fig. 9-3. Inferior joint space is entered, and the condyle is visualized through the illustrated incision of the lateral collateral ligament of the disc.

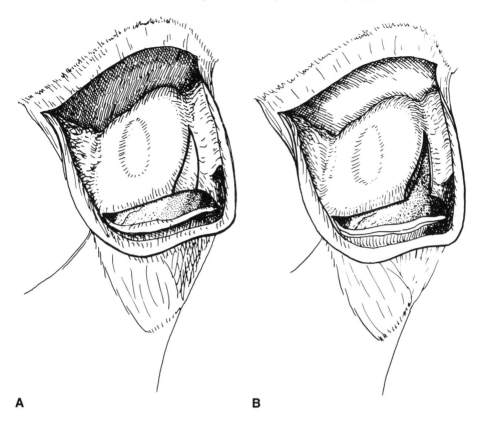

Fig. 9-4. (A) If present, amount of excess posterior tissue is estimated and outlined at the disc–bilaminar junction. (B) A wedge of posterolateral tissue is removed to facilitate posterolateral disc repositioning. The size of the excised tissue wedge is designed to provide correct postoperative disc position as well as primary closure with minimal tension.

by the surgical removal of this wedge of tissue. Whether a wedge is removed and plicated posteriorly, a lateral plication should be performed. This is done by placing a mattress suture, using a long-lasting but resorbable material, to shorten and laterally reposition the lateral collateral ligament (Fig. 9-5B). The capsule is sutured (Fig. 9-6), the wound is closed in layers, and a pressure dressing is placed over the skin.

Because patients are asked to use no chewing force for at least 3 weeks after surgery, a soft diet is necessary. Generally, no exercises are prescribed for this 3-week period; however, mild active mobility is encouraged.

Postoperative Management

In many cases, a patient will have some malocclusion, pre-existing or created by the joint surgery, after arthrotomy. A CR splint is helpful for about 6 to 8 weeks after surgery to protect the joint(s). Gradually after this, patients

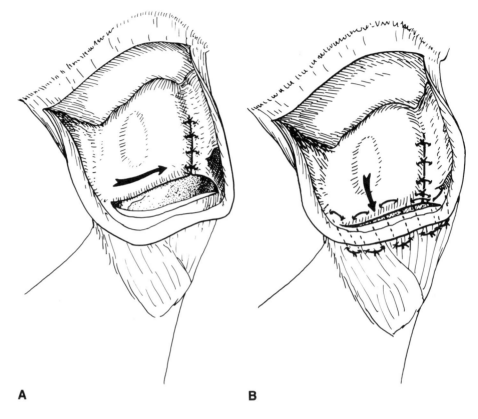

A   **B**

Fig. 9-5. **(A)** Primary closure of posterior band and attachment is accomplished using slowly resorbable suture. *Arrow* shows predominant posterior movement of the disc that results from posterolateral plication. **(B)** Similar suture is used in mattress fashion to close and plicate lateral collateral ligament, thus repositioning medially displaced disc laterally *(arrow)*. Completed disc repositioning will allow coordinated disc–condyle complex function.

are weaned off the splint, or if a major malocclusion is present, they are treated for that malocclusion.

The need for physical therapy varies widely among patients. Immediately after surgery, patients are encouraged to move the mandible easily and not to hold it still. At 1 week postoperatively, MIO and lateral excursions are checked. If adequate, 20- to 25-mm opening with 4- to 5-mm laterals, active mobilization should continue. If mobility is less which is rare, a program of passive stretching and side-to-side exercises is instituted. At 3 weeks postoperatively, MIO should be 30 mm and laterals 6 to 8 mm. If not, active formal physical therapy should begin, with the goal of achieving an MIO of 35 to 50 mm and laterals of 10 to 12 mm, depending on the patient. Patients are evaluated at 3 months, with the expectation that these goals will be met at that time. A continuation of a home

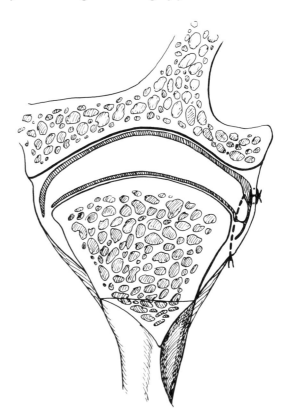

Fig. 9-6. Superior and inferior capsular flaps are primarily closed using interrupted sutures.

program may be necessary in some cases and should be customized to the particular needs of the patient.

Joint noises after arthrotomy can be confusing because they may be meaningless or they could signal relapse of the surgical correction. Postoperative joint noises should be of concern only if pain or recurrent decrease in ROM is experienced. As increased opening is achieved, it is not uncommon for some noises to emerge with wide excursions. Usually, these are of no consequence to the patient, and reassurance is indicated.

Postoperative Physical Therapy

Postoperative physical therapy can be divided into two general categories: MMD management and mobilization.

MMD Management

MMD management is similar to that used for nonsurgical patients or for preoperative management of surgical cases. This treatment can begin within 2 to 3 weeks postoperatively, depending on patient comfort. Assuming that no major stress is placed on the TMJ, any technique designed to reduce muscle pain or tension is acceptable.

Cervical spine myofascial pain that existed pre- or postoperatively must be addressed in the postoperative phase. ROM exercises, splint management, pain control, and cervical spine management to minimize myofascial pain of the cervical and shoulder musculature are essential parts of managing myofascial pain of the masticatory system.

Mobilization

Mobilization of the TMJ after intracapsular surgery is an entirely different matter. Much depends on how much mobility existed before surgery and how long the decreased mobility existed. If the patient had limited mobility for only a short time or not at all before surgery, simple stretching exercises, opening against resistance, and active lateral movement are necessary after surgery. Opening against resistance and lateral movements must be performed with caution early after surgery. How soon and to what degree will often depend on the extent of the repair and the ability of the surgeon to establish a strong surgical repair. Often, these mobilization exercises can be taught to the patient by the surgeon and may not require formal physical therapy.

If decreased mobility has existed preoperatively for several months or longer, shortening of the muscles of mastication and capsular tightness should also be expected. Also, in many cases, more severe internal damage and, thus, more extensive surgery and scarring will have compromised the joint. Therefore, the obstacles to overcome in hypomobility are both chronic muscle shortening and loss of flexibility of the TMJ capsule and ligaments. Pain is also a factor because these patients tend to have longer, more painful postoperative courses than do the simpler cases.

The dilemma faced in these severe cases is that the sooner that mobilization procedures are begun, the better the chance of overcoming capsular tightness and muscle shortening. Conversely, if a large perforation has been repaired, a longer healing period is ideal before the repair is stressed by exercise. Clinical judgment is our only guideline in deciding when to begin postoperative physical therapy.

Capsular tightness and muscle shortening that may occur after surgery should not be confused with that which existed before surgery. Any capsular tightness that occurs before surgery should simply be the result of chronic lack of mobility. After surgery, because incisions are made through the superior aspect of the capsule into the superior joint space and through the lateral collateral ligament into the inferior joint space, the resuturing and healing of these structures will undoubtedly cause scarring, contracture, and some loss of flexibility in the TMJ capsule. Muscle shortening that exists in these patients should be merely a result of decreased ROM before surgery, which has an effect on the overall muscle length and flexibility. Nothing occurs during the TMJ surgery to shorten or change muscle length.

If the disc repair is more tenuous, a longer healing period is required before stress can be placed on the joint. Again, a close communication between surgeon and physical therapist is essential to facilitate proper timing of mobilization exercises. Mobilization techniques must obviously be continued much longer in such patients, and gains will be more gradual. In the most severe cases, the mobility attained after surgery may be greater than preoperative mobility; however, it may remain less than that of the normal population. Therefore, persistence over the long term will usually provide satisfactory results.

There is a lack of clinical and basic research on postoperative adhesions. We have observed postoperative adhesions between the articular surfaces of joints after trauma or surgery. This is supposed to result from bleeding into the joint, which, because of lack of mobility, permits organization of the clot, as opposed to lysis. Studies[36] show that constant mobility after joint trauma or surgery generally causes lysis of blood clots rather than organization into connective tissue. If this organization is permitted to progress, however, adhesions may form in which strands of fibrous connective tissue exist between the disc and the fossa or condyle. In the first 3 to 4 weeks after surgery, patients commonly experience tightness on opening and during occasions of mild forced opening such as yawning, laughing, or opening for tooth brushing; patients hear a snap in an operated joint that may deliver a sharp pain but also gives them a feeling of greater ROM. This may represent the breaking of an adhesion, and even though patients may feel some discomfort, it probably represents a favorable occurrence in the mobilization and return to normal function of the joints.

Postoperative Splint Therapy

Postoperative splint therapy plays an important role in recovery from TMJ surgery.[23,35] Malocclusion is frequently present in both disc displacements of the TMJ and MMD.[37] If dental occlusion is at all contributory to the etiology or perpetuation of TMJ dysfunction, a postoperative splint is probably necessary in most cases. Even when a satisfactory occlusion is ultimately reached, it is unrealistic to expect that this occlusion will occur in the first or second week after surgery because pain, swelling of the joints, and altered muscular activity will continue. Muscular pain may very much limit joint mobility after surgery. If the CR splint is not frequently adjusted, the muscles of mastication may become extremely tender, causing limitation of opening, deviation of opening, and various other muscular influences on the position of the mandible. Persistent muscle hyperactivity and dysfunction after surgery can make it very difficult to determine normal seated condylar position and to achieve increased ROM. In certain cases, after a 6- to 8-week healing period, splints are removed and a satisfactory occlusion has occurred; in such cases, no further occlusional adjustments need to be made. Frequently, however, a significant malocclusion exists after completion of TMJ surgical and nonsurgical management, and postoperative splints are designed to compensate for this malocclusion.

The CR splint is placed in the mouth the day after surgery and is adjusted to a comfortable position for the patient. It is adjusted again at 1 week post-operatively because the mandibular position changes as swelling diminishes. This procedure is continued until a stable mandibular position is achieved. In patients with minimal MMD, this stable position is usually reached in 3 to 6 weeks. In the most severe cases, 3 to 4 months may be necessary, especially when MMD is a major factor.

Once the stable mandibular position is achieved, measures must be taken to change the occlusion of the teeth so that this mandibular condylar position can be maintained in the muscle-dictated position achieved with the postoperative splint. The methods used to alter the occlusion depend on the extent of malocclusion. In minor cases, grinding of the teeth (dental equilibration) or minor orthodontic tooth movement may be all that is necessary. Severe cases may require major orthodontic tooth movement, major dental reconstruction, or orthognathic surgery to reposition the entire lower and/or upper jaws, depending on the type of the malocclusion.

Complications

There are so many types of arthrotomy procedures that it is impossible to discuss all the potential complications involved with each. Conservative arthrotomy with disc plication has few complications as compared with other surgical procedures. Complications after conservative surgery are generally rare and of a temporary nature, including cranial nerve VII paresis involving the frontal and zygomatic branches, infection, bleeding, and numbness around the incision site. If paralysis of the orbicularis oculi muscle is profound, care must be taken to protect the eye from drying. This is accomplished with the use of artificial tears and taping of the eye at night. It is extremely rare for this complication to persist long term. The value of electrotherapy to stimulate the muscles of the interim has not been established.

Hypomobility may also be a problem postoperatively because of the patient's reluctance to exercise and an avoidance of pain. Diligence on the part of the treating practitioners and patient compliance are the best preventions.

Disc Perforation and Degeneration

Patients with perforations tend to be approximately 10 years older than the average patient receiving TMJ surgery.[23] The perforations are usually a result of chronic displacement or parafunctional stresses such as clenching or bruxism, and patients often exhibit extreme emotional involvement regarding their facial pain.[23] The significance is that these patients may continue their parafunctional and emotional targeting of the TMJ after the surgical procedure. The accompanying microtrauma that occurs in the joint will also continue over the postoperative period. Many surgeons[38,39] believe that the TMJ lacks the capability for healing and that one should, therefore, be much more aggressive in treating these patients.

When clinical and imaging examinations demonstrate that a painful joint has a degenerated or perforated disc, the surgical options include bilaminar flap repair,[17] temporalis myofascial flap,[18] auricular cartilage graft,[14] dermal graft,[16] temporary silicone implant,[38] discectomy without replacement,[19] and condylotomy.[20] Surgeon preference varies widely. I prefer the first two: the bilaminar flap repair (which is discussed later) for large perforations and areas of partial disc degeneration; and the temporalis myofascial flap for totally degenerated discs, failed implants, ankylosis, or whenever adequate intracapsular tissue is not available. Both are technically difficult, especially the former, but they can give exceptional results when performed carefully. The other procedures also give good results in experienced hands, as with so many types of TMD treatment.

Our studies[40] indicated that an experimentally induced perforation in the posterior lateral aspect of the TMJ disc of a macaque monkey generally led to degenerative changes, including proliferation of the superior surface of the condylar head and proliferation on the articular surface of the fossa. These proliferations appear to be the first stages of degeneration and resorption. The disc perforations tended to become larger mediolaterally in the postsurgical period. In two of ten joints, however, perforations healed spontaneously without any treatment.

In a subsequent study,[17] a double-layered synovial membrane flap was used to close surgically induced experimental perforations in the discs of monkeys, and the repair of the disc perforations was extremely successful. Continuity of the discs was re-established, thus preventing proliferative and degenerative changes of the articular surfaces of the condyle and glenoid fossa. Therefore, we devised a procedure inside the joint that uses available tissue. The superior and inferior lamina of the bilaminar zone together with the covering of synovial membrane and its subintimal vasculature is used to repair and reconstitute discal structures. Obviously, a badly perforated or degenerated disc will never be completely normal again. Cadaver studies[41] have indicated, however, that perforation and degenerative changes inside the human TMJ are relatively common. Therefore, a completely normal structure may not be necessary to facilitate adequate TMJ function. I believe that internally restoring the integrity of the joint using structures locally available (i.e., synovial membrane and its vasculature) is vastly superior to the introduction of either alloplastic or autogenic materials from other areas.

Our stereoscopic and histologic studies have indicated that the double-layered synovial membrane flap used to close large perforations in the discs of monkeys has led to a relatively normal reconstitution of the disc and maintenance of articular surfaces. A description follows of the technique for closure of large perforations using the synovial membrane flap and remobilization of the remaining elements of the discs.

TMJ Surgical Repair of Large Perforations

After studies on monkeys, we treated human TMJs with large perforations using a flap from the retrodiscal tissue lined with synovial membrane.[17] Rather than harvesting autologous graft materials from distance sites, we believe that a more physiologic method is to mobilize the two layers of the retrodiscal tissue and reapproximate them with the disc, allowing for healing, scar formation, and remodeling of the disc and retrodiscal tissues.

The surgical approach to the TMJ is exactly the same as described in the section on conservative TMJ surgical technique to the point of identifying a large perforation somewhere in the discs or retrodiscal tissues (Fig. 9-7). When the perforation is identified, the superior and inferior joint spaces are fully opened and the extent of the perforation is observed. An incision (Fig. 9-8A) is made through the lateral collateral ligament to expose the perforation laterally so that the entire borders of the perforation can be seen from the lateral aspect. The bilaminar zone is then carefully divided with small dissecting scissors into two distinct lamina all the way back to their origins (Fig. 9-8B). The superior lamina originates from the tympanic plate of the temporal bone. The inferior lamina originates in the neck of the condyle. The two lamina should be divided with a fine scalpel blade where they join on the medial aspect of the perforation. The anterior margin of the perforation is usually in the cartilaginous discal tissue. This is divided very carefully in a filet manner so that an incision ap-

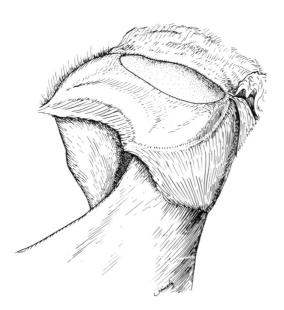

Fig. 9-7. Large perforation that may be identified after entrance into superior joint space. Extensive defect in the disc prohibits its inclusion in a conservative plication procedure. Perforations may occur in the disc (as shown), the bilaminar region, or at the junctional area.

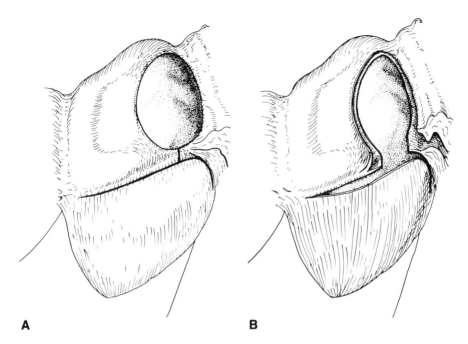

A   **B**

Fig. 9-8. **(A)** Inverted T-shaped incision is made lateral to perforation. Horizontal arm enters the inferior joint space through the lateral collateral ligament. Vertical arm connects previous incision with the perforation, allowing complete visualization of the edge of the defect. **(B)** With a fine scissors and blade, the entire perforation and vertical incision periphery is divided into superior and inferior layers. Extensive anterior dissection is accomplished to provide freedom for posterior repositioning of anterior disc segment.

proximately 1 mm deep is made in the middle of this discal tissue and brought around all the way to the lateral aspect at the junction of the condylomeniscal ligament. (This permits closure of the wound in a double-layered fashion, much as an oronasal or oroantral fistula would be closed.) The inferior aspect of the disc is often convex in these cases and does not fit well over the head of the condyle. If this is so, the surgeon may need to recontour the inferior convexity of the disc slightly with a scalpel blade so that it is somewhat more concave and fits the head of the condyle. Condyle or fossa that have irregularities should be extremely conservatively removed, with every intention of maintaining articular surface in its best integrity. The two lamina of the bilaminar zone should be maximally mobilized until the disc and the bilaminar attachments can be approximated without tension. The anterior dissection must be extensive enough to mobilize the remaining portion of the disc so that it can be removed in a posterior direction.

The inferior lamina is sutured (Fig. 9-9A) to the lower filet of the discal tissue from medial to lateral using a 5-0 vicryl resorbable suture with the knots tied on the superior side. When this has been completed, the superior lamina

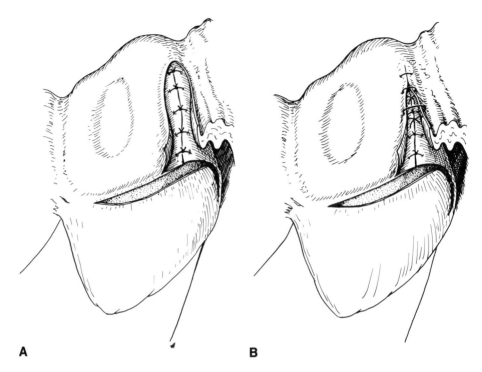

A   **B**

Fig. 9-9. **(A)** A double-layered closure is performed. First, inferior lamina and lower filet of disc are advanced and closed primarily. **(B)** Superior lamina and upper disc tissue are then opposed and sutured. Interrupted resorbable sutures with knots directed toward the center are used.

is sutured (Fig. 9-9B) to the superior aspect of the discal filet with the knots on the inferior side. Some dead space (Fig. 9-10) between the superior and inferior laminae will exist and is allowed to remain. It will fill with blood, clot, and ultimately organize into a scar of fibrous connective tissue. Often, the superior lamina may be sutured first because of access.

The remaining lateral incised tissue is plicated using horizontal mattress sutures as described for intracapsular TMJ surgery, thus securing the posterior lateral disc to the lateral portion of the condyle. The rest of the surgical closure is then performed in a manner identical to the procedure described for intracapsular TMJ surgery.

In conjunction with carefully planned CR splint and physical therapy, this technique can render most of these patients vastly improved over their preoperative situation without risking increased degenerative changes and further degeneration of the joint. In our experience, ROM is more limited. Why this is so is not entirely clear, but two reasons probably explain this phenomenon. First, many of these patients have had severe limitation of motion for many years before their surgery; therefore, a number of muscular and tendinous structures act as limiters of mandibular ROM. Second, the double-layer flap

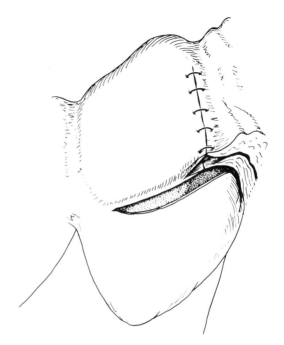

Fig. 9-10. Completed posterior repair and resultant dead space. This space will be obliterated by fibrous connective tissue formed during healing.

closure decreases the overall size of the joint, causing more tension and tightness in the joint. One would, therefore, expect ROM to return more slowly in addition to some permanent ROM loss. Whatever the reason, the decrease in ROM may not be any greater than the decrease in ROM of patients who have other types of procedures for gross disc perforation.

When large perforations have been repaired, a more gentle postoperative protocol must be adhered to because of the delicacy of the repair. Postoperative splint management is somewhat different. In large perforation repairs, the suture line may be directly superior to the head of the condyle. Therefore, an anterior repositioning splint that moves the condyle slightly forward for a period of 6 to 8 weeks after surgery probably provides the best possibility for healing of the bilaminar attachment to the disc. After 6 to 8 weeks of anterior repositioning just sufficient to prohibit pressure from the condyle on the suture line, the splint is changed to a CR splint and the same method as described above (see Postoperative Splint Therapy) is followed for seating the condyles and muscle relaxation.

No general formula can be given for postoperative physical therapy after these procedures. A close communication between surgeon and physical therapist is required to ensure proper postoperative management. Generally, the more tenuous the repair, the more cautious the approach must be to physical therapy in the early stages. After surgery, the surgeon should have some feel for the strength of the repair and should communicate this to the physical therapist so that a reasonable physical therapy program can be designed.

Autologous and Alloplastic Versus Natural Repair

The TMJ has a considerable capability for healing.[17,40,42] The cartilage in the joint is not hyaline cartilage, but fibrocartilage, and undifferentiated mesenchymal tissue in the joint is conducive to remodeling. Synovial membrane with its vasculature has a tremendous potential for repair. Therefore, much of the controversy about handling of the severely damaged TMJ centers around the opinion of the surgeon as to the healing capabilities of the joint.

An area of intense disagreement and controversy regarding surgical repair of the TMJ centers around the use of implant and alloplastic materials. It is important to divide TMJ disorders into two categories. The first category involves displaced discs without gross perforations or degenerations. The general consensus among surgeons is that a conservative relocation and plication of the disc into its most anatomic position is necessary for this group.[35] Some surgeons, however, advocate more radical measures such as meniscectomy[43] with or without alloplastic or autologous implant.[44,45] An autologous implant is a material harvested from the patient and reimplanted without its original blood supply. A good example of this is a skin graft taken from the hip and placed on the face in reconstruction of a burn injury. In such an implant system, the graft is intended to be placed on a vascularized bed that will rapidly revascularize the implant, rendering it essentially functional as a normal part of the recipient site. Autologous implants of dermis,[44] fascia,[12] and auricular cartilage[14] probably do not function as a true graft in that they are not placed in a vascularized bed, where one would expect them to "take" in classical fashion. These materials will act as a matrix for the ingrowth of fibrous connective tissue, synovial membrane, and scar formation that may function as a replacement disc.

The second category uses alloplastic implants, i.e., substances that are artificially produced, such as silicone rubber (Silastic, Dow Corning, Midland, Michigan) or Proplast/Teflon (Vitek, Houston, Texas). Animal studies[46] and our own clinical observations indicate that the use of alloplastic materials causes a degenerative process in the joint. The bone of the fossa and condylar head resorb and remodel even when the implant is placed without harming the articular surfaces. Investigators[47] have reported fraying and disintegration of the implants, with distant migration of small alloplastic particles as a result of their inability to withstand the trauma of constant occlusal forces. Giant cell inflammatory reactions have been observed around these particles, indicating a foreign body response.

Because most patients receiving TMJ surgery are in their late 20s and early 30s, use of materials that in the short term appear to cause degenerative, destructive changes would appear to be contraindicated when a normal life span is anticipated for these persons. Unlike hip prostheses that are generally placed in persons in their sixth and seventh decades of life, a TMJ implant or prosthesis may be required to function for 40 to 50 years. Therefore, I believe that in patients who have normal continuity to the disc, there is no indication for removal of the disc and replacement with an autologous or alloplastic implant material.

Failed Alloplastic Implants

A variety of alloplastic materials have been used over the past few years in TMJ surgery. Proplast-Teflon implants have met with the most dramatic complications.[48] Most recently, it has been recommended that all these implants be removed even if the patients have no signs or symptoms. Generally, patients with these implants have severe degeneration of the condyle and fossa with pain and loss of ROM. Erosion into the middle cranial fossa has been seen in several cases. Methods of reconstruction after removal are widely variable. I usually recommend removal of the implant with associated tissue, followed by interposition of a myofascial flap, consisting of the temporalis muscle and fascia, based anteriorly and rotated into the glenoid fossa medial to the zygomatic arch.[18] Others use costochondral grafts or total joint prostheses. Experience has shown this to be rarely necessary. Silicone implants have been used and have also often led to degeneration. Permanent silicone implants are no longer recommended, but some practitioners use temporary silicone implants, which are removed 2 to 6 months after placement.[49]

Osteoarthritis and Osteoarthrosis (Degenerative Joint Disease)

Osseous degeneration of the mandibular condyle may occur with or without pain. When pain is associated with intracapsular structures a diagnosis of osteoarthritis is made. If the osseous degenerative changes are not painful, the pain may be originating extracapsularly, usually from the muscles of mastication and it is referred to as osteoarthrosis. Pain in these cases is best managed by nonsurgical means because no TMJ surgical procedure presently available successfully and consistently deals with osteoarthritic pain. Frequently, the pain associated with degeneration of the joint is primarily myofascial and can be treated with splint and physical therapy. Should the degeneration include loss of vertical bony height in the condyle, a malocclusion will develop. Splint therapy will usually manage myofascial pain, and joint pain to a lesser degree, if the malocclusion is the cause of the muscle and joint pain. When faced with the situation of adequate joint mobility and minimum pain, it is wise to avoid any attempts at joint reconstruction. The resultant malalignment of the jaws can be corrected with orthodontics and/or orthognathic surgery.

Many attempts have been made to totally replace the TMJ, but, to date, no method is entirely satisfactory. The preferred techniques use costochondral grafting[50] and total joint replacement with a metal prosthesis.[51] Neither of these procedures has been successful at reducing pain, and many failures have occurred. If the goal of the surgeon is merely to replace structure and prevent ankylosis while maintaining adequate function, one of these two operations may be appropriate, but they are not indicated for the management of pain alone. The choice between these two procedures is primarily influenced by the surgeon's preference.

Ankylosis

Ankylosis is a relative term indicating a situation in which there is severe limitation of mandibular ROM caused by an intracapsular union, bony or fibrous, between the mandible and the temporal bone. In a few cases of early fibrous union, physical therapy may be sufficient to restore an acceptable ROM; however, this is rare. Usually, these patients are seen with MIOs of less than 20 mm and often less than 10 mm. If this condition has existed for more than a few months, severe muscle shortening will have occurred in the muscles of mastication, especially the temporalis, as well as capsular tightness. Arthrotomy with removal of the union and placement of an interpositional material, followed by rigorous exercising and physical therapy, is indicated for treatment of ankylosis. Coronoidectomy to release the influence of the temporalis muscle and masseter muscle myotomy is often necessary to achieve full ROM. The choice of interpositional materials varies, including temporalis muscle fascia flap, dermis, auricular cartilage, fascia graft, lyophilized dura, temporary silicone, and total joint prosthesis. The material used is not important for the sake of this discussion.

It is well accepted that surgical mobilization of the mandible is less than half of the battle in the management of ankylosis. Because reattachment of the temporalis and masseter muscles to the mandible occurs rapidly after surgical removal of the coronoid process, intense mobilization must be undertaken immediately after surgery and be as aggressive as the patient can tolerate. Patient compliance with postoperative physical therapy regimens is essential to success. The immediacy of mobilization after ankylosis surgery is a major difference between this type of surgery and other TMJ surgeries. Mobilization exercises, complete with strong active stretching using tongue blades or other mechanical devices, should begin the day after surgery and should continue at frequent intervals for 6 to 12 months. It is almost impossible to be too rigorous in the attempt to prevent reankylosis. The major deterrent to proper postoperative mobilization in these patients is pain. Strong analgesics may be necessary in the early postoperative period to achieve adequate mobility. These should be decreased as soon as possible, however, to prevent drug dependence. In these cases, the obstacles to mobility are dense scar tissue and chronically shortened muscles. Short of loosening the teeth, little harm can be done by vigorous, frequent stretching of mandibular opening. Strengthening of the depressors of the mandible (suprahyoid muscles) is also helpful in increasing mandibular opening. It must be recognized that the first 2 months are crucial to success, before scar maturity reaches a point at which no amount of exercise will help.

Trauma

For many years, the only indications for open reduction of condylar and subcondylar fractures were fractures displaced into the middle cranial fossa, inability to achieve a reasonable occlusion because of obstruction of the fractured segment, and intractable pain. With expanded knowledge of TMJ function and improved techniques and technology, open reduction of these fractures is becoming more popular. Scientific data are lacking to justify this change, but common sense would seem to support a more consistent attitude toward fractures of the condyle–subcondyle as compared with other mandibular fractures. Rigid fixation of mandibular fractures has some real advantages, but if fractures of the rest of the mandible are rigidly fixed and the condylar–subcondylar fractures are not, much of the advantage of rigid fixation is lost. Also, if practitioners who treat TMD insist on such high standards for joint function in other pathologic situations, it seems reasonable to aspire to similar goals when treating trauma.

Open reduction with internal fixation of subcondylar fractures usually involves a preauricular incision plus either a retromandibular or intraoral incision. Although a wide variety of fixation devices have been used, small bone plates, rigid enough to allow immediate mobilization, are the most reasonable. Intracapsular fractures should not be treated with intermaxillary immobilization or open reduction, but with early mandibular mobilization and physical therapy.

Arthroscopy

Enthusiasm for arthroscopy varies even more widely than in other methodologic debates; therefore, personal preference plays a stronger role. A complete discussion of arthroscopy is included in another chapter and need not be repeated. Arthroscopy involves two separate components, diagnosis and treatment. The diagnostic value of arthroscopy is subject to considerable question given the less invasive modalities available, such as history, clinical examination, radiography, arthrography, CT, and MRI. The need for biopsy of the TMJ is extremely rare, but it is occasionally valuable and is obtainable via arthroscopy. The use of arthroscopy as a treatment for TMD has greater merit but still remains entangled in controversy. Although arthroscopy and arthrotomy are often perceived as alternatives for the same group of patients, this may not be so. An analysis of the indications for both procedures reveals considerable differences, albeit with several areas of overlap. Many patients treated with arthroscopy would never be considered for arthrotomy but would be treated by more conservative methods. Among TMD patients, there is a group that would never be considered for arthroscopy due to the severity of their disease. These patients would be treated using arthrotomy for situations requiring open exposure. Many surgeons will use arthrocentesis (joint lavage) in place of arthroscopy for patients who are not responding to nonsurgical therapies but are not arthrotomy candidates.

ORTHOGNATHIC SURGERY

History

Orthognathic surgery has enjoyed a less tumultuous history than TMJ surgery. A West Virginia oral surgeon, Simon P. Hullihen, described in 1849[52] an osteotomy to correct a burn contracture of the anterior mandible. In 1859, Langenbeck[53] used maxillary osteotomies to access tumors at the base of the skull. The first real emphasis on correction of jaw deformities was in German publications on the subject in the 1930s.[54,55] Then, after World War II, a gradual interest arose, probably due to the wartime experiences of many surgeons on both sides of the military line. Orthognathic surgery flourished in Europe during the 1960s before finally migrating to the United States in the late 1960s. Until that time, most of the orthognathic surgery performed in the United States had been to correct mandibular prognathism. A variety of procedures was offered to reduce the prominence of the mandible, all of which required fixing the jaws together for 4 to 8 weeks.

In the early years of orthognathic surgery, this type of facial correction was performed primarily for esthetic considerations. However, awareness in both the professional and lay communities regarding the dental occlusion has increased greatly. We are now capable of positioning teeth, jaws, and TMJs in almost ideal positions, both functionally and aesthetically.

Since 1970, a virtual explosion has occurred in orthognathic surgery, especially in North America. Much credit must be given to the excellent orthodontics and general dentistry available in the United States, not only for the support of the practitioners but for their high level of expectation when the occlusal relationship of the maxilla and mandible is changed. The expectations require that the teeth fit together well, that the TMJs function freely and without pain, and generally that the patient look better. Although all these goals are often achievable, the quest for perfection drove many of the advances of the 1970s and 1980s through a multiplicity of maxillary and mandibular procedures.

Most recently, rigid fixation of maxillary and mandibular osteotomies has become routine, but not without problems. The demands on the surgeon, especially when rigidly fixing the mandible, are far greater than with intermaxillary fixation (IMF). As with many other innovations, the stimulus came from the Europeans, who were using rigid fixation for fractures and orthognathics long before surgeons in this country. Again, the innovative ideas from elsewhere were brought to a higher level of accuracy and precision once surgeons and orthodontists grasped the principles and began to work with them.

Whereas orthognathic surgery with IMF presented one set of problems regarding the TMJ, rigid fixation brings a new set of circumstances to the table. The superiority of one technique versus the other has not been documented, although studies are presently underway.

Indications

The functions of speech, respiration, phonation, mastication, and loving are all managed via the jaws and associated structures. Orthognathic surgery is indicated to correct malrelationships of the jaws. The effect of these discrepancies varies from patient to patient. Some patients may tolerate major disharmonies in jaw relationship, whereas others may have difficulty functioning despite a fairly minor discrepancy.

Of patients requiring TMD treatment, many have a class II (retrognathic) dental skeletal relationship.[56] Why this facial deformity exists most frequently in TMJ patients is not completely clear. Protrusion of the mandible is believed to become habitual to achieve a more appropriate incisor relationship to improve breathing and airway management, to facilitate speech, or simply for esthetic reasons. This constant protrusion of the mandible may introduce a laxity into the stabilization ligaments of the TMJ disc, contributing to a disc displacement. Whatever the reason, correlation between class II malocclusions and disc displacements is quite high. Therefore, a significant number of patients who have been treated successfully for TMJ internal derangement have a class II malocclusion after successful treatment, with or without surgery on the joints. Often, the sole possibility for correcting a class II dental skeletal relationship includes not only orthodontic management but surgical advancement of the mandible.

In patients with craniomandibular deformities, orthognathic surgery is often performed to correct a malocclusion that prevents proper TMJ function. Many patients with TMJ complaints have major malocclusions that are due to deformities of the jaws that can be corrected only by surgically altering the jaw position.

In patients that have facial skeletal discrepancies and TMD, a CR splint will often indicate the amount of influence that the jaw relationship has on TMD. If a CR splint causes a major portion of signs and symptoms to disappear for several months, correcting the jaw and occlusal position will usually give a similar degree of relief. Frequently, myofascial pain is the culprit in these cases of jaw disharmonies, which is fortunate because orthognathic surgery by itself has not been shown to reduce a displaced disc. It may be possible with orthognathic surgery to decrease pain in the joint with an improved jaw relationship, but not reduce the disc. Again, we do not know how important disc position is in the treatment of TMD. Clearly, orthognathic surgery plays an important role in optimizing jaw relationships, which in some patients will decrease stresses placed on the muscles of mastication and the TMJs. This is the primary goal of orthognathic surgery.

Esthetics plays an important role in orthognathic surgery for two reasons. First, no one would accept a poorer appearance after elective surgery, no matter how necessary. And second, esthetics and function usually go hand in hand, so that optimal goals in both can be approached.

IMF Versus Rigid Fixation

The comparative benefits of nonrigid fixation with IMF versus rigid fixation with early mobilization in orthognathic surgery are presently untested. Nonrigid fixation with IMF probably gives the best relationship between the teeth and the best condylar position at the end of surgery; however, there is less resistance to change in the early and late postoperative periods. If good bony stops are not present, the maxilla or mandible can shift, resulting in malpositioning. However, rigid fixation usually ensures that the osteotomized fragments will stay put, but if they are not accurately placed, there is little room for error. Certainly, in inexperienced hands nonrigid fixation is easier to perform and a more predictable technique in the short term. The question of long-term stability has not been resolved, but early clinical reviews suggest that rigid fixation gives slightly better stability.

The benefits of early mobilization afforded with rigid fixation would seem to be obvious. IMF in animals has revealed that there are some atrophic changes that occur during the period of fixation; however, these seem to be reversible. Whether these factors influence the long-term ROM has not yet been determined.

Maxillary surgery alone will influence the mandibular position by virtue of the new occlusion that is created. Physical therapy required to rehabilitate maxillary surgery patients is generally minimal, but some muscle dysfunction may be seen and require treatment.

Because the mandible is the movable part of the system, it gives far more concern when it is the target of surgery. Difficulties may include MMD similar to that which occurs with occlusal changes in maxillary surgery. Also, the condylar position may have been altered at the time of fixation (rigid fixation more so than IMF), resulting in a different condyle–disc–fossa relationship. Obviously, minor changes are tolerated easily, but when the changes exceed the limits of the system, difficulties with ROM may occur. Physical therapy may improve ROM in some cases, but if changes are severe, only reoperation will solve the problem. Each case must be evaluated on an individual basis.

In summary, IMF is a tried and true technique, with many cases treated successfully, albeit not perfectly. Patients must tolerate not only the period of fixation, but an additional period of rehabilitation. Rigid fixation, however, has several advantages, some real (i.e., early mobilization, comfort, improved diet, decreased anxiety, and less rehabilitation) and some theoretic (i.e., improved accuracy and long-term stability). A long-term, prospective, randomized clinical trial is presently underway investigating rigid versus intermaxillary (nonrigid) fixation of mandibular advancements to determine their relative benefits. My opinion is that rigid fixation when performed well is the superior technique and when performed poorly is definitely inferior.

Preoperative Management

Splint therapy is useful preoperatively in patients with myofascial pain that is affected by their malocclusion. Also, splints can be useful during the immediate preoperative period in achieving a seated condylar position for the workup and model surgery.

Physical therapy will improve myofascial pain in the muscles of mastication and the cervical musculature, which assists in determining the most comfortable mandibular position at the time of workup and just before surgery. Also, it familiarizes the patient with the techniques that may be necessary postoperatively.

Orthognathic Surgical Technique

Orthognathic surgery may involve surgical repositioning of the maxilla, mandible, or both. Surgical repositioning of the maxilla alone has very little effect on mandibular mobility.[57] Mandibular surgery, however, especially sagittal-split osteotomy of the mandible, does contribute to decreased mobility of the mandible.[57]

Sagittal-split osteotomy of the mandible is most often performed to advance the retrognathic mandible; however, mandibular setback and corrections of asymmetry are also performed. The technique involves an intraoral incision along the anterior border of the ramus so that the entire external oblique ridge is exposed. A subperiosteal dissection is performed along the medial aspect of the mandibular ramus inside the medial pterygoid muscle. A subperiosteal dissection is also performed on the lateral aspect of the mandible where the mandibular ramus and the mandibular body meet. This is deep to the more anterior aspect of the masseter muscle insertion. A horizontal osteotomy (Fig. 9-11A) is made on the medial aspect of the mandible just above the entrance of the inferior alveolar neurovascular bundle into the ramus. This osteotomy penetrates approximately halfway through the medial ramus cortical plate. A vertical osteotomy (Fig. 9-11B) is made on the lateral cortex of the mandible at the junction of the mandibular ramus and mandibular body. This osteotomy penetrates only the lateral cortical plate. A connecting cut is then made between the two so that the mandible can be split (Fig. 9-12) into a proximal and distal segment. After completion of this procedure bilaterally, the mandible is repositioned into a predetermined occlusion, and the teeth are wired together. The proximal and distal segments on each side are then wired (Fig. 9-13) or

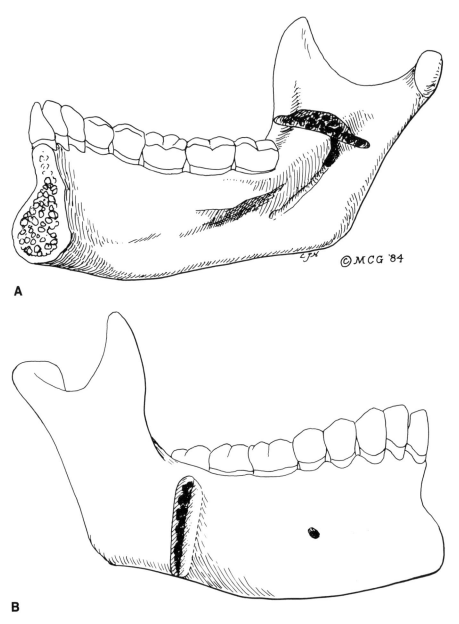

Fig. 9-11. (**A**) Initial long cut made during sagittal-split osteotomy of the mandible is a medial horizontal osteotomy through the medial cortex. It extends from the anterior border of the ramus to just posterior and above the mandibular lingula and inferior alveolar neurovascular bundle. (**B**) Vertical osteotomy is then made through the lateral cortex in the posterior body of the mandible. An access bevel is placed on the anterior lip of the osteotomy.

fixed rigidly with screws, with the condyles of the mandible unchanged from their preoperative position. Probably the most frequent complication in sagittal-split surgery of the mandible is failure to place the condyles in their preoperative position. This is especially true if a rigid fixation system is used.

To understand this inability to place the condyles in their preoperative position, one must understand the situation that exists at the time of surgery. After completion of the sagittal-split operation, one essentially has the mandible in three pieces. The distal segment includes all the teeth, the body of the mandible, and the chin. The two proximal segments include the condyles, coronoid processes, and mandibular rami bilaterally. All three segments are independent of one another. At this point in the procedure, the surgeon wires the distal segment into the desired postoperative occlusion by fitting the teeth together, using a preformed occlusal template, and wiring the teeth together. This establishes the postoperative position of the distal segment.

The difficulty lies in determining the desired positioning of the proximal segments so that the condyles will be in exactly the same position after they have been appropriately seated that they were before surgery. This issue is the subject of much controversy among surgeons. An extensive review is beyond the scope of this chapter; however, positioning of this segment can best be achieved by carefully studying the plaster model of the proposed surgery and radiographic evaluation of the cephalometric head films before the actual surgery. The surgeon should go into the operating room with a precise knowledge of the defect that will be created between the proximal and distal segments on each side (Fig. 9-13) as the mandible is advanced into its new position. If simple bony wiring and IMF for 8 weeks is to be used, this will be sufficient to permit proper positioning of the proximal segments at the time of surgery.[58] If a rigid system of fixation, such as bone screws, is to be used between the proximal and distal segments, however, it is safe to assume that some mediolateral discrepancies may exist in condylar positioning following the technique.[59]

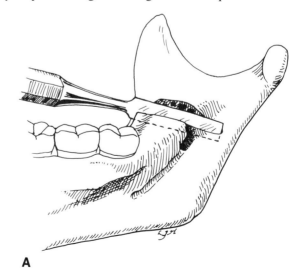

Fig. 9-12. After lateral vertical and medial horizontal cuts are connected by an osteotomy along the anterior border of ramus and external oblique line of the mandible, the distal and proximal segments are separated (split) with chisels introduced into the medial, anterior ramus, and lateral osteotomy sites. (**A**) Medial site. (*Figure continues.*)

A

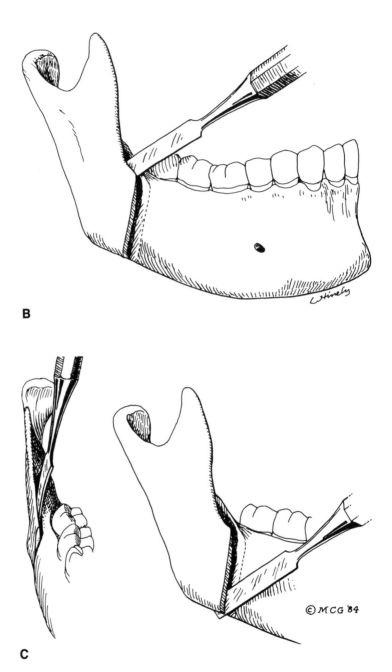

B

C

Fig. 9-12.   (*Continued.*) (**B & C**) Anterior ramus and lateral ostemysites. Gentle prying and incising movements complete sagittal splitting.

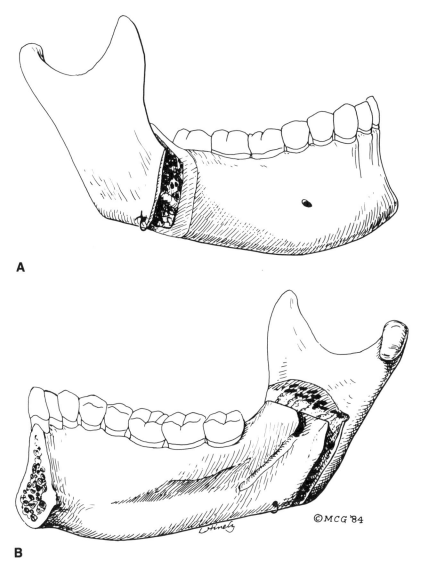

Fig. 9-13. Tooth-bearing distal segment is advanced, and the condyle of the proximal segment is postured in its preoperative position. When the resulting cortical defect is as predicted from preoperative planning, an inferior border wire may be placed for stabilization of segments: **(A)** lateral and **(B)** medial views.

Postoperative Management

Splint therapy should not be necessary after orthognathic surgery unless the occlusion is not as expected. Physical therapy is used differently based on the employment of rigid fixation, IMF, and maxillary versus mandibular surgery.

Physical therapy after rigid fixation has no specific parameters but is customized to each case. Limitations on ROM after mandibular rigid fixation cases can be due to intracapsular or extracapsular restriction. Intracapsularly, the condyle–disc–fossa relationship may be altered in any of the three planes of space or a combination of them. The condyle may be torqued bodily, moved laterally or medially, or altered vertically in the fossa. It is assumed that small changes in these planes will be tolerated and adapted. However, in exercising the joint, it must be realized that the possibility exists that the joint will not be fully able to adapt to some changes mentioned above and that it will take time to adapt to others. The most likely limitation in the extracapsular area is that of the temporalis attachment to the coronoid process and the overlying mucosal scar. This situation exists with all intraoral mandibular surgeries regardless of the fixation, but with rigid fixation, the stretching of the scar and muscle can begin earlier. It is thought that a period of at least 6 to 8 weeks is required for initial healing after mandibular rigid fixation cases. Therefore, only light ROM exercises are recommended during this period. These are accomplished by encouraging the patient to open and close routinely and to attempt side-to-side movements. A soft diet that excludes any hard or chewy foods is necessary during this period. By 6 to 8 weeks, patients should have an MIO of 30 mm or greater and laterals of 8 mm or greater. At this time, definite active and passive exercises can be instituted on an individual basis, depending on need.

With IMF cases, the clock is pushed back 6 to 8 weeks but will include similar exercises at that time. Although not proven, it is suspected that IMF cases should have less possibility of condylar changes but more problems with scarring and temporalis muscle fibrosis. Additionally, there may be some reversible atrophic changes in the joint that will take a few weeks to rebound.

After release of IMF, mobilization procedures should begin immediately and continue for at least 4 to 6 months. The probable cause for decreased mobility is scarring and contracture of the temporalis tendon. Moreover, the TMJ has been immobile, causing some decreased extensibility of the capsule and supporting ligaments. Studies[60] show that, with proper postoperative exercises performed for a sufficient length of time, mandibular mobility can be regained after sagittal-split osteotomy of the mandible.

With maxillary cases in which no mandibular surgery or IMF is used, regardless of fixation technique, the only limitation to motion would be masticatory muscle involvement related to the changed occlusion. Therefore, if a patient is experiencing significant difficulty with ROM, the treating orthodontist should be altered to the possibility of myofascial involvement, and either splint therapy or orthodontic alteration in the occlusion should be considered.

Physical therapy to assist with the myofascial limitation would be the same as for any other patient with this diagnosis except that there must be an awareness that the maxilla may not tolerate strong forces against it for 6 to 8 weeks. Modalities aimed at relaxing the muscles are important here. Joint noises after orthognathic surgery may increase, decrease, or remain the same. Each should be handled as one would with a de novo patient. If the joint noises are painful or restrictive, measures may be necessary just as with other patients; otherwise, the patient should be reassured and treatment continued. It has been very unusual in my experience for postoperative internal derangements to appear unless they were present preoperatively.

Relapse after surgical advancement of the mandible has been reported[61] by authors over the years and is believed to be caused by several factors. Clearly, previous studies[61] and my own experience show that one of the primary factors has been improper positioning of the proximal segment at the time of surgery. For instance, chronic shortening of the lateral pterygoid muscles may have occurred before surgery as the result of a patient's constant forward posturing of the mandible. This may not be detected in the surgical workup or at the time of surgery. The shortened lateral pterygoid muscles will not permit full intraoperative seating of the condyles. Therefore, if the patient is wired or fixed with rigid screw fixation in this position with the condyle slightly out of the glenoid fossa, the amount of actual bony advancement of the mandible will be insufficient. Later, once the patient is released from IMF or from training elastics, functional factors influencing jaw position may permit relaxation of the lateral pterygoid muscles, which would seat the condyles and lead to "immediate" surgical relapse. I believe that this is the overwhelming major cause for "relapse" in mandibular advancement surgery. Other factors that obviously play a role are the muscular attachments to the mandible, such as the suprahyoid musculature, that resist advancement. This is especially true when the mandible is advanced and rotated to close an open bite.[62] Devices and techniques have been developed to control these soft tissue restraints on the advanced mandible; however, no consensus has been reached on successful treatment.

After orthognathic surgery, if mandibular hypomobility occurs, a diagnosis must be made as to the cause of the hypomobility. Chronic muscle shortening, muscle or tendon scarring and contracture, fibrosis of the TMJ capsule, fibrous or bony ankylosis, and pain all contribute to mandibular hypomobility. Methods to improve mobility should be aimed at overcoming the etiology while protecting vulnerable or recently operated structures.

Complications

Complications after orthognathic surgery include hypomobility, numbness of the face in the distribution of the maxillary and mandibular branches of cranial nerve V, and some muscle atrophy caused by disuse. Hypomobility is discussed above. There is little that can be done about numbness except reassurance and time. The muscle atrophy that occurs, especially with IMF, is reversible and is usually not a problem if the patient is compliant with postoperative instructions. In some cases, long-term physical therapy may be required to return these patients to an acceptable ROM.

The TMJ–Orthognathic Patient

Many TMD patients have significant orthognathic discrepancies, and in turn, orthognathic patients may have clinical or subclinical TMD signs or symptoms. Timing and sequencing of treatment will vary according to the chief complaint and the goals of treatment. If TMD complaints are significant enough to require attention rather than observation, they should be addressed by the appropriate means before treatment is initiated to alter the occlusion. This may involve nonsurgical means or in some patients may require arthrotomy. In these cases, at least 6 months should elapse between arthrotomy and orthognathic surgery. Another subgroup exists of patients that have some TMD signs or symptoms but are primarily orthognathic. TMD conditions should be minimized preoperatively and a candid discussion held with the patient regarding the postoperative possibilities. After this, orthognathic surgery can proceed with caution.

CONCLUSION

Splint therapy plays several roles in surgery of the jaws. Anterior reposition splints can reduce a displaced disc. This may indicate whether the primary problem is intracapsular or extracapsular. If disc reduction equals pain relief, then the problem is probably intracapsular.

CR splints are most valuable in decreasing muscle pain pre- and postoperatively regardless of the type of surgery. Also if a patient has a malocclusion that is causing MMD, relief with a CR splint may indicate that correction of the malocclusion would give the same degree of relief given by the splint.

Physical therapy is an integral component of management of mandibular and cervical spine myofascial pain before and after TMJ surgery and of restoration of mandibular dynamics after intracapsular TMJ or orthognathic surgery on the mandible. The specific therapy regimen and goals are dependent on the preoperative diagnosis, the pre-existing muscular and osseous anatomic limitations, the patient's emotional status, the type and success of the surgical intervention and adjunctive therapy, and patient cooperation. The frequent and free interchange of information between surgeon and physical therapist is of paramount importance for the successful management of the oral and maxillofacial surgical patient.

REFERENCES

1. Annandale T: On displacement of the interarticular cartilage of the lower jaw and its treatment by operation. Lancet 1:411, 1887
2. Dingman RO, Constant E: A fifteen year experience with temporomandibular joint disorders: evaluation of 140 cases. Plast Reconstr Surg 44:119, 1969

3. Dingman RO, Dingman DL, Lawrence RA: Surgical correction of lesions of temporomandibular joints. Plast Reconstr Surg 55:335, 1975
4. Poswillo DE: Surgery of the temporomandibular joint. Oral Sci Rev 6:87, 1974
5. Henny FA, Baldridge OL: Condylectomy for the persistently painful temporomandibular joint. J Oral Surg 15:214, 1957
6. McCarty WL, Farra WB: Surgery for internal derangements of the temporomandibular joint. J Prosthet Dent 42:191, 1979
7. Weinberg S: Eminectomy and meniscorrhaphy for internal derangements of the temporomandibular joint. Oral Surg 57:241, 1984
8. Walker RV, Kalamchi S: A surgical technique for management of internal derangements of the temporomandibular joint. J Oral Maxillofac Surg 45:299, 1987
9. Pringle J: Displacement of the mandibular meniscus and its treatment. Br J Surg 6:385, 1918
10. Ward TG, Smith DC, Sommar M: Condylotomy for mandibular joint arthrosis. Br Dent J 103:147, 1947
11. Homsy CA, Kent JN, Hinds EC: Materials for oral implantation—biology and functional criteria. J Am Dent Assoc 86:817, 1973
12. Narang R, Dixon RA: Temporomandibular joint arthroplasty with fascia lata. Oral Surg 39:45, 1975
13. Timmel R, Grundschober F: The interposition of Lyodura in operations of ankylosis of the temporomandibular joint. An experimental study using pigs. J Maxillofac Surg 10:193, 1982
14. Witsenburg B, Freihofer HPM: Replacement of the pathological temporomandibular disc using autogenous cartilage of the external ear. Int J Oral Surg. 13:401, 1984
15. Gallagher DM, Wolford LM: Comparison of Silastic and Proplast implants in the temporomandibular joint after condylectomy for osteoarthritis. J Oral Maxillofac Surg 40:627, 1982
16. Tucker MR, Jacoway JR, White RP Jr: Autogenous dermal grafts for repair of temporomandibular joint disc perforations. J Oral Maxillofac Surg 44:781, 1986
17. Bays RA, Helmy E, Sharawy M: The synovial membrane flap for the repair of TMJ disc perforations in *Macaca* fascicularis: a stereometric study, abstracted. American Association of Oral and Maxillofacial Surgery annual meeting, Washington, DC, 1985
18. Feinberg SE, Larsen PE: The use of a pedicled temporalis muscle–pericranial flap for replacement of the TMJ disc: preliminary report. J Oral Maxillofac Surg 47: 142, 1989
19. Hall HD: Meniscectomy for damaged discs of the temporomandibular joint. South Med J 78:569, 1985
20. Upton LG, Sullivan SM: The treatment of temporomandibular joint internal derangements using a modified open condylotomy: a preliminary report. J Oral Maxillofac Surg 49:578, 1991
21. Montgomery MT, Van Sickels JE, Harms SE, Trash WJ: Arthroscopic TMJ surgery: effect of signs, symptoms, and disk position. J Oral Maxillofac Surg 47:1263, 1989
22. Conway WF, Hayes CW, Campbell RL, et al: Temporomandibular joint after meniscoplasty· appearance at MR imaging. Radiology 180:749, 1991
23. Agerberg G, Carlsson GE: The symptoms of functional disturbances of the masticatory system: a comparison of frequencies in population sample and in a group of patients. Acta Odontol Scand 33:183, 1975

24. Dolwick MF, Nitzon DW, Heft MW: TMJ disc surgery: 8 year follow-up evaluation. J Dent Res 68:310, 1989
25. Bays RA: Temporomandibular joint meniscus repair surgery: a follow-up study. Fac Orthop Temporomandib Arthrol 2:11, 1985
26. Travell JG, Simons DG: Myofascial Pain and Dysfunction: The Trigger Point Manual. Williams & Wilkins, Baltimore, 1983
27. Omnell KA: Historical review of temporomandibular joint arthrography. p. 1. In Moffett BC, Westesson PL (eds): Diagnosis of Internal Derangements of the Temporomandibular Joint. Vol. 1: Double Contrast Arthrography and Clinical Correlation. University of Washington, Seattle, 1984
28. Roberts D, Pettigrew J, Lewis B et al: Differentiation of the TMJ meniscus in CT sections. J Dent Res (special issue) 63:228, 1984
29. Wilkinson T, Maryniuk G: The correlation between sagittal anatomic sections and computerized tomography of the TMJ. J Craniomandib Pract 1:37, 1983
30. Helmy E, Bays R, Devkota J, Sharawy M: Correlation of TMJ true planes and reconstructed planes of computed tomography (CT) to anatomical sections, abstracted. American Association of Oral and Maxillofacial Surgery annual meeting, Washington, DC, 1985
31. Harms SE, Wilk RM, Wolford LM et al: The temporomandibular joint: magnetic resonance imaging using surface coils. Radiology 157:133, 1985
32. McNeill C: Nonsurgical management. p. 193. In Helms CA, Katzberg RW, Dolwick MF (eds): Internal Derangements of the Temporomandibular Joint. Radiology Research and Education Foundation, San Francisco, 1983
33. Roth RH: Temporomandibular pain dysfunction and occlusal relationships. Angle Orthod 43:136, 1973
34. Williamson EH, Steinke RN, Morse TK, Swift TR: Centric relation: a comparison of muscle determined position and operator guidance. Am J Orthod 77:133, 1980
35. Dolwick MS et al: 1984 Criteria for TMJ meniscus surgery. Am Assoc Oral Maxillofac Surg 1984
36. Salter RB: Regeneration of articular cartilage through continuous passive motion. Past, present and future. p. 101. In Staub R, Wilson PD (eds): Clinical Trends in Orthopedics. Thieme Stratton, New York, 1982
37. Krough-Poulsen W: The significance of occlusion in temporomandibular function and dysfunction. In Solburg WK, Clark GT (eds): Temporomandibular Joint Problems: Biologic Diagnosis and Treatment. Quintessence Publishers, Chicago, 1980
38. Wilkes CH: Structural and functional alterations of the temporomandibular joint. North West Dentistry 57:287, 1978
39. Silver CN, Simon SD: Meniscus injuries of the temporomandibular joint. J Bone Joint Surg 38:541, 1956
40. Helmy E, Bays RA, Sharawy M: Microscopic alterations in the TMJ of the adult monkey, abstracted. American Association of Oral and Maxiollofacial Surgery annual meeting, New York, 1984
41. Oberg T, Carlsson GE, Fajers C: Temporomandibular joint, a morphological study on human autopsy material. Acta Odontol Scand 29:349, 1971
42. Wallace D, Laskin DM: Healing of surgical defects in retrodiscal tissue of rabbit temporomandibular joint. J Dent Res 866, 1984
43. Bowman K: Temporomandibular joint arthrosis and its treatment by extirpation of the disc. Acta Chir Scand, 95(suppl):118, 1947
44. Georgiade N: The surgical correction of temporomandibular joint dysfunction by means of autogenous dermal grafts. Plast Reconstr Surg 30:68, 1962

45. Gordon S: Surgery of the temporomandibular joint. Am J Surg 95:263, 1958
46. Stewart LR: Histology of host response to alloplastic condylar implants in *Macaca fascicularis*, abstracted. American Association of Oral and Maxillofacial Surgery annual meeting, New York, 1984
47. Timmis D, Aragon SB, VanSickels JE, Aufdemorte TB: A compared study of alloplastic TMJ meniscal replacements in rabbits, abstracted. American Association of Oral and Maxillofacial Surgery annual meeting, Washington, DC, 1985
48. Wade M, Gatto D, Florine B: Assessment of Proplast implants and meniscoplasties as TMJ surgical procedures. p. 28. In: Case Reports and Outlines of Scientific Sessions, 68th Annual Meeting AAOMS, New Orleans, 1987
49. Wilkes CH: Surgical treatment of internal derangements of the temporomandibular joint. Arch Otolaryngol Head Neck Surg 117:64, 1991
50. Kaban LB: Congenital and acquired growth abnormalities of the temporomandibular joint. p. 55. In Keith DA (ed): Surgery of the Temporomandibular Joint. Blackwell Scientific Publications, Boston, 1988
51. Kent GN, Misieck DJ, Akin RK et al: TMJ condylar prosthesis, a 10 year report. J Oral Maxillofac Surg 41:245, 1983
52. Hullihen SP: Case of elongation of the under jaw and distortion of the face and neck, caused by a burn, successfully treated. Am J Dent Sci 9:157, 1849
53. Langenbeck B: Bietrage zur Osteoplastik–Die osteoplastische Resektion des OberKiefers. In Goschen A (ed): Deutsche Klinik. Reimer, Berlin, 1859
54. Wassmund M: Lehrbuch der probleschen. Cherurgie des Mundes und der Keifer. Vol 1. Meusser, Leipzig, 1935
55. Axhauser G: Zur Behandelung veralteter desloziert verheilter OberKieferbruche. Dtsch Zahn Mund Kieferheilkd I:334, 1934
56. Dibbets JM, van der Weele LT, Uildriks AK: Symptoms of TMJ dysfunction: indicators of growth patterns? J Pedodontics 9:265, 1985
57. Aragon SB, VanSickels JE, Dolwick MF, Flanary CM: The effects of orthognathic surgery on mandibular range of motion. J Oral Maxillofac Surg 43:938, 1985
58. Singer RS, Bays RA: A comparison between superior and inferior border wiring techniques in sagittal split ramus osteotomy. J Oral Maxillofac Surg 43:448, 1985
59. Spitzer W, Rettinger G, Sitzmann F: Computerized tomography examination for the detection of positional changes in the temporomandibular joint after ramus osteotomies with screw fixation. J Maxillofac Surg 12:139, 1984
60. Bell WH, Gonyea W, Finn RA et al: Muscular rehabilitation after orthognathic surgery. Oral Surg 56:229, 1983
61. Schendel FA, Epker BN: Results after mandibular advancement surgery: analysis of the 87 cases. J Oral Surg 38:265, 1980
62. Proffit WR, Bell WH: Openbite. p. 1075. In Bell WH, Proffit WR, White RP (eds): Surgical Correction of Dentofacial Deformities. WB Saunders, Philadelphia, 1980

10 | Postoperative Physical Therapy Protocols

Postarthroscopic Surgery

Jeffrey S. Mannheimer

As a physical therapist actively involved in the evaluation and treatment of patients with cervical disorders and TMDs, I have seen a significant change in the number of open joint surgical procedures performed during the past 3 years. I attribute this to the advances made in arthroscopic surgery of the TMJ.

Before the advent of TMJ arthroscopy, postsurgical referrals were usually seen no earlier than 2 weeks and at times as late as 6 weeks. This patient population was thus in the subacute to chronic stage of which a significant percentage presented with concomitant hypomobility and end-range discomfort. A longer rehabilitation process was therefore needed to restore the patient to a functional and pain-free status.

Arthroscopy has changed this course dramatically in that patients are now seen 24 to 48 hours postsurgery while they are still in the acute inflammatory stage. Intervention is thus initiated early in the postoperative course, which has resulted in a major decrease in the length of the rehabilitative process. In conjunction with this, the need for arthrotomies has also been reduced.

For the physical therapist to properly manage the patient who presents in an acute inflammatory stage, a knowledge of the presurgical status is of utmost importance. This necessitates at least one preoperative visit in which a comprehensive assessment of the patient's TMJs, muscles of mastication, and cervical spine is performed.

PREOPERATIVE VISIT

The physical therapist must have the opportunity to evaluate the patient before any surgical procedure unless it is an emergency case caused by acute trauma. When arthroscopy is to be performed for a patient whom the physical therapist has already been treating, one can assume that a definitive evaluation has already been completed.[1-3] However, a recent survey has shown that 15 of 27 physical therapists who specialize in the treatment of TMD receive greater than 50 percent of their postoperative referrals without the benefit of a preoperative visit. Twenty-five of the 27 therapists believed that a preoperative evaluation was necessary to obtain baseline data and functional status before postoperative management.[4] This is considered to be a significant hindrance to the initiation of proper postsurgical management.

Specifically, it is important for the physical therapist to have subjective and objective data relative to pain, mandibular dynamics, joint sounds, end feel, muscle function, and parafunctional habits. The feeling that an experienced physical therapist perceives when performing an intraoral joint mobilization assessment and thorough evaluation of the entire neuromuscular system is extremely valuable in the setting of short- and long-term goals after arthroscopy.

A patient who presents presurgically with a long history of hypomobility and a hard end feel will need to be managed differently in the postoperative course than one with a history of reciprocal clicking and normal mandibular range of motion (ROM) who developed an acute disc displacement without reduction. It is my experience as well as that of others that the patient with an acute disc displacement without reduction and short history of symptoms requires a much shorter postoperative course and quickly regains functional status.[5]

The patient with a long history of hypomobility not only has developed adhesions in the superior joint compartment but also presents with capsular fibrosis and contracture of the mandibular elevators. Thus, although an arthroscopic lysis and lavage of the adhesions is performed, soft tissue restriction of the capsule, temporalis, masseter, and medial pterygoids will produce a postoperative hindrance to a rapid functional restoration.

A presurgical evaluation would provide the physical therapist with all the data necessary to alter the postoperative management course with additional procedures geared to such a patient. One example that necessitates a change in the postoperative protocol relative to manual joint mobilization and therapeutic exercise techniques is the presence of a presurgical deflection or early translation involving the surgical or nonsurgical joint. Postoperatively, the patient may present with hypomobility caused by pain, inflammation, and reflex muscle guarding sufficient to minimize these abnormal movement patterns, and the physical therapist may begin to mobilize the hypermobile joint to the same degree as the hypomobile joint.

Table 10-1 outlines the main factors that need to be determined by the presurgical evaluation relative to the cause of abnormal mandibular dynamics

Table 10-1. Therapeutic Guidelines for Correction of Mandibular Deviation/
Deflection: Initial Evaluation

(Determine Etiology/Precautions/Contraindications [Precipitating Factors])

Deviation ↔ Deflection
Hypermobility ↔ Hypomobility
Anterior disc dislocation w/o reduction ↔ Muscular trismus
Structural abnormality ↔ Adhesions
Neurologic ↔ Systemic
Acute ↔ Chronic
Nonsurgical ↔ Surgical

so that an individualized postoperative protocol can be developed by an experienced physical therapist. Management precautions for this specific situation are addressed later in this chapter.

It is not uncommon for a physical therapist with extensive experience in the evaluation and treatment of TMD to perform a presurgical evaluation on a patient whom they have not previously treated and determine that arthroscopy may not be needed. This situation may arise after performing manual intraoral joint mobilization in all excursions, which is followed by having the patient actively open to end range and observing a significant increase in opening, close to functional range without joint sounds that was not seen at the beginning of the evaluation. Questioning the patient about this reveals that specific treatment including intraoral joint mobilization, manual soft tissue techniques, and therapeutic exercises were never performed. Treatment may merely have consisted of palliative modalities and/or appliance therapy. Also, the patient may not have been referred to a physical therapist with experience in the area of TMD.[4] Such a patient is an excellent candidate for a definitive physical therapy program as is discussed within this text and may not require arthroscopic surgery.

Table 10-2 outlines various other factors that may come to light during the preoperative assessment that may also negate the need for arthroscopy. Table 10-3 highlights the comprehensive management techniques that an experienced physical therapist will perform with proper dental intervention when arthroscopy is not indicated.

The therapist must also ensure that the patient has a proper joint stabilization appliance to be used postoperatively. A stabilization appliance is of utmost importance to decompress the TMJs in the presence of reflex muscle guarding, pain, and inflammation to minimize adverse effects to the TMJs. The date of surgery should be known, and the patient should be scheduled for the

Table 10-2. Indications that May Negate Need for Arthroscopy

Cervical spine disorder is a source of referred pain to the head, face, jaw areas
Active TMJ ROM increases significantly as a result of the preoperative evaluation
Patient has not had "proper" physical therapy
Cervical spine disorder is a contributing source to masticatory muscle hyperactivity
Hypermobility with end-range pain that may be able to be managed by a specific therapeutic
  exercise program

Table 10-3. Comprehensive Management Techniques In Lieu Of Arthroscopy

Instruction and education in cervical spine postural corrective techniques
Definitive hypomobility protocol of joint mobilization and therapeutic exercise
Manual muscle and soft tissue techniques to the sub-occipital and craniofacial areas
Patient compliance with home program and diet

initial postoperative visit 24 to 48 hours after arthroscopy. The therapist should also discuss the postoperative protocol with the patient and the need for compliance with the home exercise program and maintenance of a soft food diet.

INITIAL POSTOPERATIVE VISIT

When indicated, successful arthroscopic surgery increases the ability of the physical therapist to restore a functional and pain-free ROM of the TMJs. A prime hindering factor to the restoration of functional mobility of the TMJ is the formation of adhesions and soft tissue restriction.[6] The procedures most often used with TMJ arthroscopy consist of a lysis and lavage of adhesions in the superior joint compartment and a degree of mandibular mobilization under anesthesia.[7]

After arthroscopy, there are patients who rapidly regain normal TMJ motion and thus need minimal physical therapy intervention. This is most often the case with patients who had no other associated hindering factors such as cervical spine influences or masticatory muscle hyperactivity such as bruxism and did not present with long-term hypomobility.[8,9]

The initial postoperative visit optimally occurs within 24 hours after arthroscopy and preferably before 48 hours have elapsed. When a physical therapist is present in the hospital during the immediate recovery stage, intervention may commence within 2 to 3 hours of surgery.[7] Early intervention is needed to decrease the typical inflammation that occurs causing the patient to present with edema, reflex muscle guarding, and increased discomfort. These factors carry the potential for the reformation of adhesions and concomitant contracture of the mandibular elevator muscles. This will ultimately serve to prolong the postoperative course, which typically lasts 6 to 8 weeks.[10,11]

It is extremely valuable to the physical therapist to receive a telephone call or surgical notes from the oral surgeon before the initial postoperative visit to discuss the operative findings and the procedures used. Because of the recent advances in TMJ arthroscopy, procedures such as removal of loose bodies, electrocautery, anterior band release, or suturing of the disc to the posterolateral capsule may have been performed in addition to a lysis and lavage.[12] For the patient to obtain the initial postoperative treatment within 24 to 48 hours, arthroscopy should be performed early in the week. Table 10-4 lists suggestions for oral surgeons to optimize the postsurgical phase.

The physical therapist must perform a short postoperative assessment of the patient, before the initiation of treatment to establish baseline pain, edema, and ROM levels. Figure 10-1 is an evaluation form developed by this author

Table 10-4. Suggestions for Oral Surgeons

Refer the patient to a physical therapist with experience in treating craniomandibular disorders for a preoperative evaluation

Perform arthroscopic surgery early in the week to allow for intervention by the physical therapist within 24 to 48 hours

Make sure that the patient has and brings with them a joint stabilization appliance to be inserted in the recovery room

Inform the physical therapist of the arthroscopic findings and procedures performed before the patient's initial postoperative treatment

---

DELAWARE VALLEY PHYSICAL THERAPY ASSOCIATES

INITIAL TMJ POST. OPERATIVE ASSESSMENT

Surgical Procedure: _____   R   L
Surgical Date: _____
Patient: _____   Today's Date: _____

Pain	0-----------------------10
Edema	*Mild*
	Mod
	Max
Sensation	*R* *L*
Facial Nerve	
Integrity	*R* *L*
Active	
ROM	*Vert*
	R Lat
	L Lat
	Pro
Joint Sounds	

Specific Comments:_____

_____P.T.

Fig. 10-1. Evaluation form for recording initial postoperative assessment.

to record these data as well as to determine sensory changes, facial nerve integrity, presence of joint sounds, or other specific findings.

Figures 10-2 and 10-3 illustrate the degree of edema after an arthroscopic lysis and lavage procedure. Patients who undergo more extensive arthroscopic work may present with greater postoperative inflammation. Patients are initially provided with a compressive wrapping and ice packs while in the hospital and may use it for the first 24 hours to inhibit the degree of edema. Figure 10-3 (patient X) depicts the external stapling used to anchor a small Fogarty arterial embolectomy balloon placed in the anterior superior joint compartment, which is a relatively new adjunctive procedure.[13] This is used to maintain the anterior joint space, hinder the reformation of adhesions, and keep the disc from sliding anteriorly. These are removed within the first 5 to 10 postoperative days (Hoffman D: personal communication).[14] The balloon is inflated with 75 ml water. Both patients were seen within 24 hours of arthroscopy.

Patients with moderate to significant edema present indications to begin treatment with techniques that enhance fluid reduction and decrease reflex muscle guarding. The inflammatory process is compounded by retained metabolites and/or hemarthrosis. All the aforementioned sequelae can lead to impeded circulation and lymphatic drainage that will hinder the healing process, increase pain, and promote restriction to movement.[15]

The degree of irrigation that is required during arthroscopy can furthermore lead to an elevation of intracapsular pressure causing extravasation of

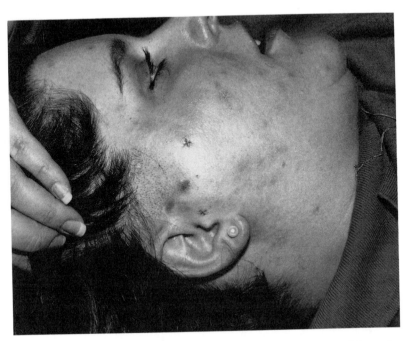

Fig. 10-2. Patient with typical degree of edema 24 hours status post-bilateral arthroscopic surgery. Note two entry portals, each with one suture in place.

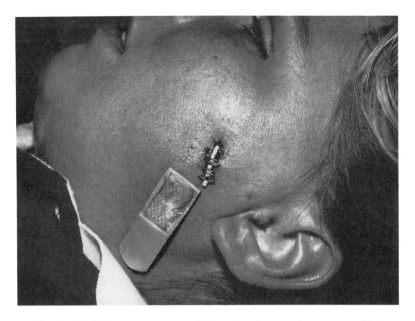

Fig. 10-3. Patient X 24 hours status post-bilateral arthroscopic surgery with temporary protective embolectomy balloon implant.

fluid into the interstitial spaces of surrounding tissues. This can create increased pain and peripheral nerve compression. The facial nerve is most commonly involved, producing functional deficit of the frontalis and perhaps related musculature. Usually fluid extravasation subsides within the first 3 to 7 postoperative days and is minimal in the hands of an experienced surgeon.[16]

Peripheral nerve compression caused by extravasation may also involve the auriculotemporal branch of the trigeminal nerve causing paresthesia or sensory loss. The lingual nerve may be involved by fluid compression in the pterygomandibular space, producing numbness of the tongue.[16] The arthroscope itself or a cannula may also damage the facial nerve.

THE SPECIFIC ROLE OF ADJUNCTIVE MODALITIES

Transcutaneous electrical nerve stimulation (TENS) and pulsed ultrasound are adjunctive modalities that have a specific role in the acute stage to increase circulation, enhance metabolite interchange, and decrease muscle guarding and pain.[15,17,18]

It is imperative that it be understood that these modalities are to be used adjunctively when indicated as part of a comprehensive treatment and not as a single modality approach. The therapeutic paradigms to be presented consist of a logical sequential approach based on patient status and treatment goals. This cannot be accomplished solely by repetitive applications of single or dual modalities.[15,17,19]

Figure 10-4 illustrates the method by which TENS can be used to provide for slow, rhythmic contraction and relaxation of the temporalis and masseter muscles bilaterally.[17,20] Small circular or square electrodes must be used that conform to the anterior temporalis and masseter on each side. Independent channels are used so that the intensity of contraction can be adjusted separately at either the right or left side. Bilateral stimulation is necessary even in the presence of unilateral surgery to ensure physiologic movement of the mandible. Resistance (impedance) to the passage of electricity through the skin is increased by edema but decreased by muscle guarding because of its hyperactive state and may also be altered by the type of electrode and interface material.[17] The intensity of stimulation will therefore vary from side to side, necessitating different amplitudes usually ranging between 10 to 30 mA because the interelectrode distance is quite small.[17] Optimal stimulation parameters consist of a frequency of 1 Hz, pulse width of 75 to 100 μsec, and amplitude to the point of mild visible and rhythmic mandibular elevation without tooth or appliance contact. These specific parameters have been shown to produce reflex vasodilation and decrease muscle guarding, thereby enhancing circulation and lymphatic drainage.[17]

TENS performed in this manner is not designed to produce pain relief as

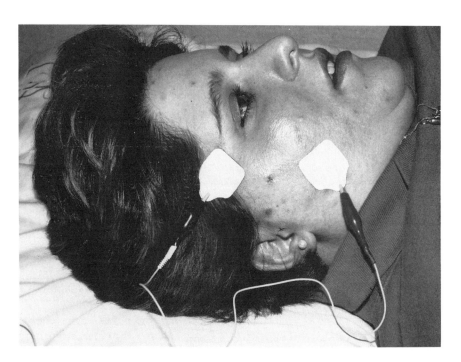

Fig. 10-4. Patient 24 hours status post-bilateral arthroscopic surgery with TENS electrodes in place on the anterior temporalis and masseter. Similiar electrode array for a second channel exists on the opposite side.

its prime goal but to enhance the healing process by reducing the effects of inflammation. Occasionally, it may be suggested for home use, but it is not necessary if the patient can properly perform mild reciprocal isometric contractions. Secondary pain relief may, however, occur. The procedure is not necessary with patients who have minimal edema or the ability to actively move the mandible without discomfort in the acute stage. It is used for 15 to 30 minutes at the start of treatment during the first to third visits if needed. The patient should be in a supine position with the head and neck properly supported. Mild stimulation of the eye musculature may occur because of the proximity of the anterior temporalis electrodes. These should be maintained as far away from the eye as possible as long as they are placed over the anterior temporalis and current overflow is minimized by the use of small electrodes about the size of a nickel or quarter.

Specific contraindications consist of epilepsy, transient ischemic attacks, and postcerebrovascular accidents. Other indications for the use of TENS, for instance as a means of pain control at home, have previously been presented.[15,17,21]

Another adjunctive modality that may be used in the acute inflammatory stage is low-intensity pulsed ultrasound. Again, the use of this modality requires parameters that negate a thermal effect and provide for a physiologic action designed to enhance the healing process. Nonthermal effects of low-intensity pulsed ultrasound are produced by the movement of fluids along cell membranes by mechanical pressure of the ultrasound wave and is called acoustic streaming.[18] Studies have shown this method to produce an increase in cell membrane and vascular wall permeability with enhanced blood flow. However, the physiologic effect of pulsed ultrasound on plasma extravasation varies with the duration and number of applications. Previous research with ultrasound and its effect on tissue repair and inflammation is mixed. Other studies have shown mast cell degranulation produced by low-intensity ultrasound in the acute stage that has been shown to enhance tissue repair or cause further damage.[17,22] Additional studies are thus needed to clarify this process.

It is clear that the physiologic effect of pulsed ultrasound is very dependent on the delivery parameters and slow movement of the soundhead. Optimally, due to the small area of application, a 5-cm or less soundhead should be used at the TMJ region to prevent sonation of the eye. A frequency of 3 MHz and low intensity of 0.5 W/cm^2 not to exceed 0.8 W/cm^2 is optimal. Because the TMJ is a superficial joint and depth of ultrasonic energy is frequency-dependent, most absorption occurs at 1 to 2 cm below the skin surface with 3 MHz.[18]

Figure 10-5 illustrates the application of 3-MHz pulsed ultrasound in the acute postoperative stage. Once inflammation has been reduced, usually after 1 week, this is discontinued. Treatment time is 3 minutes, not to exceed 5 minutes when the area of edema is greater. Care must be taken to keep the soundhead away from the eyes and to avoid usage in the presence of a malignancy or impaired circulation and over epiphyseal growth plates in children.[15,18,23] Both the application site and soundhead should be cleaned with alcohol before treatment. Sonation can be applied in the presence of postar-

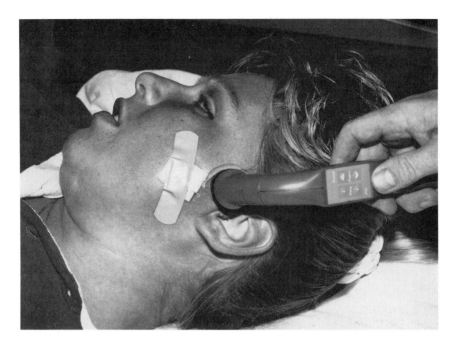

Fig. 10-5.   Application of 3-MHz pulsed ultrasound in the acute inflammatory stage in patient X.

throscopic sutures as long as the site is not weeping. In summary, low-intensity pulsed ultrasound at a frequency of 3 MHz is commonly used as an adjunctive technique for short-term application in the acute stage after TMJ arthroscopy.[4] Further research specific to this modality is, however, indicated.

Manual techniques applied to the TMJ, facial, and/or cervical spine areas can be performed in lieu of one or both modalities or immediately after them. Many times neither TENS nor pulsed ultrasound is needed, and manual treatment will commence immediately after a short postoperative assessment. Figure 10-6 (patient X) depicts the measurement of active vertical opening before the administration of 3-MHz pulsed ultrasound.

The treatment sequence continues with manual intraoral joint mobilization techniques designed to inhibit reformation of adhesions, decompress the TMJ, enhance synovial lubrication, promote muscle relaxation, and restore a functional ROM (see Ch. 7).[24,25] Joint mobilization techniques must be performed gently and slowly within the pain-free range to both TMJs even in the presence of unilateral surgery. The nonsurgical side may also have soft tissue hypomobility caused by long-standing dysfunction.

Specific techniques consist of long-axis distraction and lateral glides. Care must be taken to minimize early translation to not stress the retrodiscal tissue and collateral ligaments. Figure 10-7 depicts the initial performance of intraoral joint mobilization when vertical opening limits posterior placement of the thumb on the molar region. The specifics of joint mobilization techniques are

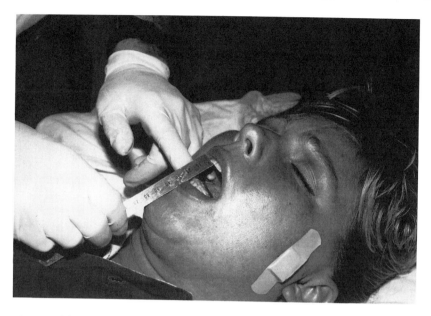

Fig. 10-6. Initial recording of active vertical opening 24 hours postarthroscopy in patient X.

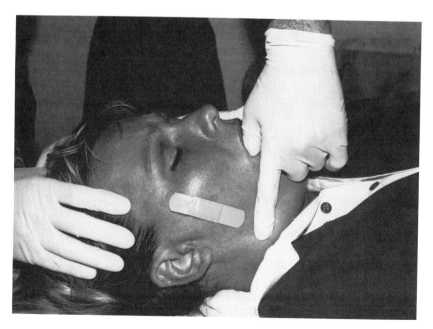

Fig. 10-7. Initial performance of intraoral joint mobilization (long-axis distraction). Decreased vertical opening limited proper thumb insertion onto posterior mandibular molars in patient X.

discussed in Chapter 7. Table 10-5 highlights specific factors relative to manual techniques.

In the presence of a significant mandibular deflection, specific precautions must be added so as not to promote this abnormal motion. A deflection is defined as tracking of the mandible to one side during active vertical or protrusive movement without correction to midline at end range. This may occur from muscle imbalance (stronger or shorter pterygoids on one side), a significant unilateral capsulitis or anteromedial disc displacement. Anteromedial disc displacement may impinge on the superior belly of the lateral pterygoid, causing pain and reflex guarding.[26] Prolonged use of an anterior repositioning appliance may also cause shortening of the superior belly of a unilateral anteromedial displaced disc producing a deflection. Table 10-6 highlights treatment considerations in the presence of mandibular deflection.

Between applications of joint mobilization techniques, gentle active exercises are performed. These must be preceded by instructing the patient in proper tongue position. It is important to also make sure that the stabilization appliance is kept in place during the performance of all procedures and adjunctive modalities, as long as it does not hinder proper thumb placement intraorally. An appliance with significant thickness may limit complete insertion of the thumb and negate positioning on the posterior arch.

One of the most important exercises is teaching the patient to open with the tip of the tongue on the palate just behind the maxillary central incisors. This serves to promote condylar rotation and inhibit early translation. It is also used to inhibit full vertical excursion during a yawn to protect the soft tissue from a fast excessive stretch. The patient is instructed to perform this exercise after each set of intraoral mobilization.

Gentle active opening and lateral exercises are performed using one or two fingers for resistance with no more than 1 lb of force. This can be taught to patients by having them press down on a letter scale. If suturing of the disc to the posterolateral capsule is performed during arthroscopy, care must be taken to minimize the degree of active lateral excursion to the opposite side

Table 10-5. Factors to Consider in Treatment of TMJ Hypomobility (Pain—Joint Sounds—ROM Changes)

Perform one mobilization technique at a time per joint
Rest inbetween with decompression techniques (active exercise, manual cranial technique, or adjunctive modality)
Limit of two to four applications of intraoral joint mobilization per treatment
Do not overtreat in office
Emphasize home program and compliance

Table 10-6. Therapeutic Guidelines for Correction of Mandibular Deflection

Do not mobilize into the direction of the deflection.
Do not strengthen into the direction of the deflection.
Perpetuation of a major deflection can lead to pathology and dysfunction of the "normal" TMJ.
The degree of correction is very dependent on the causative factors and often cannot be totally corrected.

early in the treatment course. Figure 10-8 illustrates the method of placing base plate wax around tongue depressors to minimize lateral excursion to one or both sides. The use of tubing can also be helpful in facilitating lateral movements.

There are instances when a patient has difficulty remembering how to move the mandible laterally to one side. Re-education to enhance lateral excursion can be taught by having the patient place the tip of the tongue on the last maxillary molar on the side to which movement is desired. This serves to promote movement of the mandible to the side of the tongue and is taught with the patient facing a mirror.

The application of cryotherapeutic agents also may be used adjunctively when needed for pain control or to act as a counterirritant during stretch and spray techniques. Figure 10-9 shows the placement of an Elasto-Gel pack (Southwest Technologies Inc., Kansas City, Missouri), which can easily be applied during the treatment sequence for quick pain relief. The use of a Cryostim Probe (Pelton Shepard Industries, Stockton, California), as illustrated in Figure 10-10, allows the patient to also obtain comfort at any time during the initial postoperative sessions. The specific physiologic effects of cold and its methodologies have previously been presented.[15,19]

The initial postoperative treatment ends with instruction in a home program of exercises, maintenance of a soft food diet, and postural control of the head and neck. I do not encourage any stretching beyond active exercises at home

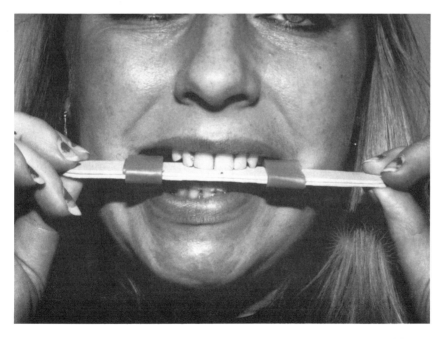

Fig. 10-8.   Performance of lateral excursion exercise with base plate wax limiting range as a safety feature.

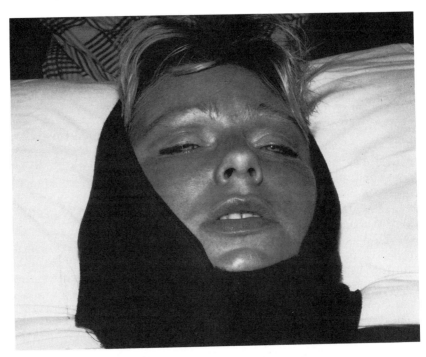

Fig. 10-9. Elasto-Gel soft ice pack.

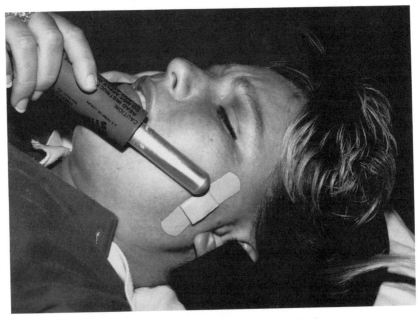

Fig. 10-10. Application of Cryostim Probe.

during the first week, except for bidigital stretching or use of the Therabite device (Therabite Corp., Bryn Mawr, Pennsylvania). Tongue-up opening and rhythmic stabilization exercises (gentle isometrics) are stressed. Patients initially perform the home program three to six times per day. Table 10-7 reviews the prime therapeutic procedures used in the management program. Table 10-8 outlines the home program, which should include a written description or illustration of each exercise. At the beginning of the postoperative course, patient X illustrated in Figure 10-6 demonstrated active vertical opening of 18 mm with 3 mm of right and 2 mm of left lateral excursion and protrusion to the edge-to-edge position. The complete initial treatment then consisted of 3-MHz pulsed ultrasound to each TMJ followed by three applications of intraoral joint mobilization and therapeutic exercise, interspersed with cold applications plus manual techniques to the facial and cervical spine muscles. The patient should also be taught various TMJ decompression techniques besides tongue-up opening, such as the "TMJ mantra." This consists of the following phrase: "tongue up (resting on the palate), teeth slightly apart, and lips together." They should repeat this phrase throughout the day to help maintain TMJ decompression.

The physical therapy armamentarium consists of many other modalities that may also be used to decrease inflammation, edema, reflex muscle guarding, and pain. These include phonophoresis, iontophoresis, and biofeedback. The specific application techniques of these procedures have previously been discussed.[15] Microcurrent electrical nerve stimulation (MENS) is a new modality that may also be used in the acute inflammatory stage. It can be administered via intraoral probes or surface electrodes to the muscles of mastication or

---

Table 10-7. Prime Therapeutic Procedures After Arthroscopic Surgery

Appliance decompression
Active—passive—resistive ROM exercise
               Extraoral
             /
Manual joint mobilization technique
            \
             Intraoral
Manual cranial and soft tissue release technique
Tongue repositioning
Postural correction of the head and neck
Soft food diet, stifle yawns, TMJ mantra
Definitive home program

Table 10-8. Day 1 Home Program (three to six times per day)

Low rate or modulated TENS (only if needed in the presence of significant edema and reflex muscle guarding)
Intermittent bidigital gentle stretching/mobilization or use of Therabite
Isometric exercises/tongue-up opening
Graded lateral excursion with one or two tongue depressors
Stabilization appliance
Postural corrective exercises for the head and neck

surrounding the area of edema for reduction of muscle guarding and inflammation, respectively.[11]

My preference for achieving therapeutic value and cost control is to make optimal use of the adjunctive modalities that are available in the respective clinics. There obviously are various therapeutic means of accomplishing physiologic goals, and an intimate knowledge of the modalities on hand should be acquired and administered in a logical sequence.

The addition of one or more adjunctive modalities is not always necessary. However, in the presence of an acute inflammatory state after arthroscopy, 3-MHz pulsed ultrasound followed by low-rate TENS is suggested as previously described. MENS may be substituted in lieu of pulsed ultrasound and TENS. To my knowledge, no study has compared the effectiveness of one method versus the other in the acute inflammatory stage, although both have shown benefit.

When muscle hyperactivity is a hindering factor, both low-rate TENS and MENS can be used. Again, however, studies have not been performed comparing one against the other in a similar patient population. Because the physiologic effects of each modality are different, research is needed to establish efficacy as well as versatility of one over the other.

SECOND AND THIRD POSTOPERATIVE VISITS

The second and third postoperative visits may either occur successively after the initial one or on the third postoperative day. I most often see the patient twice during the first week and occasionally three times if they are experiencing great discomfort and/or have significant edema with reflex muscle guarding.

The goals of the second and third postoperative visits are unchanged from the first unless a significant reduction of edema, pain, and reflex muscle guarding has occurred. Patient X presented on the third postoperative day with 14 mm of active vertical opening. She was reporting continued discomfort with a lot of bilateral craniofacial pain in the parietal, temporal, and frontal regions. Treatment was initiated with 3-MHz pulsed ultrasound followed by manual craniofacial and suboccipital techniques. Intraoral joint mobilization then was able to be performed, followed by therapeutic exercise. I have found gentle craniofacial techniques very effective in providing a quick reduction of discomfort and facilitating performance of intraoral joint mobilization.[27] They can also be performed as the patient actively moves the mandible or during stretching techniques with tongue depressors or the Therabite.

The temporary balloon implants in patient X were removed 8 days after arthroscopy, at which time minimal edema remained. The patient demonstrated active vertical opening of 25 mm at the end of treatment on the tenth postoperative day (Fig. 10-11). Intraoral joint mobilization, however, revealed that end feel was hard, and on questioning the patient about compliance with the home program that now included stretching with tongue depressors, she stated

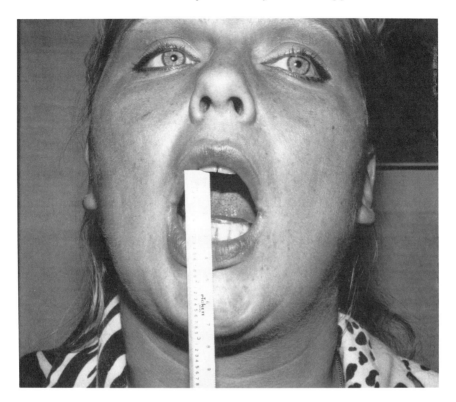

Fig. 10-11.   Recording of active vertical opening on tenth postoperative day.

that she could not perform this more than two times per day because of her home situation. I thus suggested use of the Therabite, a device that is easily inserted and can be used by the patient for short applications frequently throughout the day.

The patient continued to be seen on a two times per week basis for the next 4 weeks, with increased emphasis on compliance with her home program.

SUBACUTE STAGE

In the subacute stage, treatments may be reduced to twice per week or less depending on progression of ROM and pain reduction. The more compliant the patient is with the home program, the shorter the rehabilitation course becomes. Most patients can be discharged within 6 to 8 weeks once the goals have been reached.

I strive to obtain a pretreatment active vertical range of at least 35 mm, with 6 to 8 mm lateral and 2 to 3 mm of protrusion beyond the edge-to-edge position. In patients who have significant retrognathia or an overjet, the protrusive goal is merely to reach an edge-to-edge position. On nearing the ROM goals, stabilization exercises are increased, as is discussed elsewhere in this chapter.

In the presence of hypomobility with a relatively hard end feel, collagen bonding provides resistance to stretch. It has been shown that by heating the involved tissue to 40 to 50° C, collagen bonding decreases and stretching is easier when performed simultaneously with heat. Ultrasound is the modality of choice for this approach but must now be administered continuously for 3 to 5 minutes at an intensity between 1.0 to 1.5 W/cm², keeping the frequency for the TMJ region at 3 MHz.[15,18] Figure 10-12 illustrates the use of tongue depressors to provide a stretch during the application of continuous ultrasound. The patient uses the least number of tongue depressors needed to produce only a mild stretch and is instructed to remove or reduce the number of tongue depressors periodically if discomfort occurs. This procedure is much easier to perform with the Therabite device, as the patient can easily alter the degree of stretch if discomfort occurs or relaxation increases. Figure 10-13 illustrates the heat and stretch technique with the Therabite.

The use of moist heat before the application of the stretch is also beneficial, as depicted in Figure 10-13.[28] Stretching of this nature for periods ranging from 1 to 3 minutes is recommended in the presence of long-standing nonsurgical or postsurgical situations in which a hard end feel persists. Because of capsular fibrosis and elevator muscle contracture, home use of the Therabite has demonstrated greater compliance and ROM progression as compared with tongue depressors.[29,30]

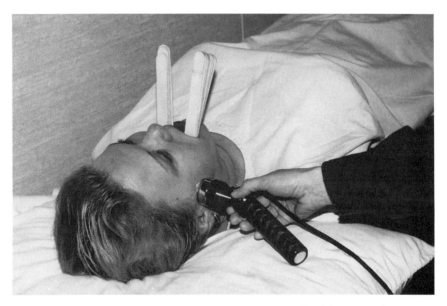

Fig. 10-12.   Continuous 3-MHz ultrasound under stretch with tongue depressors.

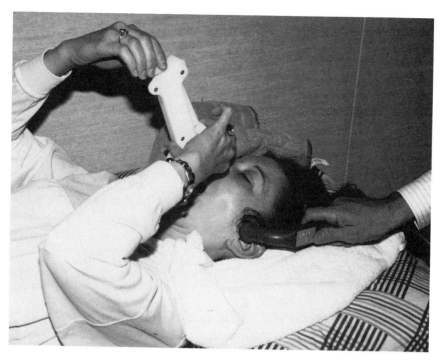

Fig. 10-13. Continuous 3-MHz ultrasound under stretch with Therabite unit. Note moist heat pack still in place on opposite side.

Home instructions for the use of the Therabite consist of gentle contract–relax then stretch techniques, or slow controlled opening to the point of mild stretch, at which point it is maintained for 3 to 10 seconds and performed for six repetitions at least three to six times per day. The patient is also instructed to perform tongue-up opening exercises before and after each set, as well as lateral and protrusive movements as needed. By adjusting the range setting arm, the therapist can ensure that vertical opening during home exercise will be limited to the point of mild stretch. This is an excellent safety feature. Figure 10-14 illustrates use of the Therabite for home exercise.

Patient X continued treatment twice per week for the first 6 weeks, after which time treatments were reduced to once per week. A root canal procedure during the rehabilitation course and continued stress at home interrupted treatment and hindered progress, but she was discharged pain-free with pretreatment ROM of 36 mm of active vertical, 6 to 7 mm of right and left lateral excursion, and 2 mm of protrusion beyond the edge-to-edge position after 3 months and 20 treatments. Figure 10-15 shows the active ROM at the time of discharge. She was instructed to continue with her home exercise program and contact me for recheck in 3 months.

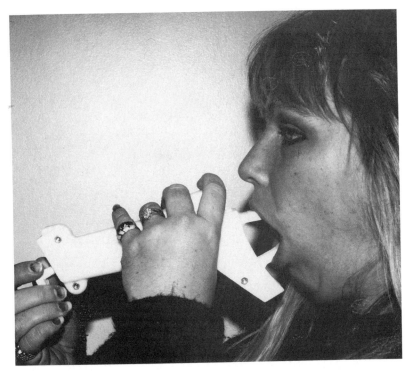

Fig. 10-14. Use of Therabite. Patient adjusting opening by use of control screw.

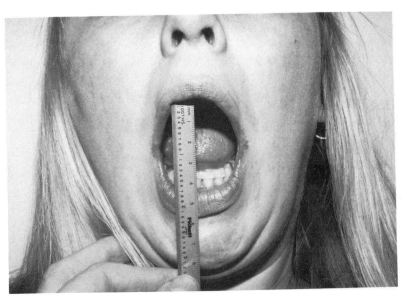

Fig. 10-15. Active vertical opening at time of discharge.

FACTORS THAT INHIBIT POSTSURGICAL PROGRESSION

Patients who do not demonstrate continuous progression usually are those with major muscle hyperactivity of both the muscles of mastication and cervical spine, which hinders normal mandibular rest position or active movement. Other factors that can hinder the rehabilitative process consist of stress, clenching or bruxism, and poor sleeping and working postures, promoting cervical and shoulder girdle strain with pain referral to the craniofacial region.[8] Occlusal abnormalities that may have been present before or that may have developed from prolonged appliance therapy are additional hindering factors.

On discharge, the patient should be instructed to contact the therapist by telephone after 3- and 6-month intervals. The soft food diet is gradually decreased, and chewing foods that do not require power strokes or wide opening is added. In addition to rhythmic stabilization exercises, a patient who has difficulty chewing because of weakness of the mandibular elevators or fatigue with slow but repetitive chewing may be placed on a conditioning program using eccentric contractions with the Therabite device. This consists of a releasing or lengthening contraction to gently inhibit the Therabite from opening. Only 1 to 2 lb of force should be applied initially by the elevator muscles as the patient slowly opens with the device. Patients who have undergone only a lysis and lavage procedure may be able to use greater elevator muscle contraction on a progressive basis if needed. In many cases, a simple graded food change or addition program may suffice. Conditioning may be facilitated more easily by gentle eccentric contractions via the Therabite, which is limited to the pain-free active vertical opening of the patient.

CONCLUSION

The treatment of patients after arthroscopic surgery requires the therapist to manage the patient in an acute stage with a mild to maximal degree of inflammation. Additional hindrances to treatment thus exist, and the use of adjunctive techniques and different management approaches is needed. Specific guidelines to enhance the rehabilitation process for the physical therapist and oral surgeon have been presented. Professional communication between both clinicians is necessary in the pre- and postoperative stage for the patient to obtain optimal benefit from this surgical procedure.

Postarthrotomy Surgery

Tom Keith

Although it is desirable, it is often not feasible for a patient to have preoperative physical therapy treatment and/or education. However, I strongly encourage therapists to develop a rapport with their referring dentists/oral surgeons to promote preoperative visits to the physical therapist. Unfortunately, preoperative visits may be restricted because of managed health care policies limiting the number of physical therapy visits.

Whenever possible, the physical therapist should see the patient within the first 3 or 4 days postoperatively to use appropriate anti-inflammatory modalities and to begin active or passive range of motion (ROM) activities when indicated.

An operative report that accurately describes the procedure performed should be requested even if a verbal conversation has been held with the surgeon. Also, a specific effort should be made to observe each of the most common surgical procedures performed by the referring oral surgeon. Operative procedures that alter muscle attachments are of particular interest in postoperative treatment. If a procedure results in detachment of a pterygoid muscle in particular, it is vital that the treating therapist be aware of this to ensure realistic goals are determined.

Contraindications for physical therapy treatment using exercises either passive (i.e., intraoral mobilization) or active are as follows:

1. Acute inflammation
2. Nonunion of fractures or reconstructive procedures of bony structures that have had inadequate healing time
3. Infection of incision site or synovial joints
4. Malignancies involving the mandible and/or temporal area
5. Hypermobility
6. Rheumatoid arthritis

Contraindications for modalities may be

1. Allergic reactions to iontophoresis and/or associated drug delivery systems
2. Seizure activity that may be initiated by electrotherapy procedures (i.e., transcranial electrical stimulation)
3. In the presence of known cardiac arrhythmias, or installed pacemaker, electrotherapy should not be performed
4. Ultrasound use may be restricted or eliminated when the patient is too young, as growth plates may be affected

Treatment aggressiveness is determined by the extent of the arthrotomy, patient age, stage of healing, degree of inflammation, and structure repaired. The individual surgeon's guidelines must be followed. If such guidelines are not available, the TMJ postarthrotomy protocol that follows will be a catalyst for discussion between the physical therapist and oral surgeon.

If a disc has been reconstructed or retrodiscal tissue repair performed, motion may be quite limited, initially allowing only condylar rotation. Usually after the fifth or sixth week postoperatively, condylar translation will be progressively and aggressively obtained.

Goal setting must be determined through consultation with the individual surgeon, which may vary significantly between practitioners. Basic goals must include reduction of pain and swelling, along with restoration of maximum function in all planes of mandibular movement. Also, duration and frequency of active physical therapy and long-term follow-up must be coordinated with maximum patient understanding of the condition and compliance with the proposed treatment plan.

Historically, when a "failure" occurs in patient care, it is often caused by an incomplete physical therapy evaluation and treatment plan. It is tempting to identify what appears to be the primary problem rather than the complex of several problems that complicates overall treatment. For example, when a patient lacks adequate central incisal opening, biomechanical function has not been restored. This may be mistaken as a problem of rotation of the condyle when instead it is a problem of a lack of translation with the condyle. Specific exercise, either passing or active, will be directed toward restoring condylar translation.

Splint therapy is usually an integral part of the patient's overall treatment. Depending on the oral surgeon's instructions, the appliance is removed only when it prevents access to intraoral mobilization procedures. Otherwise, the appliance should be used to enhance occlusal function and to minimize the effects of parafunctional activity.

In summary, when receiving a referral for postarthrotomy physical therapy, the following information is necessary:

1. Operative report
2. Any structural or anatomic changes that alter function
3. Presence of residual or possible neurologic impairment
4. Short-term and long-term goals
5. Predicted duration of treatment to achieve established goals
6. Medical history that may alter treatment

TMJ POSTARTHROTOMY PROTOCOL

Physical therapy treatment guidelines will be discussed for the following arthrotomy procedures: (1) discectomy with and without implant; and (2) disc repair including retrodiscal tissue.

Modalities commonly used with either of the above arthrotomy procedures may include any one or combination of cold packs, hot packs, ultrasound, iontophoresis, high-volt galvanic electrical stimulation (probe), and interferential electrical stimulation.

Guidelines to follow in the use of the above modalities can be found in the previous section of this chapter and in Mannheimer: Physical Therapy Concepts in Evaluation and Treatment of the Upper Quarter. In Kraus S (ed): TMJ Disorders, Management of the Craniomandibular Complex, 1st Ed., Churchill Livingstone, 1988.

Discectomy With or Without Implant

Discectomy may be performed a variety of different ways. Common procedures may include complete removal of the disc, disc replacement by Silastic implant, or auricular graft. Also, costochondral grafting may be performed.

Overall goals are to achieve at least 42 mm of central incisal opening with 12 mm of lateral excursions bilaterally. Proper biomechanical function should include rotation and translation symmetrically of the condyles.

Treatment Guidelines

One-Week Postoperative

1. Cold packs to reduce joint swelling
2. High-volt galvanic or interferential electrical stimulation to decrease pain and swelling
3. Hot packs to masseters, temporalis, and suboccipital musculature to decrease muscle tension
4. *Gentle* joint mobilization (inferior distraction only) to stretch lateral capsular structures (Fig. 10-16)
5. Active opening and closing with rotation only, beginning within pain-free range (Fig. 10-17)
6. Instruct patient in mandibular distraction, "jaw pull" (Fig. 10-18).
7. Instruct patient in self-mobilization of scar (Fig. 10-19).
8. Treatment frequency is three times per week.

During this first week, the oral surgeon may prescribe anti-inflammatory and muscle relaxant medications. An intraoral appliance may also be prescribed by the dentist for occlusal problems and for control of parafunctional activity.

Two-Week Postoperative

1. Pulsed ultrasound (10 cm^2 soundhead), 20 to 50 percent of pulsed, 8 W, for 8 minutes to masseter and TMJ (parameters apply to a Richmare unit)

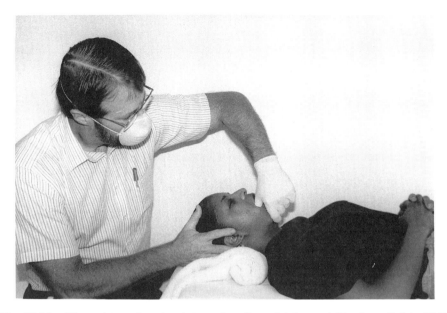

Fig. 10-16. Therapist performing intraoral unilateral joint mobilization of right TMJ capsule. Right condyle lateral pole is being palpated to ensure distraction. Supine position used with neck roll for stability of cervical spine. Appropriate protection for the therapist is used for communicable diseases. OSHA guidelines require gloves, mask, and eyewear.

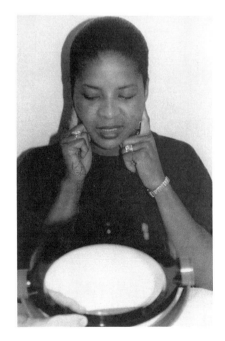

Fig. 10-17. Beginning position for active rotation only. The tongue is up in the "clucking" position, and finger pads are palpating the condyle to ensure symmetry of movement and no translation. The mirror is for visual feedback to ensure no lateral excursions.

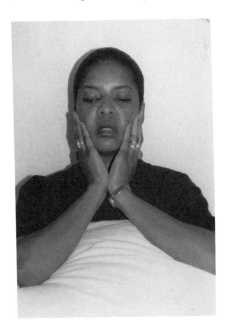

Fig. 10-18. "Jaw pull." Mandibular distraction being performed by the patient for decompression of TMJ. Force is being directed anteriorly and inferiorly. Patient instructed to "rest the upper arms on the chest, gently squeeze the face and pull forward and downward." Patient is to concentrate on being "slack jawed."

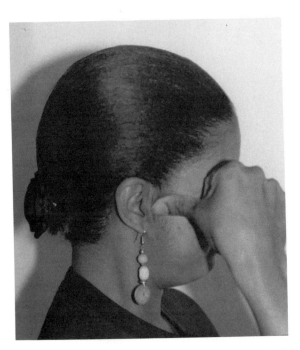

Fig. 10-19. Patient performing transverse friction massage on incision site. Mobilization is performed in all directions ("around the clock") and is always directed toward the incision line.

2. If central incisal opening is less than 25 to 30 mm, use tongue blades between posterior molars to distract TMJ, while applying ultrasound (Fig. 10-20).

3. If patient has greater than 30 mm of central incisal opening, commence intraoral mobilization techniques of translation and lateral glide (see Ch. 7).

4. If inflammation is present in the TMJ, iontophoresis or phonophoresis may be applied.

5. Continue self-mobilization of scar (Fig. 10-19).

6. Treatment frequency is three times per week or less.

Third and Fourth Weeks Postoperative

1. Increase aggressiveness of joint mobilization both intraorally by the therapist and with tongue blades by the patient

2. Initiate muscle re-education of masticatory muscles.
    a. Tubing for lateral excursions (Fig. 10-21)
    b. Resisted opening (Fig. 10-22)
    c. Resisted lateral excursions (Fig. 10-23)
Use mirror for visual feedback for all the above exercises.

3. Treatment frequency is two to three times per week.

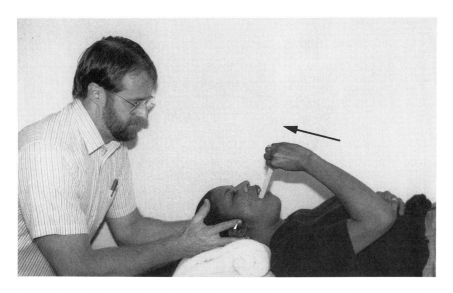

Fig. 10-20. The therapist is palpating the condyle to ensure appropriate distraction of the condyle from the fossa. The patient is instructed to push tongue blades with hand while relaxing jaw muscles. The stretch is to be maintained 10 to 20 seconds if tolerated. If sustained stretch is not tolerated, perform oscillating "pump" stretch for pain modulation. Ultrasound may also be applied during this procedure.

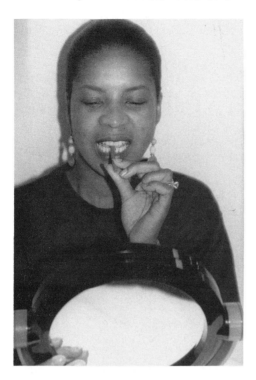

Fig. 10-21. Tubing being used for active lateral excursion with central incisors being maintained at end-to-end position. Mirror is for visual feedback to ensure no retrusion occurs.

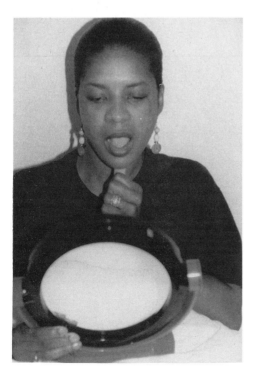

Fig. 10-22. Resisted opening at midline with concentric contraction of the muscles that depress the mandible. Used when patient is progressed well into the translatory phase, with emphasis placed on straight, midline, mandibular depression and protrusion.

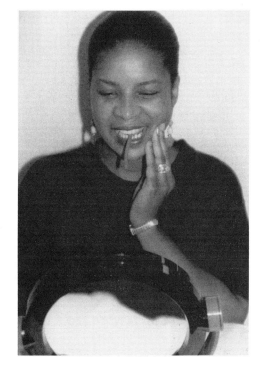

Fig. 10-23. Lateral excursion submaximal isometrics being performed while maintaining end-to-end central incisors at the midline. This is performed in this photograph for strengthening of right pterygoids and inhibition of left pterygoids.

The oral surgeon may decrease use of anti-inflammatory modalities as joint irritability and pain subsides.

Fifth and Sixth Weeks Postoperative

1. Joint mobilization becomes more aggressive, ensuring proper sequence of rotation and glide with symmetry of condylar movement
2. Do not allow patient to alter normal biomechanics by failure to translate adequately. Emphasize use of mirror for biomechanical function
3. Treatment frequency is one to two times per week

More Than 6 Weeks Postoperative

1. Continue with emphasis on home exercises previously described to sustain function and or until the goal of 42 mm of central incisal opening is reached
2. Treatment frequency decreases to one to two times per month for the next 2 months

Disc Repair and/or Retrodiscal Tissue Repair

The goals of disc repair and/or retrodiscal tissue repair are to achieve good biomechanical function without damage to the repaired disc and its associated soft tissues. Lateral excursions to the opposite side of the repair need to be obtained more slowly, otherwise, rupture may occur in the repair.

Because of adaptive shortening of the superior head of the lateral pterygoid muscle, re-education of this musculature is important for successful rehabilitation.

If joint hypermobility was present before surgery, then opening must be controlled. Maximum central incisal opening is in the 40- to 45-mm range, with lateral excursions no more than 10 mm.

Treatment Guidelines

The protocol for the first to fifth weeks postoperative is the same as that for discectomy. Guidelines for the sixth week postoperative are as follows:

1. Ensure opening does not progress beyond the 40- to 45-mm range. Often these patients progress to hypermobility because of adaptive shortening of the lateral pterygoid that has occurred secondary to long-standing disc displacement without reduction.

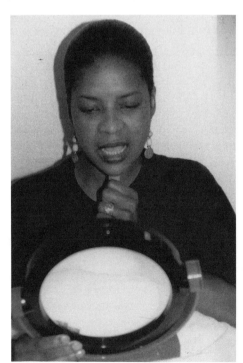

Fig. 10-24. Resisted opening at midline with isometric muscle contraction. Instructions the same as Figure 10-8.

2. Home program should include
   a. Resisted mandibular opening (Figs. 10-22 and 10-24)
   b. Lateral excursions with theratubing (Fig. 10-21 and 10-23)
   c. Controlling overopening when yawning (tongue tip against roof of mouth)

CONCLUSION

The preceding protocols have extreme variability. They are meant as guidelines and are readily modified according to the individual patient's condition.

Postorthognathic Surgery

Jennifer J. Osborne

Orthognathic surgery by its very nature of alterations in the skeletal system forces changes in the muscles and associated tissues. This is accompanied by changes in mobility, function, and overall symmetry. The surgical trauma may involve the maxilla, mandible, dentition, TMJ, masticatory muscles, and associated soft tissues. The expected response to any type of trauma, whether accidental or the unavoidable trauma of surgery, is limitation of movement of the structures.[31] Physical therapists have long dealt with these limitations as well as the alterations in function of traumatized structures in other areas of the body. After surgery, the body is forced to adjust to a "new" homeostasis.[32] Whether the changes were accomplished in the maxilla, mandible, or both areas, the changes must be evaluated and addressed in both a preoperative and postoperative state. The goal of physical therapy is to guide the new condition as far as possible toward a "normal situation."

Many studies mention the use of physical therapy to avoid or deal with adverse responses to surgery.[31–34] These complications include hypomobility, decreased bite force, paresthesias and hypoesthesias, residual pain, and muscular imbalances, which can not only affect function but aesthetics as well. After orthognathic surgery, hypomobility can be the result of a scar band of the temporalis tendon, coronoid impingement secondary to autorotation of the proximal segment of the mandible, muscle contracture, or psychological problems such as fear of pain. Compromised bite force can be attributed to rotation of the proximal segment during the surgery, muscular imbalance, pain, or a combination of factors but is often accompanied by mandibular hypomobility.[33] Sensory disturbances are extremely common after orthognathic surgery, secondary to compression or stretch of the inferior alveolar nerve and injury to the lingual nerve when holes are drilled in the distal segment for rigid fixation.[33] Any of the above complications can cause residual pain and muscular imbalance. Appropriate rehabilitation can greatly diminish these side effects.

Although therapy is often recommended, it is often limited to restoring oral mobility. "Function" is too often considered to be only maximum opening and lateral and protrusive excursions rather than a combination of pain-free and maximum ranges and the biomechanics of chewing and swallowing. Range of motion (ROM) must be evaluated with the idea of functional as well as maximum ROM, functional being 75 to 80% of the maximum range. When the connective tissue functions beyond this, abnormal tension is placed on the ligaments, intrajoint pressure increases, and irritation can occur at the synovial membrane and joint receptors. Protective muscle spasm can also occur. The final 20 to 25 percent of the range is "leeway" to protect the joint, disc, ligaments, synovium, etc., which can be adversely affected if the joint is allowed to function in the end ranges.[35] Quality and quantity of the motion, as well as the aforementioned factors, must also be considered for full normal function.

A preoperative evaluation is essential for differential diagnosis.[33,34,36] Signs and symptoms of pre-existing TMJ and/or cervical dysfunction must be recognized and addressed. In situations in which this surgery is performed to stabilize the joint by a surgeon experienced in TMJ dysfunction, these problems are not usually missed. However, if the surgery were performed purely for cosmetic reasons, immobilization of an unrecognized dysfunctional joint by an uninitiated surgeon can increase the chances of postoperative joint complications. There are multiple causes of relapse in orthognathic surgery including surgical technique, complexity of surgery, method of fixation, rotation of the proximal segment, and muscle pull from the hyoids and pterygoids primarily.[37] Much study needs to be performed to determine the extent of each factor's role in relapse, but physical therapists are probably best trained to evaluate the muscle function. Changes in the cervical spine have been noted after mandibular advancements, and changes in the hyoid position have been noted after mandibular setback procedures.[38–40] Although the long-term clinical significance of these changes needs further study, it would seem logical that any abnormalities in this area need to be addressed. If the surgical corrections are superimposed on existing dysfunction, it not only increases the magnitude of the pre-existing problem but also makes it more difficult to rehabilitate. Therefore, an assessment of muscle strength, balance between right and left side muscle function, muscle length, parafunctional activity, and the cervical spine is important to help predict outcome. Realistic expectations for rehabilitation must be based in part on the preoperative status of the patient in these areas.[34] Other specific variables that appear to affect the outcome include the osteotomy design, the stabilization technique (i.e., intermaxillary or rigid fixation),[31] and, of course, patient compliance. Modifications in the surgical procedures including the use of rigid fixation in mandibular surgery have allowed for earlier mobilization after orthognathic surgery[31] and have lessened some of the postoperative complications but not eliminated them. Consultation with the oral surgeon regarding all these factors is necessary for planning and optimum outcome of the physical therapy program.

Preoperative Evaluation and Planning

Every patient should be made aware, at the beginning of the process, that physical therapy will be a part of the overall protocol.[36] Initial referral to the therapist should be made at the time of the oral surgery evaluation or sooner by the orthodontist if any problems of pain, parafunction, or joint or muscle dysfunction are noted. Because of the wide range of variability in patients, an early referral can be helpful in treating the conditions noted in the previous section (i.e., muscle, joint, etc.), thereby preventing complications.

At the first visit, a complete subjective history will be taken. This must include the entire upper quarter as well as the orofacial region. Asymptomatic predisposing factors can be noted at this time that may relate to the outcome of the surgery. These include difficulty with function (e.g., chewing, yawning), history of joint noises, trauma to head or neck, and diagnosis of degenerative joint disease (DJD) in the head or neck. Although a previous automobile accident without residual pain may not seem important to the patient, it will make the therapist aware that there may be underlying cervical problems that should be addressed. Specific questions regarding the functional level of the TMJ, muscles of mastication, and cervical area must be asked. Quite frequently, a long-term, slow-developing decrease in function will not be acknowledged by the patient. They may have adapted and be unaware of the extent of their problem, whereas the therapist should be able to note these problems. These factors may not influence the surgery itself, but a pre- and postoperative comparison should be made.

Any complaints of pain in the upper quarter should be taken seriously. Referred pain patterns must be assessed, especially those related to facial pain, to determine if they are truly related to the facial region or referred from the facet joints, muscles, or soft tissues of the upper cervical spine.

Parafunctional activities such as bruxism, clenching, and nail biting should be investigated. Postural alignment such as forward head position and rotated shoulders, as seen with poor work and sleep habits, may affect the head and neck region. Habitual posture during work and all activities of daily living (ADL) should be assessed. Observation while the patient is in the waiting room can be very helpful, as well as monitoring facial activity during the interview. Evidence of nail biting is usually obvious. An inexperienced therapist can turn to the dental professionals for assistance in identifying tooth wear secondary to bruxism. Although not common, thumb sucking can be an adult habit as well as a pediatric one and should not be overlooked.

The objective portion of the evaluation is similar to that presented in Chapter 3, with particular attention to the following areas. During this time, coordination with the oral surgeon and other health care practitioners is essential for differential diagnosis.

Range of mandibular motion should be measured for maximum and pain-free opening, and lateral and protrusive movements with any deviations/deflections from normal should be noted. Overbite and overjet must be accounted for in opening and protrusive measurements. These measurements are important in the postoperative planning. If, for example, a patient must protrude the mandible greater than 10 mm to reach an end-to-end position before a mandibular advancement, it means that the translatory component of movement may already be excessive preoperatively and will need to be specifically stabilized to prevent hypermobility and continued overstretch of the ligamentous structures. Although in some instances a mandibular advancement may eliminate or significantly reduce the translation, this is not always the case. Excessive overbite can mean that the elevator muscles are shortened and may be of particular concern in midface vertical augmentation surgery. Passive end feel should be "springy" without any sensation of pain or mechanical block. Once again, therapists unfamiliar with these aspects should consult with the dentist/surgeon.

Joint auscultation in some form will help in the differentiation of internal derangement, but it must be kept in mind that joint noises are typically of two types: popping and crepitus. Popping can come from many sources such as deformation of the disc or ligamentous hypertrophy. A pop or click that occurs at the same location in the range, especially without limitation of movement or deflection on opening, may be an irregularity in the path of the disc–condyle complex. These noises must be evaluated in conjunction with the other members of the team.

Palpation of the structures in the orofacial and cervical areas must include not only the muscles and their structures but also the ligaments on the lateral area of the condyle. Intraoral palpation of the masseter, medial pterygoid, lateral pterygoid region, and the temporalis tendon insertion on the coronoid process may give warning signs of parafunction.

Muscle testing of the individual facial and mandibular muscles is difficult and can elicit false-positives secondary to the degree of difficulty in isolating a single muscle to test, pain, fear of "popping" or joint noise, or poor proprioception. However, an attempt should be made to resist functional movements to determine if any muscle weakness exists. These should be dealt with preoperatively if possible.

Postural alignment should be examined from the side, front, and back. Ideally, when viewed laterally, the malar bone should line up with the manubrium of the sternum and amount of lordosis in the cervical spine and kyphosis in the thoracic spine should be noted. Anteriorly, the clavicles should approach a horizontal plane, and there should be no tilt or rotation of the head. Posteriorly, winging of the scapula, scoliosis, and elevation or rotation of the shoulder girdle are evidence of varying degrees of skeletal imbalance and affect the position of the head on the spine and, subsequently, the mandible on the maxilla and the associated structures.[41–43]

A complete cervical evaluation should not be limited to ROM and general palpation. It must include tests of ligamentous stability of the upper cervical spine: occiput to atlas, occiput to axis, and atlas to axis. Segmental testing of the entire cervical spine must also be performed. It is not uncommon to have full ROM with significant segmental restrictions. It is important to remember that any changes in the cervical spine may affect the position of the mandible and vice versa.[41–43] The clinical importance of this has not been fully documented. Any mobility and positional changes that can be made in the cervical spine should be done before skeletal changes in the face.

Preoperative Instruction

An explanation by the surgeon and reinforced by the physical therapist of possible difficulties (i.e., hypomobility, muscle weakness, pain, numbness, etc.) that may occur and possible mechanisms of dealing with them will make it easier for the patient postoperatively. Although not all patients will need to take advantage of all the pre- and postoperative treatment, it is better for the patient to be prepared. Instruction in the use of the following techniques before surgery gives the patient the power to deal with the pain. Written instructions can be given, or a review after surgery can be given.

Muscle spasm and pain can occur in any area of the face or neck after surgery regardless of the type of surgery or mechanism of stabilization. Instruction in self-help techniques that will not affect the stability of the segments should be given. These include the thermal modalities of heat and ice, which can easily be used on a home basis. Soft tissue mobilization of the masseter, temporalis, suprahyoid region, and cervical spine can often reduce pain significantly. In the cases in which intermaxillary fixation (IMF) is not used, small pain-free range active movements can provide a pumping action to reduce swelling and decrease muscle spasm. These should be given in coordination with the oral surgeon with regard to the type of surgery planned.

Full instruction in a neuromuscular control program should be given at this time and reviewed periodically throughout the entire process. This includes tongue positioning against the palate, a normal nasal breathing pattern, and swallowing with the tongue up and back.

Patients should be informed during the preoperative phase that if self-help techniques are not sufficient to control the pain, further use of modalities may be indicated. These include ultrasound, electrical stimulation, and transcutaneous electrical nerve stimulation (TENS). The proper use of these pain relief methods can decrease the use of pain medications and promote healing. The specific use of modalities is addressed elsewhere,[44] but the metal used in rigid fixation should be considered, particularly with the use of deep heating modalities.

The final area of preoperative instruction is the explanation regarding difficulties with eating and speech. Once again, this will vary with the type of fixation used, and consultation with the oral surgeon is needed. In cases of allergies, diabetes, or other nutritional difficulties, a referral to a registered dietician is indicated to provide appropriate guidance.

When IMF is used and a full liquid diet is necessary, cookbooks are available to help the patient with a variety of healthy liquid meals.[45] There is a need to increase the seasonings used for better flavor. Patients should be warned against only increasing the amount of high-fat, high-sugar foods such as ice cream. Protein supplements are often indicated and can be added to average foods to boost the nutritional value.

When only maxillary surgery is performed or when rigid fixation allows for earlier mobilization, a soft diet may be prescribed. This allows for much more variety, but the patient should be warned against chewing when the segments are unstable. This diet usually allows for most foods to be finely chopped and/or partially liquified.

Speech difficulties in the immediate postoperative period are often overlooked but can be a significant frustration for the patient and the family. This is especially evident with IMF. Even when speech is achieved during the period of IMF and when rigid fixation is used, volume of the voice is decreased and long conversations can be fatiguing. Making not only the patient but also the family aware of these difficulties can significantly decrease the frustration level.

A full explanation regarding the postoperative physical therapy program is helpful. Because of the great variability in patient response, not all postoperative treatment is of the same length.[34] Flexibility in the program is necessary, and an understanding by the patient regarding the importance of compliance is essential. It should be explained that as long as the patient progresses with a home program and no difficulties arise, the time period will be very short and consist more of updates and follow-up visits rather than long-term hands-on treatment. However, the patient should not be misled into thinking that hands-on treatment, the use of modalities, etc., will not be needed. A philosophy of "hope for the best and prepare for the worst" is generally a good tactic.

Postoperative Physical Therapy

Postoperative physical therapy can be divided into two stages: (1) the immediate postoperative period when fixation is used or, in the case of maxillary surgery or rigid fixation, when active movement therapy is not indicated but passive soft tissue techniques and modalities are used; and (2) the subsequent period when the segments have been determined to be stable and, with the approval of the surgeon, when increased motion and function are desirable.[35]

The first phase of treatment is usually on an "as-needed" basis, but I believe that a routine visit during this time to review the discussion of the preoperative evaluation is helpful. Patients often think that they should "live with the pain" instead of dealing with the discomfort. Reminders and general support can be very helpful at this time. As noted in the section on Preoperative Instruction, self-help techniques and modalities should be used as needed for muscle spasm and pain relief. In the event that a preoperative evaluation was not performed, it is up to the surgeon to make the patient aware that this help is available.

As soon as the segments have been determined to be stable by the surgeon or when IMF has been removed (average 6 to 8 weeks), the second, more aggressive stage of therapy begins. The initial visit should include a re-evaluation of the mandibular dynamics, muscle strength to resistance of functional movements, subjective complaints of pain and response to palpation of areas of the face and jaw, any paresthesias or hypoesthesias, and cervical evaluation.

Instruction should begin at this time in a home program to increase ROM and strengthen any muscular imbalances that are noted. I believe in using Rocabado's "6 × 6" method of exercises for most of the home program. This involves doing the exercises for six repetitions six times a day.[35] The patient is given stickers to place in frequently seen places as reminders. The exercises should be kept simple to encourage compliance.

Soft tissue mobilization of the affected tissues will make the stretching techniques more tolerable and more effective. Massage of temporalis and intraorally of the masseter, in particular, will allow for a better stretch. One of the most common causes of hypomobility is scarring of the temporalis tendon. Cross-friction massage in this area will help to soften the tissue also.

The simplest method of self-stretch is to use the thumb crossed over the index finger forming an "X." The index finger is placed on the lower teeth and the thumb on the upper teeth, as far posterior as possible. This technique should be performed bilaterally to avoid compression of one joint while trying to stretch the other side. Gentle pressure is given into opening until a stretch is felt. This is held for 6 seconds and repeated six times (Fig. 10-25).

Lateral excursions and protrusive movements are accomplished by having the patient hold six or seven tongue blades between the anterior teeth and gliding bilaterally and forward (Fig. 10-26). Lateral movement is also greatly helped by holding surgical tubing between the anterior teeth and rolling it side to side (Fig. 10-23). Proprioception is often diminished in these cases, and the use of a mirror can be helpful for visual input.

I believe with any technique, but especially with a home program, that the patient should understand the sensations that should be expected. If the technique is performed too vigorously, an increase in soreness and inflammation can occur and result in a decrease in range. The patient may also then be afraid to continue with the program. Self-mobilization should be performed only to the point of a stretching sensation and only in the muscles associated with that technique. Pain in other areas is a sign of compensation and should be avoided.

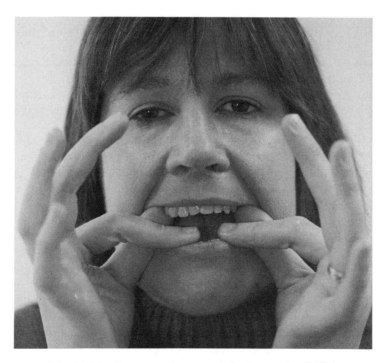

Fig. 10-25.   Postoperative stretch for increasing ROM.

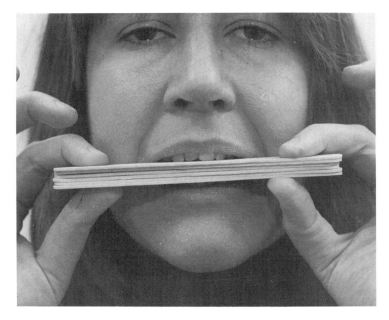

Fig. 10-26. Exercise for lateral excursions and protrusive movements.

Before patients leave after the first visit at this stage, they are given one of two methods of evaluating their opening. The first is to use their knuckles (Fig. 10-27). These are preferable to the fingertips because there is less soft tissue give, and therefore it is more reproducible. The patients mark how many knuckles they are able to fit in. The second method is to cut a tongue blade to the distance they are able to open and one to the distance you want them to achieve before their next visit (Fig. 10-28). These methods give patients immediate feedback regarding their efforts.

A discussion regarding the patient's ability to chew within the surgeon's restrictions will give the therapist a baseline of bite force and overall function in the new position. Although difficulty with chewing may only be related to decreased lateral movement initially, as time and movement progress, so should the ability to chew without fatigue.

The patient continues at this time using the self-help modalities as needed in addition to the new exercises. The program for neuromuscular control must also continue.

As mentioned previously, some patients need only to be monitored for their progress. One week should lapse between the first two appointments to give patients time to increase range and function on their own. If, at that time, an increase of 5 mm of interincisal opening and 2 to 3 mm of lateral excursions is noted, then continued rechecks and increases in the intensity of the home program are given every 7 to 10 days and should include the stabilization program described below. If, however, there has not been the expected progress

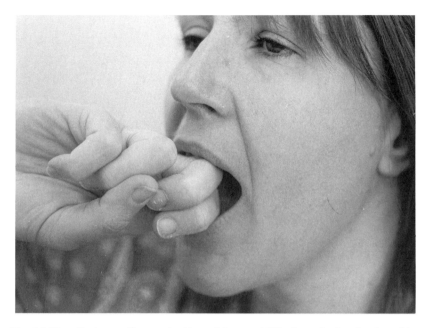

Fig. 10-27.   Postoperative evaluation of jaw mobility (opening) using knuckles.

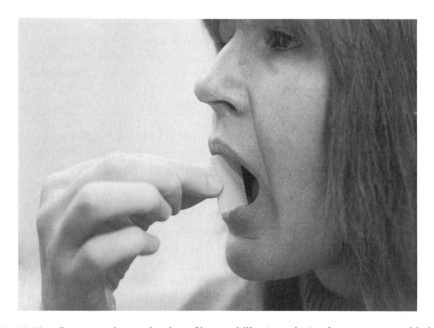

Fig. 10-28.   Postoperative evaluation of jaw mobility (opening) using a cut tongue blade.

or if pain is present or increasing, then regularly scheduled visits of two to three times a week should be set up.

The more aggressive treatment should still be within the patient's tolerance and will include the various modalities described elsewhere in this chapter. They should be used with a specific goal in mind (i.e., muscle relaxation and lengthening, scar tissue realignment and softening, and joint mobilization to increase capsular extensibility). The various forms of electrical stimulation noted in this chapter are indicated in the case of sensory/motor nerve symptoms. Manual therapy techniques are essential in these situations. These are necessary to restore the normal biomechanics in the joint that cannot be accomplished with forceful active movements. The techniques of long-axis distraction, translation, and lateral glide are performed as described in Chapter 7.

During this time, the use of a Therabite unit (Therabite Corp., Bryn Mawr, Pennsylvania) should also be considered (Fig. 10-14). It allows for a bilateral stretch with a greater but still controllable force into opening. Continued reinforcement of the lateral and protrusive movements is necessary with the tongue blades (Fig. 10-26) or surgical tubing. In my opinion, use of the Therabite under controlled situations can begin within the first 2 weeks with the approval of the surgeon. It should be adjusted to not allow for forceful opening beyond the patient's maximum in these early stages. If the opening is extremely limited (i.e., less than 10 mm), the use of the Therabite will not be possible.

The use of continuous passive motion (CPM) units can help in situations in which it is known that excess scar tissue is a problem, in repeat surgeries, or in cases in which patient compliance is a problem. The involvement of the physical therapist in using CPM devices varies greatly. Although some surgeons wish to fit and monitor the device themselves, others prefer to involve the physical therapist secondary to their more frequent visits with the patient. Regardless, the therapist should become aware of all the devices available. The TheraPacer unit (KVM Rehabilitation, Inc., Houston, Texas) allows for continuous movement many hours a day and is generally comfortable enough for the patient to sleep with. It works only with opening, so it is necessary to continue mobilization for lateral movements. It has a counter that allows for a printout of patient compliance (Fig. 10-29). My experience with the Therapacer has been very positive, and I believe that, as the oral surgeons become more comfortable with the concept of CPM, we will increase its use.

The FMA Translator (Great Lakes Orthodontics, Ltd., Tonawanda, New York) is not, strictly speaking, a CPM device, as its recommended use is up to 12 minutes four times a day. It has the advantage of working on lateral and protrusive movements. Its basis is that if the patient can regain the translatory component of movement, then the rotary movement will follow (Fig. 10-30). As with the Therapacer, my experience with the FMA Translator has been positive. It is simple to use, and a therapist can make the splint needed with a little practice. In situations in which time to use the unit is limited or the patient is claustrophobic and does not tolerate the continuous use of a CPM device, the Translator should definitely be considered. Each of these units has

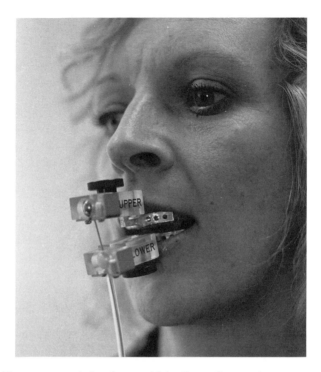

Fig. 10-29.   Therapacer unit in place, which allows for continuous movement many hours a day and is generally comfortable enough for a patient to sleep with.

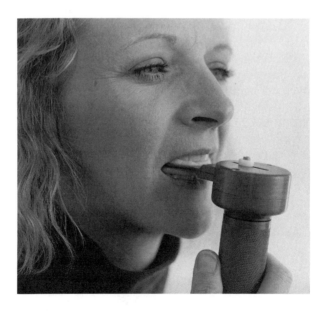

Fig. 10-30.   FMA Translator in place. It has the advantage of working on lateral and protrusive movements.

advantages and disadvantages, and as the therapist becomes familiar with them, they will better be able to choose which one is appropriate for each individual.

The use of these relatively new devices has a basis in orthopaedic surgery, but modification is required for use with the TMJ. As research and development continue, the therapeutic value of these motorized devices for the TMJ will be determined.

If, at any point in the treatment, progress decreases or stops, there should be no delay in an effort to determine the cause. When pain is involved and is localized to the joint region, disc displacement must be considered, especially in the case of mandibular advancements. During that type of surgery, difficulty maintaining control of the proximal (condylar) segment can cause a displacement. A return to the oral surgeon is indicated in these situations. Although fibrous or bony ankylosis is an uncommon complication, it is severe and very difficult to deal with. Manipulation under anesthesia can be used to evaluate these situations and, unfortunately, subsequent surgeries, including coronoidectomies and the use of temporary implants. Rib grafts or, as a last resort, total joints may be indicated in an attempt to correct the problem.

Nonpainful restrictions in movement must be assessed for possible excessive scar tissue formation in the area of the temporalis tendon. In this situation, the end feel will be hard and a thick band of scar tissue will be palpable in the area of the coronoid process, but you should still feel some movement of the condyle when palpated in the preauricular area. Scarring in the superior joint space will hold the disc to the fossa and may also present as a nonpainful restriction; however, in these cases, no distraction of the condyle can be accomplished. Often, an attempt to manipulate the mandible with the patient under sedation will help with a differential diagnosis. Small adhesions may be released in these situations, but larger bands will continue to provide resistance.

If the above-noted problems are ruled out, patient compliance must be questioned. A review of the total program and the reasoning behind it should be carried out and may be done as part of a conference including the patient and the team.

The goals of the physical therapy program are set before the surgery in accordance with the preoperative findings but may need to be adjusted if any of the above complications arise. In general, a maximum interincisal opening of at least 40 mm with a functional, pain-free opening of 35 to 38 mm, 4 to 5 mm of lateral excursion, and 2 to 3 mm of protrusion beyond the end-to-end position of the central incisors is desirable. The mandibular movement should be balanced, without deviations in opening, or protrusion and lateral movements should be equal. These goals should be reached within 3 months, and the stabilization program should continue beyond that for at least 6 months with periodic checks. It has been shown that some instability can be present for up to 2 years after surgery.[46] Muscular changes can therefore continue for the same amount of time.

The stabilization program consists of continued reinforcement of the neuromuscular control with the addition of rhythmic stabilization exercises (Fig. 10-31). These should be performed in a pure isometric manner. Small amounts

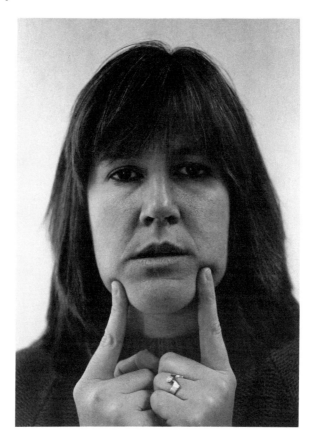

Fig. 10-31. Example of rhythmic stabilization exercise.

of resistance are applied into opening, closing, and lateral excursions, and all pressures are performed with the mouth slightly open and the tongue against the palate in an effort to avoid excessive compression to the joint. In situations in which increased translation is present, an isometric contraction into retrusion is indicated. Any other ongoing muscular imbalances should be addressed with specific resistance for that motion. Stabilization of the cervical spine is indicated also at this time.

CONCLUSION

A consistent protocol agreed on by the orthodontist/oral surgeon team in coordination with the physical therapist is important for the optimum result after orthognathic surgery. Oral surgeons not familiar with working with a physical therapist should seek out someone with postgraduate training in upper quarter and, specifically, in the management of TMJ disorders. They, in conjunction with the orthodontist, must work together to agree on the specifics of the protocol. In these situations, a referral for the protocol is all that is needed. If the therapist is not as familiar with these cases, they must look to the surgeon for guidance and make an attempt to contact other therapists for additional help. Using their basic knowledge of orthopaedics and physiology of joints and soft tissue should allow the more inexperienced therapist, with caution, to treat postoperative orthognathic surgery cases. Although it may seem that most patients may not need an extensive program of therapy, the range of changes that can and do result from this type of surgery indicate the need for at least a minimal amount of monitoring in all cases. The overall expertise of physical therapists trained in the treatment of upper quarter dysfunction makes them the logical choice to address the muscular and skeletal changes involved. A close working relationship will allow the therapist to continue to modify the treatment and exercises accordingly, allowing for the individual differences between patients.

REFERENCES

Postarthroscopic Surgery

1. Mannheimer JS, Dunn J: Cervical spine evaluation and relation to temporomandibular disorders. In Kaplan A, Assael LA (eds): Temporomandibular Disorders: Diagnosis and Management. WB Saunders, Philadelphia, 1991
2. Widmer CG: Evaluation of temporomandibular disorders. In Kraus SL (ed): TMJ Disorders: Management of the Craniomandibular Complex. Clinics in Physical Therapy (18). Churchill Livingstone, New York, 1988
3. McNeill C: Craniomandibular Disorders: Guidelines for Evaluation, Diagnosis and Management. Quintessence Publishing Co., Chicago, 1990
4. Mannheimer JS: Physical therapy management of the arthroscopic surgery patient: a retrospective analysis focusing upon therapeutic paradigms, outcomes and concerns. Presented at the third International Conference on Arthroscopy of the Temporomandibular Joint, New York, 1991
5. Sanders B, Buoncristiani RD: Diagnostic and surgical arthroscopy of the temporomandibular joint: clinical experience with 137 procedures over a 2-year period. J Craniomandib Disord 1:202, 1987
6. Bewyer DC: Biomechanical and physiological processes leading to internal derangement with adhesions. J Craniomandib Disord Oral Fac Pain 3:44, 1989
7. Sanders B, Buoncristiani RD: Temporomandibular joint arthrotomy: management of failed cases. Oral Maxillofac Clin North Am 1:443, 1989
8. Mannheimer JS, Rosenthal R: Acute and chronic postural abnormalities as related to craniofacial pain and temporomandibular disorders. Dent Clin North Am 35:185, 1991
9. Zislis MW, Wank HA, Gottehrer NR: Temporomandibular joint arthroscopy: a preoperative and post-operative rehabilitation protocol. J Craniomandib Disord Fac Oral Pain 3:218, 1989
10. McCain JP, De La Rua H: Principles and practice of operative arthroscopy of the human temporomandibualr joint. Oral Maxillofac Clin North Am C1:35, 1989
11. Bertolucci LE: Physical therapy: post arthroscopic temporomandibular joint managment (update). J Craniomandib Disord 10:130, 1992

12. Hoffman D, Mosses J, Topper D: Temporomandibular joint surgery. Dent Clin North Am 35:89, 1991

13. Fogarty TJ: A method for extraction and removal of arterial emboli and thrombi. Surg Gynecol Obstet 116:241, 1963

14. Hoffman D: Presentation at scientific session on management of internal derangements. AAOMS annual meeting, Chicago, 1991

15. Mannheimer JS: Physical therapy concepts in evaluation and treatment of the upper quarter: therapeutic modalities. In Kraus SL (ed): TMJ Disorders: Management of the Craniomandibular Complex. Churchill Livingstone, New York, 1988

16. Carter JB, Schwaber MK: Temporomandibular joint arthroscopy: complications and their management. 1:185, 1989

17. Mannheimer JS, Lampe GN: Clinical Transcutaneous Electrical Nerve Stimulation. FA Davis, Philadelphia, 1984

18. Michlovitz S: Thermal Agents in Rehabilitation. FA Davis, Philadelphis, 1991

19. Mannheimer JS: Non-medicinal and non-invasive pain control techniques in the management of rheumatic disease and related musculoskeletal disorders. J Rheumatol 14:28, 1987

20. Hoffman D, Mannheimer JS, Attanasio R et al: Management of the temporomandibular joint surgical patient. Clin Prev Dent 11:28, 1989

21. Mannheimer JS: TENS: uses and effectiveness. In Michel TH (ed): Pain: International Perspectives in Physical Therapy. Churchill Livingstone, Edinburgh, 1985

22. Dyson M, Luke DA: Induction of mast cell degranulation in skin by ultrasound. UFFC 33:194, 1986

23. Sokoliu A: Destructive effect of ultrasound on ocular tissues. In Reid JM, Sikou MR (eds): Interaction of Ultrasound and Biological Tissue. DHEW Pub (FDA) 73-8008, 1972

24. Kraus SL: Physical therapy management of TMJ dysfunction. p. 139. In: TMJ Disorders: Management of the Craniomandibular Complex. Ch. 6. Churchill Livingstone, New York, 1988

25. Rocabado M: Physical therapy for the post surgical TMJ patient. J Craniomandib Disord Fac Oral Pain 3:75, 1989

26. Piper MA: A rationale for microsurgery. In Kaplan AS, Assael LA (eds): Temporomandibular Disorders: Diagnosis and Treatment. WB Saunders, Philadelphia, 1991

27. Gehin A: Atlas of Manipulative Techniques of the Cranium and Face. Eastland Press, Seattle, 1985

28. Lentell G, Hetherington T, Eagan J et al: The use of thermal agents to influence the effectiveness of a low-load prolonged stretch. J Ortho Sports Phys Ther 16:202, 1992

29. Cohen SG, Fletcher M: Comparison of jaw mobilization regimens. J Dent Res 70:329, 1991

30. Buchbinder D, Currivan R: Evaluation of mobilization regimens for jaw hypomobility. Presented at 73rd Annual Meeting AAOMS, Chicago, 1991

Postorthognathic Surgery

31. Boyd SB, Karas ND, Sinn DP: Recovery of mandibular mobility following orthognathic surgery. J Oral Maxillofac Surg 49:924, 1991

32. Ellis E, Carlson DS: Neuromuscular adaptation after orthognathic surgery. Oral Maxillofac Surg Clin North Am 2:811, 1990

33. Epker BN, LaBanc JP: Orthognathic surgery: management of postoperative complications. Oral Maxillofac Surg Clin North Am 2:901, 1990

34. Bell WH, Gonyea W, Finn RA et al: Muscular rehabilitation after orthognathic surgery. Oral Surg Oral Med Oral Pathol 56:229, 1983

35. Rocabado M, Iglarsh ZA: Musculoskeletal Approach to Maxillofacial Pain. JB Lippincott, Philadelphia, 1991

36. Osborne JJ: A physical therapy protocol for orthognathic surgery. J Craniomandib Prac 7:132, 1989

37. Will LA: Mandibular advancement using bilateral sagittal osteotomy past, present and future. Oral Maxillofac Surg Clin North Am 22:717, 1990

38. Valk JWP, Zonnenberg JJ, vanMaanen C, vanWonderen OG: The biomechanical effects of a sagittal split ramus osteotomy on the relationship of the mandible, the hyoid bone, and the cervical spine. Am J Orthod Dentofac Orthop 102:99, 1992

39. Yasuaki T, Gamble JW, Proffit WR, Christiansen RL: Postural change of the hyoid bone following osteotomy of the mandible. Oral Surg Oral Med Oral Pathol 23:688, 1967

40. Wickwire NA, White RP, Proffit WR: The effect of mandibular osteotomy on hyoid position. J Oral Surg 30:184, 1972

41. Goldstein DF, Kraus SL, Williams WB, Glasheen-Wray M: Influence of cervical posture on mandibular movement. J Prosthet Dent 52:421, 1984

42. Darling DW, Kraus SL, Glasheen-Wray MB: Relationship of head posture and the rest position of the mandible. J Prosthet Dent 52:111, 1984

43. Kraus SL: TMJ Disorders: Management of the Craniomandibular Complex. Churchill Livingstone, New York, 1988

44. Mannheimer J: Physical therapy concepts in evaluation and treatment of the upper quarter—therapeutic modalities. p. 311. In Kraus SL (ed): TMJ Disorders: Management of the Craniomandibular Complex. Churchill Livingstone, New York, 1988

45. Wilson JR: Nonchew Cookbook. Wilson Publishing Inc., Glenwood Springs, Colorado, 1985

46. McDonald WR: Stabilization of mandibular lengthening: a comparison of moderate and large advancements. Oral Maxillofac Surg Clin North Am 2:729, 1990

11 | Cervical Spine Influences on the Management of TMD

Steven L. Kraus

Management of the symptomatic and dysfunctional TMD patient requires an understanding of the cervical spine that is not commonly realized by many patients, health professionals, and third party payers. The clinician who can differentiate signs and symptoms of cervical spine involvement from the signs and symptoms of TMD and/or masticatory muscle hyperactivity (MMH) will be less likely to make an error in determining the primary source(s) of dysfunction. Chapter objectives include a discussion on:

1. Prevalence of symptoms associated with cervical spine involvement.
2. Local, distal, and cephalic symptoms originating from cervical spine involvement.
3. Mechanisms by which the cervical spine may influence the mandible. Effects of the cervical spine upon mandibular position and mobility may influence the attending dentist to alter the sequence of treatment to include physical therapy treatment of the cervical spine prior to, during, and/or following surgical or nonsurgical intervention for TMD and or MMH.
4. The dilemma of diagnosing. Patients, clinicians, and third party payers often place a great deal of importance on the diagnosis. Unfortunately, they assume that the diagnosis is correct and is the source of the symptoms, which may lead patients to say; "I now know what is wrong with me," clinicians to say; "I now know what to treat," and third party payers to say; "I now know how much it will cost and how long it will take." If the diagnosis is important, then hopefully it is the correct diagnosis.

5. Overall management of cervical spine involvement from a physical therapist perspective.

This chapter does not intend to question the expertise of the medical, dental, and psychological professions in diagnosing and managing the symptomatic and dysfunctional patient. However, in an attempt to discuss reliability and validity issues surrounding diagnosis and management of the cervical spine, the reader will become aware of inconsistencies. This chapter attempts to place in better perspective the essential role of the physical therapist, as well as the medical and dental professions, in the team approach to patient care.

PREVALENCE OF CERVICAL SPINE INVOLVEMENT

Reliable epidemiologic data on the incidence and prevalence of neck pain is lacking, as most studies have been on low back pain. Throughout this chapter, various studies on low back pain or spinal pain are cited. Based upon these studies, inferences to the cervical spine will be postulated.

It has been estimated that some 40 to 50 percent of the general population will experience neck pain with limitation of mobility at some time during their lives.[1] Although most patients improve with time, as many as one-third of them may continue to have moderate or severe pain that interferes with the patient's life-style 15 years later.[2] The etiology of neck pain, unlike other musculoskeletal conditions, is multifactorial. This spectrum emphasizes the frequency of symptoms often originating from the cervical spine, which can occur from but not be limited to the following events and syndromes.

Motor Vehicle Accidents

Of the 3,800,000 rear-end collisions that occur annually in the United States, relatively few result in death or quadriplegias.[3] The majority of motor vehicle accidents (MVA) result in neck and shoulder pain secondary to soft tissue injury without objective neural or osseous spinal involvement.[4] At speeds of less than 15 mph a forewarned driver may escape significant injury caused by being hit from behind by bracing himself against the steering wheel.[4] In rear-end collisions that exceed 20 mph, however, the unrestrained driver may experience facet joint loading and excessive stretching to the anterior cervical tissues.[4] In either case, rebound cervical flexion may occur with reflex contraction of the neck muscles.[4]

Statistics on the prevalence of cervical spine related symptoms as a result of MVA reveal an ever increasing patient population. Canadian MVA statistics in 1986 revealed an increase of 15 percent in bodily injuries as opposed to a 4 percent decline in deaths over the previous 3 years.[5] In addition to these "new" injuries, one must take into account previous MVA in which the symptoms have not resolved. According to Ameis,[6] 15 percent of MVA victims fail to recover full function while 40 to 70 percent have some mild to moderate symptoms persist. It is reported that 50 percent or more of patients after injury may experience symptoms 5 to 10 years after settlement of litigation.[7,8]

Repetitive Motion Injury

Repetitive motion injuries, also known as cumulative trauma disorders, repetitive strain injuries, or overuse injuries, occur in various professions as well as during sporting and recreational activities. Repetitive motions place individuals at a higher risk of developing musculoskeletal problems due to the duration and position in which they are performed.[9,10] Hagberg and Wegman,[11] following their review of 21 articles, state that there is an association between occupation and diseases of the shoulder and neck that suggest that "highly repetitive shoulder contractions, static contractions, and work at shoulder level are hazardous exposure factors." Several authors report correlation between psychosocial factors and musculoskeletal disorders.[12,13] Anxiety, nervousness, and mental strain are suggested to increase static muscle activity and provoke pain.[12,13]

Repetitive motion injury affects as many as 70 million Americans, according to a study by the National Institute for Occupational Safety and Health.[14] Examples include the use of the hand and/or wrist, elbow, shoulder, and neck while using a computer terminal,[14] working on an assembly line,[14] long distance driving to and from work, or professional and amateur musical instrument playing.[9]

Musculoskeletal pain and discomfort among dentists was investigated based on questionnaires distributed in 1987 and again 2.5 years later in 1990.[15] The results of this prospective study showed the prevalence of musculoskeletal pain and discomfort had increased between 1987 and 1990. From the answers in 1990 it was shown that frequency of headaches and pain and discomfort in the neck, shoulders, and/or lower back was relatively high. Such symptoms were believed to be associated with work environment and work tasks (repetitive motion injury).

Fibromyalgia

Fibromyalgia, a controversial diagnostic syndrome, has been estimated by Goldenberg to afflict between 3 to 6 million patients.[16] Fibromyalgia has been referred to by different names over the years, such as rheumatic pain modulation syndrome,[17] nonarticular rheumatism,[17] and interstitial myofibrositis,[18] to mention a few. Twenty percent of outpatients who see a rheumatologist are diagnosed with fibromyalgia.[19] Myofascial trigger points in a population of patients with spinal pain represent a primary source for clinical symptoms, according to Travell and Simons.[20-22] Differentiation between fibromyalgia and myofascial pain syndrome will be discussed below.

Cervicogenic Headache and Other Cephalic Symptoms

The prevalence of cervical spine symptoms would be greater if past epidemiologic studies included symptoms not commonly associated with the cervical spine. This list of ignored symptoms related to cervical spine involvement includes cervicogenic headaches and dizziness. In the field of headache research, the cervical spine has been a largely unexplored frontier until recent years. Bogduk states,[23]

> Although disorders of the neck are acknowledged as possible causes of headache, there are no established guidelines whereby, on clinical grounds, cervical headache can be reliably differentiated from other forms of headache. . . . It is possible that 'cervical headache' has been avoided as a diagnosis by neurologists dealing with headache problems, and its actual incidence underestimated.

Summary

If the "numbers" are close to being accurate, the prevalence of symptoms associated with cervical spine involvement is indeed high. A patient who is seeking help for their TMD and/or MMH-related symptoms will more than likely have a complaint associated with a cervical spine involvement that may require further investigation.

CERVICAL SPINE AS A SOURCE OF LOCAL AND DISTAL SYMPTOMS

Cervical spine tissues can be the source of local and distal (upper extremity) symptoms. Empirical evidence suggests that if certain tissues are found to be involved, they suggest or indicate the cervical spine as the source of symptoms and limitation in function. Some clinicians may be biased toward one tissue based upon their educational background and what they are capable of evaluating and treating. Such a bias will prevent the clinician from recognizing not only other tissues that might be involved, but also the complexity of the patient's clinical presentation.

Muscle

It is well documented that muscles of the cervical spine and shoulder girdle areas can be a major source of local and referred symptoms into the upper extremities.[24-29] Palpation examination is a procedure used to determine the presence of muscular involvement.[30] Patients may have full pain-free range of motion, normal strength, and normal neurologic reactions but still have muscular involvement.[30] A patient may complain of referred pain in the absence of pain at the primary site of origin. Silent primary pain is discussed in the section on History.

Muscular involvement is commonly identified as either fibromyalgia or myofascial pain syndrome. The criteria to diagnose fibromyalgia have varied as much as the name. Today's general criteria for diagnosing fibromyalgia include multiple tender points (four or more), diffuse musculoskeletal aches, pain, stiffness at many sites, and easy fatigability.[21,31,32] Fibromyalgia is often confused with myofascial pain syndrome.[22] The hallmark of myofascial pain syndrome is a trigger point that is located in one or two muscle(s) as a taut band of exquisite tenderness in response to manual pressure, and a characteristic pattern of referred pain.[22,24] Tender points associated with fibromyalgia are areas of tenderness that may or may not be in muscle tissue, do not have palpable taut bands, and do not refer pain to adjacent areas.[21]

Both fibromyalgia and myofascial pain syndrome cause pain and tenderness and exhibit similar histologic changes, and both conditions are noted to exhibit increase pain with activity.[33] Simons and others suggest that multiple or generalized myofascial trigger points or tender points are in the spectrum of fibromyalgia.[25–28,32] No attempt to differentiate between fibromyalgia or myofascial pain syndrome will be made in this chapter. Managing either fibromyalgia or myofascial trigger points by suggested procedures and/or techniques covered in the section on management should yield satisfactory results (see also Ch. 13). For the rest of this chapter, the term "muscular involvement" will be used to indicate symptoms associated with either fibromyalgia or myofascial pain syndrome.

Facet Joint

A significant source of pain associated with cervical spine involvement originates from facet joints, also known as zygapophyseal joints. Each vertebral segment of the cervical spine has a pair of facet joints starting from occiput and C1 (atlantooccipital) through C6/C7. With the exception of occiput/C1 and C1/C2 (atlantoaxial) facet joints, the remaining paired facets from C2/C3 through C6/C7 are located laterally and posteriorly to each side of the vertebral body (Fig. 11-1). Another set of joints located only in the cervical spine are the joints of von Luschka, also known as the lateral interbody joints (Fig. 11-1). These joints extend upward from the lateral margins of the upper surfaces of the vertebral bodies of the lower five cervical vertebrae.[34] Only the facet joints will be discussed as a primary source for joint pain, mainly because of available documentation. For further information about the joints of von Luschka the reader is referred to the references.[35]

Research into lumbar spinal pain syndromes has shown that the lumbar facet joints can be a major source of low back pain, referred pain into the lower extremity, and even neurologic signs.[36–39] Even though Wyke and co-workers describe in detail the articular neurology of the facet joints in the cervical

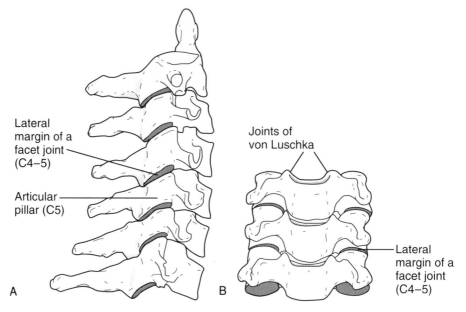

Fig. 11-1. Typical cervical vertebrae. (**A**) The 2nd to 7th cervical vertebrae viewed from the right side. (**B**) The 3rd, 4th and 5th vertebrae viewed from in front.

spine,[40,41] little attention has been given to the cervical spine facet joints as a source of neck and upper arm pain until recently (Fig. 11–2).[42] Dwyer and co-workers[43] mapped out pain patterns evoked by stimulation of normal cervical facet joints by injecting about 1 ml of contrast medium into the facet joint, distending the joint capsule (see Ch. 12, Fig. 12-2). As a follow-up to this study, Aprill and co-workers[44] tested the predictive value of segmental pain charts in patients with suspected cervical facet joint pain. This study concluded that pain charts used for locating the segmental location of a symptomatic joint were accurate in each patient on the basis of the alleviation of pain with diagnostic joint blocks.[44] Inflammation and/or edema is a likely cause of facet joint pain and limited movement since the facet joints are true synovial joints. To identify inflammation and edema occurring at a cervical facet joint, a manual procedure of palpating the lateral margin of the facet joint (Fig. 11-1) will be mentioned in the physical examination. Jull and co-workers[45] evaluated one manual therapist's ability to identify cervical facet joint syndrome in 20 patients, all of whom had complained of chronic neck pain or headaches for at least a year. The authors concluded that manual examination by a trained manual therapist is as accurate as radiologically controlled blocks in the diagnosis of symptomatic cervical facet joints.[45]

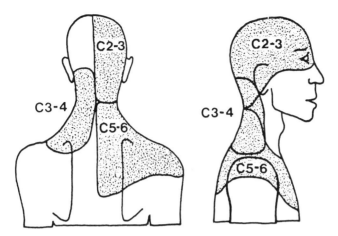

Fig. 11-2. Facet joint pain distribution. Distribution of presenting symptoms in the patients with positive responses correlated with the offending level revealed by the diagnostic blocks to the facet joints.

Neck pain and limited neck movement due to facet joint involvement have also been related to a torn or trapped menisci of the facet joint.[46-49] The form, incidence, and disposition of menisci in facet joints have been studied by several authors.[50,51] The menisci is a peripheral ring of tissue covering from a small fraction up to 50 percent of the articular cartilage of the facet joint, depending upon the vertebral level and age of the subject.[52] The inner margin of the meniscus contains dense collagenous tissue whereas the outer margin contains collagen and fatty tissue attaching firmly to the facet joint capsule.[50] The primary role of the menisci in the cervical facet joints is said to be providing uniform distribution of pressure.[53] Other secondary functions, including compensation for joint incongruency, preservation of articular facet edges, and occupation of cavities or spaces left open during motion, have been suggested.[47] The presence of menisci invites speculation about their causal role in pain and limitation of neck movement if torn or trapped.[54,55] Clinically, certain neck and distal symptoms can be resolved if proper manual techniques are applied to the restricted facet joint(s) (see Fig. 11-22H).

Peripheral Nerve

Peripheral entrapment neuropathy is another source of neck an distal symptoms related to cervical spine involvement. Kopell and Thompson define the term *entrapment neuropathy* as "a region of localized injury and inflammation in a peripheral nerve that is caused by mechanical irritation from some impinging anatomical neighbor."[56] A peripheral entrapment neuropathy occurs lateral to the intervertebral foramen. An entrapment neuropathy occurring inside the intervertebral foramen and medially will be considered a central entrapment neuropathy involving the nerve root. A peripheral or central entrapment occurs because the nerve is unable to move in relation to neighboring structures. There are a number of potential sites where a peripheral nerve can become entrapped.

Brachial Plexus

A common peripheral entrapment neuropathy associated with the cervical spine occurs at the interscalene triangle involving the brachial plexus. The interscalene triangle boundaries are the first rib inferiorly, the scalene medius muscle posterolaterally, and the scalene anticus muscle anteromedially.[57] The dimensions of the interscalene are not static. Movement or positioning of the cervical spine can affect the dimensions, especially the anteroposterior dimensions. Scalene muscle hypertrophy linked to physical demands of certain occupations and recreational activities may also alter interscalene dimensions.[57] Contents of the interscalene triangle that are potentially at risk of impingement include the brachial plexus and the subclavian artery. The majority of symptoms are related to neurogenic involvement but the most serious, yet rare, are vascular.[58] To some clinicians an entrapment occurring at the interscalene triangle may be considered a part of the thoracic outlet syndrome (TOS), which would not be an inaccurate assumption. However, no attempt will be made by this author to discuss TOS because of the confusion and contradiction in the literature that underscores our poor understanding of this syndrome.[59]

At the point of nerve entrapment either compression or friction can cause a reaction in a nerve.[60] The degree of such a reaction is proportional to the intensity and duration of the entrapment pressure.[61] Since the connective tissue components of nerves are innervated by pain fibers, inflammation may result in pain reactivity.[61] Based upon the amount of compression, nerve injury can range from the mildest degree of injury involving interruption of conductivity (known as demyelination),[61,62] to severe injury involving destruction of the nerve components (known as axonal degeneration).[61,63] Clinically, most nerve injuries at the interscalene triangle are related to inflammation and mild nerve injury giving rise to the patient's neck and upper extremity symptoms. Once inflammation and compression is removed from the nerve, symptoms and function are restored.[62]

Greater Occipital Nerve

Although the greater occipital nerve (GON) contributes to cephalic symptoms it will be discussed in this section, since it is a peripheral nerve in the cervical spine. The greater occipital nerve is the main sensory nerve in the occipital area, deriving most of its fibers from the C2 nerve root.[64] Involvement of the C2 nerve root or GON has been collectively referred to as "occipital neuralgia."[65] C2 or GON compression or irritation has been attributed to various causes, ranging from post-traumatic lesions or cervical degenerative arthrosis, to muscle spasm in the upper cervical spine.[66,67] Diagnosis often depends on pain location and the exclusion of other causes. Jansen and co-workers state; "There are no radiological or electrophysiological maneuvers for demonstrating compression or irritation of the C2 root."[68] Unlike the C2 nerve root, the GON is superficial, so compression or irritation may be more verifiable. For over 40 years, occipital nerve zone tenderness has been known to be a feature of GON entrapment.[67,68] Bovim and coworkers examined 20 unselected adult autopsy cases without a history of headache according to the hospital files.[70] They found variations in the anatomic relation of the GON to muscles and tendons. Such variations may contribute to predisposition to entrapment in certain individuals. On the basis of this study, it can be inferred that the semispinalis muscle of the neck most often is penetrated by the GON.[70] Nerve penetration to the trapezius was also a frequent finding, although a greater variation in the course of the nerve was present.[70] Bovin and co-workers indicate that these findings contrast with some classic anatomy books that describe the GON as circumscribing these muscles to reach the occipital insertion of the trapezius.[70] It is speculated that entrapment of the nerve may occur from an increase in muscle tone (guarding, spasm, etc.) of any one or two of the muscles names above.[70] Symptoms associated with GON entrapment may be relieved by physical therapy management.

Location of symptoms associated with GON entrapment would be in the area innervated by cutaneous branches of the GON. Cutaneous branches and their innervation of the GON include:[64]

Medial branch. Innervates the occipital skin.
Lateral branch. Innervates the region above the mastoid process and behind the pinna (the projecting part of the ear lying outside of the head).
Intermediate branches. Run rostrally and ventrally across the top of the skull as far as the coronal suture. At the coronal suture, the GON is traditionally regarded as communicating with terminal branches of the supraorbital nerve.

Based upon the cutaneous innervation, complaints may be located in the occipital area, the top of their skull and/or around or in the ear or TMJ. A burning dysesthesia, described by the patient as "my hair is on fire," may also be a clinical presentation of GON entrapment.[4]

During manual palpation over the GON, certain symptoms may occur that cannot be explained by the GON's cutaneous innervation. Unilateral hemicranial, fronto-ocular or dysaesthesias located in areas innervated by the trigeminal nerve may still be attributed to GON and or C2 involvement.[68,71–73] Symptoms located in these areas are best explained by the convergence of cervical and trigeminal afferents on common neurons in the trigemino-cervical nucleus. This neuroanatomic connection will be described in more detail in the section on Cervical Spine as a Source of Cephalic Symptoms.

Nerve Root

Nerve root involvement will be referred to as *radiculopathy*. Radiculopathy is a central nerve root entrapment of any portion of a nerve root from the intervertebral foramen and medially. As with peripheral entrapment neuropathy, a central entrapment neuropathy can occur by mechanical irritation or compression from some impinging anatomic neighbor. *Stenosis* is a frequent term meaning a narrowing or stricture. Stenosis can involve any anatomic opening, one of which can be the intervertebral foramen. Various causes have been attributed to stenosis of the intervertebral foramen possibly resulting in radiculopathy.[74] Stenosis of the intervertebral foramen has often been attributed to pathologic change of the intervertebral disc.[75] Symptoms of radiculopathy may range from localized neck symptoms to referral of symptoms into the shoulder and upper extremity. Neurologic assessment may show varying degrees of neurologic deficits.

Intervertebral Disc

Symptoms associated with discogenic involvement resulted from the discovery by Mixter and Barr that the nucleus pulposus in the lumbar discs can "herniate" through the annular fibers to occlude the nerve root within the intervertebral foramen.[76] In the cervical spine, a herniated nucleus pulposus as a *direct* cause of radiculopathy is not as likely as it is in the lumbar spine.[77] The nucleus pulposus of cervical discs are initially very small in the child and, in adults, have only a relatively brief existence as a soft central gel.[78–81] Horizontal fissuring of the annulus begins toward the end of the first decade, usually accompanied by an associated loss in disc height.[81] Horizontal fissuring is universal in the adult cervical disc, completely dividing the posterior two-thirds of the disc in late adult life.[78,82] Progressive and slow loss of nuclear material continues with the central gel converting to firm fibrocartilage.[83] In the adult cervical spine the nucleus pulposus is usually absent at most levels. In many adult discs, the anterior annulus is the only intact part of the disc.[81] The progression of cervical disc degeneration is a relatively linear function of age in that 90 percent of the population is afflicted by age 60 and 50 percent severely so.[82] Thus *nuclear* protrusion and herniation, which has long been a feature of descriptions of lumbar pathology, is not a major problem in the cervical spine.[81,83]

The end product of this nuclear pulposus degeneration is referred to as *cervical spondylosis*. Cervical spondylosis as defined by Parke "is not a single temporal or pathologic entity, but the result of a concatenation of degenerative events of which the initial lesion is the deterioration of the intervertebral disc."[83] The end product of cervical spondylosis can be radiculopathy or myelopathy. The evaluation for cervical spondylosis can be through x-rays, identifying disc space narrowing, osteophytosis of both the facet joints and joints of von Luschka, and hypertrophy of the ligamentum falvum.[83] The highest incidence of cervical spondylosis is at the level of C5–6.[84] A more in-depth discussion of cervical spondylosis is provided in Chapter 12.

Radiculopathy secondary to cervical spondylosis may require a different physical therapy approach to management. Depending on other clinical and paraclinical findings (Ch. 12), additional medical involvement may be in order. Fortunately, degeneration of the cervical disc is insidious and most often asymptomatic unless suddenly exacerbated by a traumatic stress[83] or dramatic changes in occupational or recreational activities. Studies on neck pain and disc degeneration seen in imaging studies have shown that there is only a weak correlation between symptoms and degeneration.[85,86] A host of medical diagnoses such as disc degeneration, bone spurs, degenerative arthritis, arthrosis, etc., fall under the spectrum of cervical spondylosis. This host of cervical spondylitic diagnoses should not misdirect the clinician's attention away from addressing the other tissues previously covered (muscle, facet joint, peripheral nerve) that could instead be the primary source of the patient's neck and distal symptoms.

In conclusion, cervical radiculopathy appears to be related to degenerative changes secondary to loss of nuclear material rather than from a *direct* herniation of a soft nucleus pulposus. A major study has demonstrated that spinal pain is rarely derived from structural abnormalities such as a herniated disc or stenosis; such conditions exist in only 1 percent of the target population.[87] It remains to be seen whether or not the disc itself can be a *significant* source of symptoms. In a recent study, Mendel and co-workers[88] confirmed previous reports that no nerves are to be found in the nucleus pulposus. Nerves were found throughout the annulus, however, and provide further evidence that human cervical discs are supplied with both nerve fibers and mechanoreceptors.[88,89] It has been suggested that in severe traumatic cases that did not result in death, pain originating from the nerve endings located in the annulus of the disc is possible.[89] Hence, the disc may be implicated as a source of a patient's symptoms. Further discussion on the disc as a source of pain will occur in the section on Management by the Use of Cervical Collars.

Summary

This section addressed key tissues that can be the cause of the patient's neck, shoulder, and upper extremity symptoms. All tissue components can be managed through physical therapy intervention. Depending upon the mechanism of injury, chronicity, patient's irritability, and degree of degeneration, medical management may be necessary (see Ch. 12, 13). Clinicians will recognize that a pure entity of tissue involvement is not common; instead, the patient's symptoms are often of diverse etiologies.

CERVICAL SPINE AS A SOURCE OF CEPHALIC SYMPTOMS

It is evident that cephalic symptoms can be due to serious disease or pathology and require a thorough neurology and often otolaryngology examination. It is just as evident that the cervical spine has not been sufficiently recognized as being a source for nondiseased or pathologic cephalic symptoms.

Neuroanatomy

The following is the documented neuroanatomic pathway explaining how nociceptive activity originating in the cervical spine tissues is perceived by the patient as symptoms in the head, face, and jaw areas (Fig. 11-3).[90]

> The spinal nucleus of the trigeminal nerve consists of three parts: pars oralis, par interpolaris, and pars caudalis. The pars caudalis extends cau-

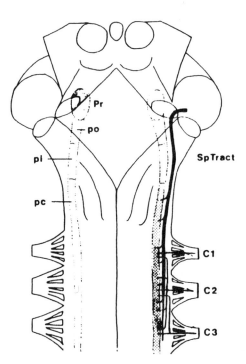

Fig. 11-3. A posterior view of the brainstem illustrating the disposition of nuclei of the trigeminal nerve. The principle nucleus of the trigeminal nerve (Pr) lies at the level of the pons. Below it extends the spinal nucleus of the trigeminal nerve which is subdivided into pars oralis (po), pars interpolaris (pi), and pars caudalis (pc). On the right, the continuity between the pars caudalis and the spinal grey matter is indicated by the shading. This column of grey matter receives afferents from the spinal tract of the trigeminal nerve (Sp Tract) and from the C1, C2, and C3 nerve roots.

dally to merge with the grey matter of the spinal cord. The spinal tract of the trigeminal nerve descends to the level of at least C3 level and possible as far as the C4 level. Fibers from the spinal tract terminate in the pars caudalis and in the upper three segments of the spinal cord. In the spinal cord, termination of the spinal tract of the trigeminal nerve overlaps those of the upper cervical nerves.

From the above description, Bogduk summarizes[90]: ". . . terminals of the trigeminal nerve and the upper three cervical nerves ramify in a continuous column of grey matter formed by the pars caudalis of the spinal nucleus of the trigeminal nerve and the dorsal horns of the upper three cervical segments." Bogduk states that this region of grey matter can legitimately be viewed as a single or combined nucleus, for which he prefers to use the term *trigemino-cervical nucleus*.[90] Thus, the anatomic basis for cervical headache appears to be the convergence of trigeminal and cervical afferents in the trigeminocervical nucleus.[90–95] Trigeminocervical nucleus incorporates the essential central nervous structures responsible for the transmission of pain. The trigeminocervical nucleus receiving afferents from the trigeminal and upper cervical nerves is viewed by Bogduk as the nociceptive nucleus for the entire head and upper neck.[90] Essentially, nociceptive information from cervical spine tissues is transmitted to the trigeminocervical nucleus, which in turn gives the patient the perception of symptoms in the head, face, and jaw areas.[90–95] (Figs. 11-4, 11-

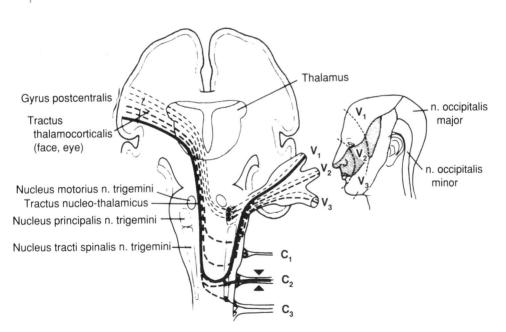

Fig. 11-4.   Transference of pain from C2 innervated tissues or greator occipital nerve or C2 nerve root compression into the fronto-ocular region—a hypothesis. (From Jansen et al.,[68] as modified from Jansen and Spoerri,[380] with permission.)

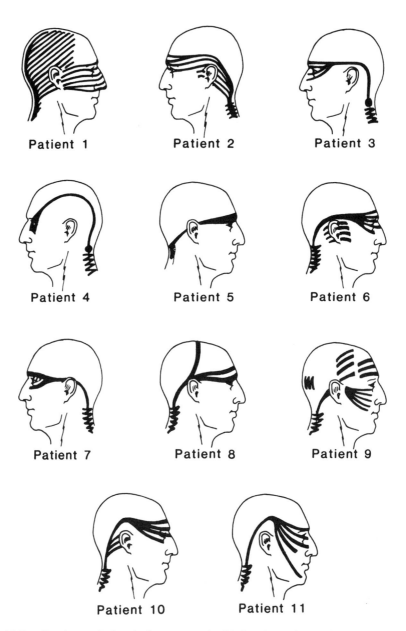

Fig. 11-5. Cervicogenic headache pattern in 11 female patients. See Table 11-1 for explanation. (From Fredriksen et al.,[109] with permission.)

5, Table 11-1). Those tissues with sensory innervation from the upper three cervical nerves are:[90]

C1 Sensory Distribution
Suboccipital tissues and muscles
Atlantoccipital and atlantoaxial facets joints
Paramedian dura of the posterior cranial fossa and dura adjacent to the condylar canal
Upper prevertebral muscles (longus capitis and cervicis and the rectus capitis anterior and lateralis)

C2 Sensory Innervation
Skin of the occiput
Upper posterior neck muscles; semispinalis capitis, longissimus capitis and splenius capitis, the sternocleidomastoid, trapezius, and prevertebral muscles
Atlantoaxial facet joint

Table 11-1. Cervicogenic Headache Pattern in 11 Female Patients[a,b]

Description	No. of Cases
Accompanying symptoms and signs	
Nausea	7
Vomiting	6
Piloerection	7
Photophobia	5
Phonophobia	10
Reduced hearing, subjectively	2
Dizziness	9
Tinnitus	2
Irritability	10
Discomfort in the throat	6
Rhinorrhea, symptomatic side	4
Tearing, symptomatic side	4
Blurred vision, symptomatic side	9
Redness of eye, symptomatic side	4
Edema of eyelids, symptomatic side	8
Head movement leading to precipitated attacks[c]	
Turning of the head	8
Bending forwards	5
Bending backwards	5
Location of "pressure" points[d]	
Midway between external occipital process and mastoid process	8
C_2 area—that is, behind and just below the mastoid process	8
Transverse processes of the C_3/C_4	8
Muscle insertion of the external occipital protuberance	1

[a] See Figure 11-5 for diagrams.
[b] Mean age of 43 years. Durations of headaches were: 5 patients, <5 years; 2 patients, 5–10 years; 1 patient, 10–15 years; 2 patients, 15–20 years; 1 patient, >20 years. The pain was very constant in duration when considering the single patient.
[c] A total of ten patients could precipitate attacks by one head movement or another.
[d] In a total of 10 patients attacks could be provoked from the pressure points. (Modified from Fredriksen et al.,[109] with permission.)

Paramedian dura of the posterior cranial fossa
Lateral walls of the posterior cranial fossa

C3 Sensory Distribution
Multifidus, semispinalis capitis, sternocleidomastoid, trapezius, and pre-
vertebral muscles
Suboccipital skin
C2/3 facet joint
Cervical portion and intracranial branches of the vertebral artery

Numerous studies over the years have confirmed the trigeminocervical connection. Kerr, through electrical stimulation of the rootlets of the C1 dorsal nerve, produced pain in the orbit, frontal region, and vertex.[94] Cyriax injected 4 percent saline into various posterior neck muscles, which produced local and referred pains to the forehead and temporal regions.[96] Campbell and Parsons injected 6 percent saline in the basal occipital, occipitocervical, and C1/2 areas, which produced frontal pain.[97] Feinstein et al.[98] induced forehead pain by stimulating the midline soft tissues between occiput and C1, and occipital pain by stimulating the upper cervical interspinous spaces. Bogduk and Marsland, through electrical stimulation of the C3 dorsal ramus, evoked referred pain to the occiput, mastoid region, and forehead.[99]

Clinical experiments clearly demonstrate the capacity of experimental painful stimuli in the upper neck to produce referred pain in the head.[90] It is therefore proposed that cervical spine involvement of any of the tissues and/or structures innervated by the upper cervical nerves is equally capable of producing referred pain into the head.[90,100]

Cervicogenic Headache

The dental explanation of the etiology of headache is often TMD.[101] The medical explanation of the etiology of migraine headache is often vascular, and of a tension-type headache is often psychosomatic.[102] In 1988 the Ad Hoc Committee on the Classification and Diagnostic Criteria for Headache Disorders recognized the cervical spine as an etiology for headache.[103]

John Edmeads[104] points out that in order for the cervical spine to be a source of headaches, the following three conditions must be obtained:

1.   There should be pain-sensitive structures within the neck
2.   There should be identifiable pathologic processes or physiologic dysfunctions within the neck capable of serving as an adequate stimulus to the pain receptors in the cervical structures
3.   There should be identifiable neurologic pathways and mechanisms through which pain originating in the cervical structures may be referred to the head.

It appears that all of Edmeads' criteria are present for the cervical spine to be a source of headaches. Referring to #2 above, in the absence of disease processes, the role is less clear when understanding dysfunction. Controversy over this point is inevitable because of the difficulty and, at times impossibility, of demonstrating in a reliable and valid way certain types of dysfunction, other than to say "it is clinical opinion." The reader needs to keep this in mind during the upcoming discussion on diagnosis and management. I believe that the ensuing management for cervical spine involvement can be extremely effective in alleviating local, distal, and cephalic symptoms. The reason for such therapeutic responses may not always be apparent.

Several names have been used to incriminate the cervical spine as the source of headache such as "syndrome cervical sympathique posterieur"[105] and "cervical migraine."[106] The term *cervicogenic* was first used by Sjaastad et al. in 1983.[107] The previous two terms used to describe a headache of cervical origin have been replaced with the term *"cervicogenic headache."*[107] "Cervicogenic" only indicates the region, it does not indicate the structure primarily affected.[107] Since 1983, numerous articles have appeared in the literature providing documentation on the existence of a cervicogenic headache.[71,108–117]

The following is a description of the clinical features of a cervicogenic headache:[109]

> Predominately unilateral symptoms (at times bilateral) always on the same side of a non-excruciating, non-continuous character, without cluster pattern. Unilateral symptoms are combined with signs of neck involvement in the form of ipsilateral pain/stiffness and a decrease range of motion of the neck. Variable presence of ipsilateral shoulder or arm pain are also part of the clinical picture. Precipitation of the headache occurs either by neck movement or pressure on certain tender spots on the neck. Tender spots on the neck [as originally described by Sjaastad[107]] are over the C2 nerve root, greater occipital nerve and over the transverse process of C4/5. The attack typically lasts from 1 to 3 days, and the pain free interval (or at least a period with clearly reduced pain) typically varies from 1 to 3 weeks.

The Ad Hoc Committee on the Classification and Diagnostic Criteria for Headache Disorders makes the following comment on cervicogenic headache[103]:

> Cervical headaches are associated with movement abnormalities in cervical intervertebral segments. The disorder may be located in the joints or ligaments. The abnormal movement may occur in any component of intervertebral movement, and is manifest during either active or passive examination of movement.

The radiologic investigative methods (cervical myelography, cerebral angiography, cerebral computed tomography (CT), cervical CT, plain x-rays of the cervical spine, x-rays of the cranium, and x-rays of the paranasal sinuses) utilized by Fredriksen and co-workers[114] did not offer any clear evidence regarding the etiology of cervicogenic headache. The etiology for cervicogenic headache, as suggested in this chapter, will be any one or combination of muscle, facet joint, and neural tissue (peripheral and or central) involvement.

Cervical spine involvement needs to be considered even when other forms of headache have been implicated. There is no doubt an overlap of diagnostic categories since most headaches are diagnosed by location of symptoms.[117] The cervicogenic headache is not suggested to replace a more popular headache label (i.e., common migraine or tension-type headache) but at the very least, cervical spine involvement should be considered as a primary or secondary feature or epiphenomena. The following are several classifications of the more frequently seen headaches that may be mistaken for headaches originating from the cervical spine. The reader is referred to the references for further information on this vast topic of headache.[118]

Migraine

Migraine has been considered a disorder of cerebral or extracranial blood vessels, blood constituents, or possibly a primary disorder of the brain itself.[119] Semantically, the term *migraine* derives from the Latin *hemicrania* which ipso facto should designate a unilateral headache.[113]

Classic Migraine. *Premonitory* symptoms apply to changes in mood (i.e., elation, hyperactivity, depression, and/or irritability) which occur up to 24 hours before the attack.[113] *Prodromal* symptoms such as the visual aura, especially the scintillating scotoma, are part of the migraine attack and usually last less than 30 minutes, followed by headache. Nausea and vomiting may also occur with the aura.[113,120]

The certainty of diagnosing a classic migraine usually exceeds that with which one of common migraine can be made.[113] Walters[121] indicated that the symptoms most frequently diagnostic of classic migraine (prodrome, unilateral onset, and nausea) occur together only a little more frequently than by chance, thereby making the diagnosis of classic migraine questionable. Bakal and Kaganov[122] demonstrated that muscle contraction and migraine headache patients were equally familiar with head pain locations thought to be diagnostic of each group. Migraine patients also experienced muscle contraction symptoms more frequently than migraine symptoms according to Bakal and Kaganov.[122] Olesen[123] raised the question, "Is the muscle tenderness which develops in association with a migraine attack caused by the migraine pain (reflex spasm) or is it a primary event causing the migraine?" Kaganov et al.[124] concluded that "There was a strong trend for increasingly problematic/severe headache to be accompanied by an increasing presence of both muscle contraction and migraine symptoms." The question still remains unanswered as to whether or not muscle contractions precipitate a migraine like attack.

Common Migraine. This headache is differentiated from classic migraine by the absence of a visual aura.[113] Common migraine can be easily confused with cervicogenic headache because of the lack of typical visual disturbances and the fairly long-lasting nature of attacks.[71] There are no scientifically acceptable diagnostic tests for common migraine, so an admixture of cervicogenic headaches could be overlooked and treated as though they were common migraine.[113]

Tension-Type Headache

The clinical features describing cervicogenic headache are close to those of tension-type headache. A tension-type headache is based on the criteria that the headache appears almost daily as a constant tight pressing or bandlike sensation in the occipital, temporal, and/or frontal areas.[118] Tension headache is bilateral but not necessarily symmetrical. The patient cannot provoke a tension headache by head movements and there is no painful limitation of neck mobility.[102,125] The cause is believed to be emotional stress. Cervicogenic headaches that involve the muscles of the cervical spine could also be triggered by emotional stress. The possibility that a patient could experience a cervicogenic headache bilaterally, ("unilaterality on both sides") has been suggested.[126] As was the case with common migraine, an admixture of symptoms originating from the cervical spine could be overlooked and treated as though the symptoms were all caused by a tension-type headache.

Post-Traumatic Headache

The organic source of post-traumatic headache has been thought to be localized in the brain, in the scalp, or in the soft tissue of the neck.[127] Head trauma invariably implies some traumatic impact to the neck. As discussed in the section that follows on dizziness, various visual disturbances and ear symptoms following head trauma could be part of a cervical spine-related headache.[127,128] It is suggested that therapy directed to the cervical spine can influence headaches that are of post-traumatic origin.[127,128]

Summary

In the following quote by Frykholm (1983),[129] if one substitutes "cervicogenic headache" for "cervical migraine" many of the preceding chapter concepts about this type of headache classification are well summarized:

> In my experience, cervical migraine is the type of headache most frequently seen in general practice and also the type most frequently misinterpreted. It is usually erroneously diagnosed as classical migraine, tension headache, vascular headache, hypertensive encephalopathy or post-traumatic encephalopathy. Such patients have usually received inadequate treatment and have often become neurotic and drug dependent.

Dizziness

Dizziness "is a general term, implying only the sense of a disturbed relationship to the space outside oneself."[130] Vertigo is the illusion of motion or position, either of the patient or the patient's environment, and has been used more specifically to connote rotation.[131] Both dizziness and vertigo refer to a false sensation of motion of the body and will be considered synonomously in this chapter.[132] Dizziness often is described by the patient as unsteadiness, imbalance, floating, light headedness, spinning and as those features of ataxia noted subjectively.[130–132] Dizziness results from discrepancy or conflict in positional information from the cerebellum, vestibular nuclei, ears, eyes, proprioceptors, and other peripheral receptors.[90,132] Uemura and co-workers[133] state that "if a patient can stand on either leg with eyes closed, he may be regarded as essentially normal, and other vestibular tests are not necessary." Troost[134,135] lists the cause of vertigo as either a peripheral or central disorder. A brief discussion of peripheral disorder will aide the therapist to appreciate and respond accordingly to patients who may get dizzy when manual therapy to the cervical spine is administered. Pertinent to this discussion are central disorders contributing to dizziness in which one of the various etiologies can be cervical spine involvement.

Peripheral Disorders

Benign paroxysmal positional vertigo (BPPV) is the most common diagnosis of the peripheral disorders.[136] BPPV bears discussion since it may often be confused with cervical vertigo. Common clinical findings of BPPV are vertigo and nystagmus when the patient is moved from a sitting to a supine position with the head over the edge of the table and the neck in 30 to 45° of extension and 30 to 45° of rotation, referred to as the Hallpike-Dix maneuver or Nylen-Barany test.[137] Vertigo usually appears after a 1- to 5-second latency period once the patient's head has been placed in the provoking position previously described. In order to observe the nystagmus, the patient must be lowered quickly. Vertigo along with nystagmus increase in intensity and disappear in 30 to 60 seconds while the provoking position is maintained.[138] The cause is usually dysfunction of the vestibular end organ—semicircular canals, utricle, and saccule.[138] Treatment is based on two theories—"cupuloithiasis" and "canalithiasis."[137] Cupulolithiasis theory proposes that degenerative debris from the utricle fall onto the cupula of the posterior canal, making the ampulla gravity-sensitive.[139] Canalithiasis theory proposes that the degenerative debris is not adherent to the cupula of the posterior canal but instead is free-floating in the endolymph.[140] A specific physical therapy exercise program has become a common treatment for BPPV.[136,141–143] The exercise treatment approach purports to dislodge embedded debris in the canals or to habituate the central nervous system (CNS) response to movement-provoked vertigo.[136]

Central Disorder

The most common central disorder involves the vestibular nuclei.[90] The vestibular nuclei are often involved through ischemic processes,[144] or through disturbances of the tonic neck reflexes often referred to as cervical vertigo or reflex vertigo.[134,145]

Ischemic Vertigo. Ischemic vertigo involves the basilar artery or the vertebral artery. Vertebrobasilar artery occlusion can be the first sign of vertebrobasilar insufficiency.[144] Many additional signs and symptoms (nausea, vomiting, faintness, ataxia, and blurred vision) so often accompany dizziness of any origin that they cannot be used as reliable indicators of ischemic vertigo.[144] However, the presence of diplopia, drop-attacks, dysarthria and/or dysphagia in association with dizziness is *highly indicative* of vertebrobasilar occlusion.[146] The serious consequences of ischemic vertigo are obvious and cannot be overlooked. If in doubt, the clinician must have the patient consult with a neurologist or otolaryngologist. Ischemic vertigo can be caused by intrinsic or extrinsic factors that can decrease blood flow to the vestibular nuclei.[90] The clinician who performs manual procedures to the cervical spine must be alert to both intrinsic and extrinsic factors. Emphasis will be on extrinsic factors since the involvement of extrinsic factors can be more readily tested by the physical therapist and, if positive, may become a contraindication for manual therapy to the cervical spine.

Intrinsic factors may involve such conditions as atherosclerosis of the vertebrobasilar system. If this is suspected, secondary to the *highly indicative* symptoms associated with vertebrobasilar occlusion as mentioned above, a referral to medical personnel is forthright.

Extrinsic factors involve the vertebral artery. The close relationship between the cervical spine and the vertebral artery can predispose the vertebral artery to injury.[147] Congenital anomolies altering the spine and route of the vertebral artery as well as spondylitic cervical changes may adversely influence the integrity of the vertebral artery. It is recommended that prior to active/passive cervical spine exercises, the cervical spine be moved or positioned so as to test for vertebral artery symptoms, primarily dizziness.[148,149] A general screening maneuver for vertebral artery symptoms (i.e., dizziness, as related to extrinsic factors) will be discussed in the section on Diagnosis.

Reflex Vertigo. Reflex cervical vertigo can also effect the vestibular nuclei activity and cause dizziness.[90,145] Often the diagnosis of BPPV is confused with reflex vertigo.[145] Both cervical vertigo and BPPV may have a history of trauma and both can induce dizziness by head movement.[145]

Bogduk states that "along with the eyes and labyrinths, the cervical vertebral column is an important source of proprioceptive information that influences the sense of balance, and it is well known, on clinical grounds, that cervical disease or injury can be accompanied by vertigo, but of a nature that does not imply vertebrobasilar insufficiency."[90]

Neck proprioception consists of the muscle spindle reflexes and tonic neck reflexes (TNR).[150,151] Recognition of the role that muscle spindle receptors play in providing abundant proprioceptive feedback cannot be overlooked.[152,153] The proprioceptive outflow from the muscle spindle is a result of gamma motor neuron activity, which is influenced greatly by the TNR.[40,154] The TNR, with its influence over muscle spindle activity, can be considered a main source for neck proprioception. The TNR originates in the facet joints of the upper cervical spine and will be discussed further in the section on Cervical Spine Influences on Mandibular Position and Movement.

Although orientation of the head in space is the special role of the vestibular apparatus, there is, as Cohen states,[155] "no conceivable way by which the semicircular canal or the otoliths can, by themselves, inform the brain of the angle formed by the head and the body." Orientation of the head to the body can only be achieved by neck proprioception. To have information from the vestibular system indicating a position of the head in space without information from the neck proprioceptors indicating relationship of head on neck, would prove greatly insufficient to function.

Vestibular catastrophes such as vertigo and nystagmus can be caused solely by abnormalities related to neck proprioceptors.[155] Various studies show that damage to deep cervical tissues, including neck muscles, produce a generalized ataxia, with symptoms of imbalance, disorientation, and motor incoordination.[153,157–159] Vertigo, ataxia, and nystagmus were induced in animals and humans by injecting local anesthetic into the neck.[160] The injections presumably interrupted the flow of afferent information from neck muscles and joint receptors. Ataxia in humans was associated with a broad-based staggering gait, hypotonia of the ipsilateral arm and leg, and a strong sensation of ipsilateral falling or tilting.[160] Hinoki,[161] through his experiments and clinical studies, suggests that vertigo following a whiplash injury may be due to overexcitation of the cervical soft tissues, such as muscles, ligaments, facet joints, and sensory nerves. Other seemingly unrelated symptoms such as vomiting, tinnitus, and diminished hearing could be related to cervical spine involvement.[145] Several studies have also shown that proprioceptive impulses from various neck receptors influence eye movements.[162–164]

In conclusion, cephalic symptoms such as headaches and dizziness can have a variety of origins and may require input from a variety of health professionals. In all instances, however, the attentive clinician must address cervical spine involvement as one of the primary sources of cephalic symptoms.

CERVICAL SPINE INFLUENCES ON MANDIBULAR POSITION AND MOVEMENT

This section analyzes and outlines the effects of cervical spine involvement on mandibular position and movement. The rest position of the mandible is primary to this analysis. Mandibular rest position and trajectory of mandibular closure as effected by cervical spine dynamics are reviewed. Ways in which the vertical dimension of an intraoral orthotic appliance potentially alters cervical spine dynamics are highlighted. Clinical observations pertaining to cervical spine influences upon mandibular dynamics complete this section of the chapter.

The Rest Position of the Mandible

The rest position of the mandible is the position at which all functional mandibular movements of the mandible start and end.[165,166] When the mandible is in its rest position, a freeway space exists between the upper and lower arch of teeth.[167] The average freeway space is 3 mm and is measured between the tips of the central upper incisors and central lower incisors.[168] The freeway space has also been referred to as interocclusal distance, interocclusal clearance, interocclusal gap, or the interocclusal rest space.[169] The rest position of the mandible has also been referred to as the clinical rest position, tonic rest position, and rest relation.[170] A more appropriate term to describe the position of the mandible at rest is the *upright postural position of the mandible* (UPPM).[171] The term itself implies the essential interrelationship of the jaw, head, and neck in the upright posture.

In previous terminology the postural position of the mandible at rest implies a state of quiet or repose. However, in the UPPM, there is tonic contraction of the muscles attaching to the mandible.[172] Kawamura and Fujimoto[173] found spontaneous motor activity in masticatory muscles in the clinical rest position. Thus two "rest" positions have been stated to exist with the mandible: the clinical UPPM and the EMG rest position.[174] The mandibular EMG rest position has an average 11-mm freeway space and is not the same as or near the UPPM, which has an average 3-mm freeway space.[172,175,176] In the clinical setting, the diagnosis of an EMG rest position is difficult to arrive at (see Ch. 4) and does not influence treatment options. Clinically, it is therapeutic to decrease the amount of time a patient stays in occlusion and increase the amount of time the patient spends in the UPPM.

Dentistry often uses the UPPM as a guide to determine vertical dimension of occlusion (VDO) for diagnostic and therapeutic purposes in both edentulous as well as dentulous patients.[177,178] Dentistry has and continues to improve scientific evaluation of the UPPM other than by clinical judgment.[177] Conventional methods using a physiologic approach to arrive at an UPPM have involved swallowing, phonetics, and esthetics and are still used today.[179] Electromyography (EMG) with or without biofeedback, the myomonitor/kinesiograph,[180] and the use of cephalometric analysis[181] have been use to evaluate the UPPM. In the final analysis, judgement and clinical trial are still the common choices of the dentist when determining the UPPM.[178]

Numerous subtle factors can influence the UPPM from person to person as well as interpersonally from day to day and moment to moment.[182] Anatomic factors (weight and number of teeth) physiologic factors (tongue positioning and breathing), and pathologic factors (ridge resorption under dentures) may all influence the UPPM.[169,170,183,184] Other influences such as age, drugs, and emotions have been suggested as influencing the UPPM.[185] Identifiable yet imprecise, the UPPM is still a position to which reference is made as a basic datum in many procedures in clinical dentistry.[176-178]

Cervical Spine Dynamics Influencing Mandibular Position

A variable influencing the UPPM that has not received much consideration is the cervical spine. Effects of cervical spine dynamics on mandibular tissue elasticity and mandibular muscle tone will be considered as factors that influence mandibular dynamics. Before pursuing this discussion, an overview of cervical spine dynamics is offered.

Cervical Spine Dynamics

The term *cervical spine dynamics* will be interchanged with the term *head-neck posture*. The term *altered cervical spine dynamics* will be interchanged with the terms *forward head posture* and *cervical spine involvement*. Cervical spine dynamics infer regional (flexion, extension, rotation, and sidebending) and segmental (movement between vertebrae) movements required to achieve and maintain a given head-neck posture. Terms such as "forward head posture" and "upright posture" can be misleading. Clinicians may mistakenly think a "forward head" posture necessitates a problem. On the other hand "good" head-neck posture may mistakenly suggest an absence of cervical spine dysfunction. Studies that investigate static cervical spine relationships without considering cervical spine dynamics will most likely arrive at invalid conclusions.[186] In the presence of good cervical spine dynamics, a forward head posture may be normal. Focus should be on the patient's posture and on the presence or absence of normal regional and/or segmental cervical spine dynamics. The status of cervical spine dynamics can only be determined by doing a physical examination that considers active and passive mobility assessment.

Achievement and maintenance of head posture in humans is an interaction of numerous factors; factors that are not totally understood and have not yet been recognized. Evolution, heredity, congenital growth and development, and pathologic factors influence the head-neck posture. Once musculoskeletal maturity is reached, other factors such as the aging process[187] and a decline in health[188] will create changes in function and performance capabilities and contribute to a deterioration of head-neck posture. Whereas these factors are recognized as exerting a long-term effect on head-neck posture, the achievement and maintenance of head-neck posture on a moment-to-moment basis will be accomplished through the peripheral and central control system.

Peripheral System

The peripheral system includes the vestibular, occular, and proprioceptive systems. Pertinent to the cervical spine is the proprioceptive system, which would include the muscles (muscle spindles) and tonic neck reflex (TNR). TNR pertaining to reflex vertigo has been previously addressed. Involvement of the proprioceptive system can have a significant impact on cervical spine dynamics in the achievement and maintainence of posture.[159,160,189–192] TNR will be mentioned again as a variable that can influence masticatory muscle tone.

Central Control System

The central control system (the brain) also influences the achievement and maintanence of posture on a continual basis.[193,194] Determination of head position is an interaction between the peripheral system and central control system[193,194] The central control system is comparing feedback from the peripheral system with pre-existing data that is based upon the central control's past and current proprioceptive experiences. Only when the feedback that the central control system anticipates is matched with the peripheral system's feedback does a certain head-neck posture exist.[195] This designates a type of reverse action of one system's dependence upon another. This reverse action of interdependence is the concept of reafference, promoted by the Nobel lauriate Nikolaas Tinbergen.[195,196] This concept of reafference strongly indicates that at various levels of integration from single muscle units up to complex behavior, the correct performance of many movements and positions is continuously checked by the central control centers.[196]

Peripheral and central control mechanisms constantly adjust, fine tune, and maintain the infinite number of head-neck postures used to fulfill the task at hand. Muscles and facet joints in the upper cervical spine provide important proprioceptive feedback for the peripheral system. Empirically, cervical spine management, especially manual therapy techniques, can influence the proprioceptive system in a therapeutic way. Empirically, the central control system is influenced by general and/or specific exercise programs that are designed to "put into touch" the patient's awareness on body movement and positioning.

Cervical spine dynamics are suggested to have the most immediate and long-lasting effect on the UPPM.[165,198–200] Patients present with various combinations and degrees of head-neck postures that may be flexed, extended, rotated or side bent. A three-dimensional model that displays the various effects the cervical spine can have on the UPPM is not available. What is available are conclusions derived from normal subjects in which the effects of head-neck postures in extension and flexion upon mandibular position and movement were investigated. Conclusions regarding cervical spine influences upon mandibular position and movement in a patient population are based entirely on empirical observations.

Tissue Elasticity Tone Affecting The UPPM

Tissue elasticity tone refers to the elastic tissue properties found in connective tissues both outside the epimysium and within each muscle.[201] The epimysium is the connective tissue sheath surrounding each muscle. Elastic properties consist of the connective tissue of the muscles, namely the fascial sheaths and the fibrillary muscle protein molecular aggregates (myosin and actin) within the individual muscle fibers.[201,202]

Tissue elasticity tone is present in all muscles. Slow closure of the mandible from a fully opened position to occlusion has been shown to take place without any change in muscle activity of the jaw closing muscles.[203] A study investigating jaw closing from a fully opened position showed that the closing was controlled by the elastic qualities of the digastric muscles.[204]

Cervical spine dynamics may affect tissue elasticity tone in muscle or connective tissue extending from the cervical spine or cranium to the mandible. During active or passive extension of the head on the neck, an increase in tension occurs in the supra and infrahyoid musculature that would result in depression of the mandible, thereby increasing the freeway space.[203,205] Ultimately, changes in head-neck relationships affect tissue elasticity tone about the mandible so as to alter mandibular position at rest.[206]

Muscle Tone Affecting The UPPM

The continuous state of tonic muscle activity occurring in the mandibular elevator muscles, namely the masseter, temporalis, and the medial pterygoids can influence UPPM. Resting muscle tone is primarily an expression of the number of firing motor units.[207,208] The motor unit consists of the anterior horn cell, the cell's axon, and all the muscle fibers innervated by the axon.[209] The anterior horn cell's activity will be influenced by both peripheral and corticospinal (central control) activity.[208] Under normal circumstances, the number of active motor units of the mandibular elevators should be minimal when the mandible is in the UPPM. The TNR can influence mandibular muscle activity.[210]

The role of the TNR in reflexly orienting the limbs in relationship to the head-body angle was described by Magnus in 1912.[211] Magnus,[212] in his classic work, analyzed the postural reaction of the decerebrate quadrupeds when their heads were experimentally turned to an extreme right or left position. He found extension of the forelimb on the side toward which the head was turned and flexion of the opposite forelimb.

Localizing the origin of the TNR to a specific area and tissue began with Magnus and DeKleijn,[213] who had limited the receptive field for the TNR to the first three cervical segments of the spine. They showed that the decerebrate cat possessed TNR that were not labyrinthine in origin but occurred secondary to activation of neck proprioceptors. The neck proprioceptors that are implicated consist of the facet joint receptors (the mechanoreceptors) and muscle spindle receptors. McCouch et al.,[214] showed in 1951 that the TNR of the decerebrate labyrinthectomized cat were not abolished when the muscle mass of the neck was sectioned. The TNR was abolished only after the facet joints in the upper cervical spine were denervated, demonstrating that facet joint mechanoreceptors in the upper cervical spine are the origin of the TNR.

The TNR affects mandibular muscle tone through the trigemino-neck reflex. The trigemino-neck reflex has been demonstrated to occur via motor neurons located in the subnucleus caudalis and probably in the dorsal horn of the upper cervical spine. (Table 11-2)[40,215,216] This is verified when electric stimulation is applied to the central end of the ablated first cervical nerve and electromyographic activity is recorded from the masticatory muscles.[215] There appears then to be a closely organized neurophysiologic reflex relationship between TNR activity and trigeminal motor neuron activity. In the same study, EMG responses were abolished after the first three cervical nerves supplying the facet joints were cut.

Extension of the head on the cervical spine produces an increase in jaw muscle activity in the temporalis, masseter, and anterior digastric.[215,217] An investigation measuring anterior digastric and masseter muscle activity in response to head extension showed a marked increase in the masseter and a decrease in the anterior digastric muscle activity.[210]

Flexion of the head on the cervical spine causes a general decrease in jaw muscle activity, especially in the temporalis and masseter muscles.[215,217] Anterior digastric activity consistently increases with head flexion.[218,219]

In a study involving 30 normal adults, EMG was used to determine masticatory muscle activity in response to extension and flexion. Incremental movement of the head by 5°, 10°, and 20° into extension and flexion induced changes in EMG recording for the muscles under investigation (i.e., anterior temporalis, masseter, supra and infra hyoid muscles).[218]

The above studies conclude that during extension of the head on the neck, an increase in tone occurred in the supramandibular muscles under investigation. Flexion of the head on the neck caused a decrease in the same supramandibular muscles. Changes in head-neck relationships effects mandibular muscle tone, which will alter how the mandible is positioned at rest.

Cervical Spine Dynamics Influencing the Trajectory of Mandibular Closure

Mohl states:[219]

> we must logically conclude that, if rest position is altered by a change in head position, the habitual path of closure of the mandible must also be altered by such a change."

Table 11-2. Morphological and Functional Characteristics of Cervical Articular Receptor Systems[a]

Type	Morphology	Location	Parent Nerve Fibers	Behavioral Characteristics	Functions
I	Thinly-encapsulated globular corpuscles (100 μm × 40 μm) in clusters of 3 to 8	Fibrous capsule of joint (superficial layers)	Small myelinated (6–9 μm)	Static and dynamic mechanoreceptors; low threshold, slowly-adapting	(a) Tonic reflexogenic effects on neck, limb, jaw and eye muscles (b) Postural and kinaesthetic sensation (c) Pain suppression
II	Thickly-encapsulated conical corpuscles (280 μm × 100 μm), singly or in clusters of 2 to 4	Fibrous capsule of joint (deeper layers). Articular fat pads	Medium myelinated (9–12 μm)	Dynamic mechanoreceptors; low threshold, rapidly-adapting	(a) Phasic reflexogenic effects on neck, limb, jaw and eye muscles (b) Pain suppression
IV	Three-dimensional plexus of unmyelinated nerve fibers	Entire thickness of fibrous capsule of joint. Walls of articular blood vessels. Articular fat pads	Very small myelinated (2–5 μm) and unmyelinated (<2 μm)	Nociceptive (pain-provoking). High threshold, nonadapting	(a) Tonic reflexogenic effects on neck, limb, jaw and eye muscles (b) Evocation and pain (c) Respiratory and cardiovascular reflexogenic effects

[a] Please note the functions (a) of Type I, II, and IV receptors. (From Wyke,[40] with permission.)

A change in the UPPM will influence the trajectory of jaw closure to the initial tooth or teeth contact. Altered cervical spine dynamics affects the UPPM, which results in a change in the trajectory of jaw closure.

McClean[220] studied changes in occlusal contact points during changes in body position by inclining the subject on a tilt table from a supine to upright posture while maintaining a constant head-to-thorax position. Electrical stimulation of the elevator muscle was done while the body position was changed from a supine to an upright posture. The results showed that in the supine position, contact points were more retruded. As the upright position was approached, the contact points moved forward into maximum intercuspation. Changes in occlusal contact patterns reflects changes in the trajectory path of mandibular closure during involuntary jaw closure. It was postulated that changes were due to gravitational influence on tissue elasticity tone and masticatory muscle tone. The position of the head-neck in the earth's gravitional field has been shown in other studies to change the UPPM and trajectory of jaw closure.[207,221]

The sound (acoustic energy) of occlusal contacts as maxillary and mandibular teeth come together provides information regarding the end-point of jaw closure.[220] The sound of occlusal contact is picked up via bone conduction by a contact microphone placed on the forehead of the subject. As the teeth meet, the sounds are recorded on tape, which constitutes the occlusogram. This technique is referred to as *gnathosonics*.[222] During voluntary and involuntary (electrically stimulated) jaw closure, occlusogram findings display either premature tooth contacts or prolonged intercuspal sliding contacts when present. Premature tooth contact occurred more often and in a more posterior position when subjects were in the supine position verses the upright position. Changes in occlusograms reflected changes in the trajectory of involuntary and voluntary mandibular closure. Graded changes in body position, from the supine to the upright position, appear to alter the function of the afferent-efferent loop that controls the finite and discrete neuromuscular coordination of a voluntary jaw closure to centric occlusion.[220,221,223,224]

Mohl[197] demonstrated habitual closing pathways are posture-dependent with subjects in the upright position. Extension of the head on the neck produces more posteriorly placed habitual closing pathways, with the initial occlusal contact occurring behind the maximum intercuspated position. Conversely, flexion of the head on the neck produces more anteriorly placed habitual closing pathways. Postural effects on occlusion in the upright position similar to Mohl's study were also found by Brenman and Amsterdam.[225] One study investigated the effects of normal subjects assuming different degrees of anterior to posterior positioning of the head-neck while maintaining the eyes in the horizontal plane. Vertical and anterior components of mandibular position and movement were altered.[226]

In summary, UPPM and trajectory of mandibular closure was altered in normal subjects when head-neck posture was moved from a supine to an upright posture, when the cervical spine was moved into extension, flexion, and anteroposterior movement with eyes kept horizontal in the sagittal plane.

Cervical Spine Dynamics and Vertical Dimension of Occlusion

Vertical dimension of occlusion (VDO) is the distance designated from the base of the nose to the base of the chin, when the teeth are in maximum intercuspation.[178] The freeway space encompasses the space between the UPPM and VDO. The freeway space is a physiologic necessity that allows the muscles of the oral-masticatory system to relax.[227] If the freeway space is infringed upon by increasing VDO, this may cause disturbances in the oral-masticatory system.[227]

Contrary to what has just been said, most patients adapt to changes in vertical dimension. The determination of the height of occlusion might not be a critical procedure as has often been stated.[228,229] However, these views may change if VDO is increased in patients with altered cervical spine dynamics.

There are many ways in which dentistry can change VDO. Pertinent to this discussion is the intraoral orthotic appliance, which will increase the vertical dimension. Appliance thickness may range from thin to thick according to the dentist's individual judgement and the various theories indicating use of an appliance.

Several studies support the view that the head is maintained by synergistic activity of the anterior head-neck and posterior head-neck muscles, as documented by EMG confirmation.[230,231] Studies have shown a close correlation between trigeminal inputs and neck muscle activity,[232,233] suggesting some degree of synergy exists between these two areas. Neural communication also has been shown to exist between the trigemino-neck reflex and the jaw opening reflex.[234] Research has shown[172,235] that as VDO is increased, EMG activity of mandibular muscles decreases until a resting range of approximately 11 mm is achieved. Speculation that a decrease in cervical spine muscle activity may occur as a response to the increase in VDO is inviting. I am not suggesting that intraoral orthotic appliances should be at a vertical dimension of 11 mm in order to decrease neck muscle activity. The preferred way to decrease neck muscle activity is to address the cervical spine directly through physical modalities and manual procedures.

Using a bite wedge that increased vertical dimension by 8 mm, Daly demonstrated the occurrence of cervical extension in 90 percent of his subjects (30 male students) within one hour.[236] This finding is sequential to the observation of Vig et al.[237] Two studies showed that when vertical dimension was increased, there was a tendency for the head to be raised from the horizontal plane, as measured by lateral cephalometric analysis.[238,239]

I hypothesize that the following head-neck posture events occur in response to an increase in VDO. In order to receive an object between the teeth two responses will occur. The most obvious response is depression of the mandible. The second and less obvious response is extension of the cranium on the cervical spine. When yawning, one will experience that opening the mouth is accompanied by extension of the head on the neck. Placing a thick object between the teeth (i.e., a half-inch wooden dowel), would result in depression of the mandible and extension of the head on the neck. Extension of the head directs the eyes above the horizontal plane. The peripheral system (i.e., neck proprioceptors) will attempt to bring the eyes back to the horizontal plane. To return the eyes to a level position, the head-neck will either self-correct into an axial head-neck posture or move forward and slightly down, bringing the eyes level. Which way the patient self-corrects will often depend on the condition of the cervical spine (Fig. 11-6). A more dynamic cervical spine will experience less adverse reaction to any thickness of an intraoral orthotic appliance. In a more involved cervical spine, even a thin appliance can increase or reproduce the patient's symptoms.

Changes in cervical spine dynamics in response to the vertical dimension of an appliance may provide yet another explanation for symptomatic changes (improvement or aggravation) in response to an appliance. The anterior repositioning appliance used to "recapture" a disc displacement, often overcorrects jaw position in both the horizontal and vertical dimensions. The more the jaw is advanced anteriorly, the more the vertical dimension is increased. Williamson[243] relieved the symptom of vertigo (dizziness) in 25 patients (for 11 of the 25 patients, vertigo was the chief complaint) who had internal de-

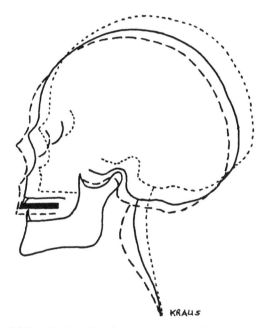

KRAUS

Fig. 11-6. The solid line depicts head-neck posture prior to a change in vertical dimension. Not shown is the initial response of the head extending on the cervical spine in response to an increase in vertical dimension by an intraoral orthotic appliance. Following the initial response of extension of the head on the cervical spine, in order for the eyes to return to the horizontal plane, one of two head postures may occur. The dotted line depicts an axial head-neck posture that would bring the eyes to the horizontal plane. The dashed line depicts a head-neck posture that is more forward and slightly down that would bring the eyes to the horizontal plane.

rangement with an anterior repositioning appliance.[240] He presented two hypotheses implicating the TMJ in the association of vertigo (dizziness) with internal derangement. In my opinion, a third explanation could be that the VDO of the anterior repositioning appliance altered cervical spine dynamics. The reader is reminded of an earlier section discussing dizziness, reflex vertigo, originating from the cervical spine. In this same study, dizziness reoccurred in 6 patients when they were taken off the anterior repositioning appliance after 3 months of wear. These same 6 patients underwent remission of their vertigo when placed back on the anterior repositioning appliance. It would be interesting to know if these 6 patients had cervical spine involvement. If cervical spine involvement was present it would be interesting to see if cervical spine management would have relieved the dizziness so as to avoid the continuation of the anterior repositioning appliance and subsequent occlusal work.

A patient's positive or negative response to the vertical dimension of an intraoral orthotic appliance will be dependent upon (1) the degree of cervical spine involvement, (2) thickness of the intraoral orthotic appliance, and (3) patients' individual physiologic adaptive range. The clinician should be aware that an intraoral orthotic appliance will effect mandibular posture which in return may directly or indirectly effect the cervical spine.

Clinical Significance of Cervical Spine Dynamics Influencing Mandibular Dynamics

The clinical interrelationship between the vertical dimension of an appliance and the cervical spine has been addressed. Attention will now focus on the clinical significance of the trajectory of jaw closure effected by an intraoral orthotic appliance and cervical spine dynamics. A discussion of this clinical hypothesis will begin with the occlusion, since it is the occlusion to which the appliance is fabricated.

The occlusion has been considered a popular etiology for the development and progression of TMD and/or MMH.[241] Reduction of MMH with an intraoral orthotic appliance is often used to minimize further aggravation to the TMD.[242,243] Appliance designs vary depending on the patient's occlusion, degree of TMD and/or MMH, and the dentist's preference. Although an intraoral orthotic appliance fits over an arch of teeth (mandibular or maxillary), symptomatic improvement from wearing an appliance may have nothing to do with the occlusion. A review of *intercuspal occlusal relationships* and *functional occlusal relationships* concluded that the etiologic role of occlusal factors has been overstated in the past, and in recent published research.[241,244] Intercuspal and functional occlusal interferences are too common and variable to offer sensitivity or specificity for defining a present or potential TMD population.[244] Intercuspal investigations consisted of skeletal anterior open bite, overbite, overjet, symmetry of retruded contact position, crossbite, and posterior occlusal support.[241] *Functional occlusal relationships* are occlusal contacts occurring when the teeth *are not in maximum intercuspation but contact is occurring during specific mandibular movements.*[244] Functional occlusal relationships reviewed by Seligman consisted of balancing and working occlusal contacts, retruded contact position-intercuspal position (RCP-ICP) slide length and symmetry, occlusal guidance patterns, parafunction, and attrition.[244]

Although the role of occlusion in the development of TMD and/or MMH signs and symptoms remains controversial,[245-248] intraoral orthotic appliances have been and will no doubt continue to be a popular treatment choice offered by the dentist.[242,243,249]

Understanding the role of the cervical spine influencing *functional mandibular movements* may help in understanding yet another aspect of *functional occlusion*. Functional mandibular movements have been defined as "all natural, proper, or characteristic movements of the mandible made during speech, mastication, yawning, swallowing, and other associated movements."[250] The following discussion pertains to a single aspect of functional occlusion involving occlusal interference(s) as maximum intercuspation is approached. This aspect of functional occlusion is suggested to be influenced by cervical spine dynamics.

Searching/Avoidance Phenomenon

Regardless of cervical spine dynamics, the first contact between the upper maxillary teeth and the lower mandibular teeth during a series of jaw closures to maximum intercuspation is postulated to be a "searching" maneuver.[251] There is a registration of an afferent "engram" in the sensory cortex arising from the periodontal mechanoreceptors (the proprioceptors of the teeth).[251] The periodontal mechanorecepters are stimulated by the impacts and gliding contacts of the occlusal surfaces as the teeth move towards a position of maximum intercuspation. The afferent signals arising from the contacting occlusal surfaces interact with proprioceptive elements in the mandibular musculature to form a central sensory-motor "feedback-loop" that modifies the occlusal behavior of the individual.[223] Other investigators[252-254] demonstrated that the existence of occlusal interferences resulted in altered patterns of neuromuscular activity that tended to *circumvent* the occlusal interferences, and which were typified by *increased* EMG activity.

Similar to the searching maneuver, the "avoidance phenomenon" (Ch. 6) is believed to be a protective mechanism to prevent or minimize overloading of the joints or teeth. The avoidance of or the circumventing of occlusal interferences is done at the expense of altered (increased) muscle activity. A study investigated the introduction of an occlusal interference in 12 healthy subjects for a 1-week period.[255] The individual response to the interference varied substantially with regard to muscle tenderness to palpation. However, at the end of the experimental period, adaptation of the neuromuscular system to the interference was evident.

Avoidance maneuvers may be secondary to a "malocclusion" or "pseudomalocclusion." A pseudomalocclusion will infer an occlusal interference occurring prior to maximum intercuspation, resulting from altered cervical spine dynamics. Therefore, it would seem as though altered cervical spine dynamics may trigger the "searching maneuvers"/"avoidance phenomenon" as maximum intercuspation is approached. This postulated series of events is as follows: (expanded from Mohl).[197,219]

Cervical spine dynamics affects the UPPM through alteration of tissue elasticity tone and mandibular muscle tone.

A change in the UPPM affects the trajectory of jaw closure.

A change in the trajectory of jaw closure results in tooth/teeth contact prior to maximum intercuspation (the pseudomalocclusion).

Teeth contact prior to maximum intercuspation are avoided but at the expense of altered (increase) muscle activity (searching/avoidance phenomenon).

Avoidance of tooth/teeth contact prior to maximum intercuspation continues as long as the patient's *physiologic adaptive range* is not exceeded.

An unlimited number of head-neck postures can be achieved throughout the day and night. Varying degrees of cervical spine involvement will accompany each individual patient. Therefore, it would be futile to attempt to predict a specific way that the mandibular posture and movement will be effected by cervical spine involvement.

The postulated series of events listed above can be experienced in the following exercise:

1. Sit or stand straight with jaw relaxed and begin to slowly look up and down. As previously described, tissue elasticity tone and muscle tone are affecting mandibular posture in response to extension and flexion of the neck.

2. Return the head to a neutral head posture. Now slowly and lightly tap the back teeth together. Be sure to relax and not allow cortical influences to dictate how the muscles move the mandible.

3. With the head straight continue tapping. Notice that in some individuals, occlusal contacts may be occurring in maximum intercuspation while others may be experiencing the initial occlusal contacts to be forward, back, left, or right to maximum intercuspation.

4. Continue tapping, and slowly look up and then down. What should be experienced is a change in the initial occlusal contacts from those contacts made in the neutral head posture.

5. Continue to tap with the head extended or flexed. Now avoid the initial tooth/teeth contacts and close straight into maximum intercuspation. The avoidance of occlusal contacts prior to maximum intercuspation can be done regardless of the head-neck posture. However, the avoidance of the pseudoocclusal interference(s) is done with an increase in masticatory muscle activity.

It can be surmised in the previous exercise that altered cervical spine dynamics, regardless of the occlusal state, may be a source of masticatory muscle hyperactivity. I know of no studies confirming the previous observations in a symptomatic cervical spine patient population. The clinician, however, should be suspicious that MMH is originating from cervical spine involvement when (1) the history and physical examination is positive for cervical spine involvement, (2) the history indicates that the patient's cervical spine complaints preceded mandibular complaints, and (3) the patient's response to an intraoral orthotic appliance has been unfavorable.

Historically, bruxism is believed to be a result of occlusal prematurities and interferences[256] or stress.[257] However, both the etiology and the pathology are unknown. Could a symptomatic cervical spine be added to the list of multiple causes of bruxism? Is it possible for a patient to experience physical stress because of "neck pain," causing the patient to respond by clenching and/or bruxism?

There is speculation regarding the effects of cervical whiplash injury on the TMJ and MMH. Recent studies have shown that patient populations with a cervical spine whiplash injury have a higher incidence of signs and symptoms of TMD compared to a matched controlled group.[258,259] Unless there is a reported direct trauma to the mandible during a traffic accident, I have difficulty in accepting that jaw whiplash/jaw lash[260]/internal derangement whiplash[261] causes traumatic tearing of the posterior attachment at the time of the cervical spine whiplash. The high incidence of jaw-related symptoms to cervical whiplash may be explained by the patient clenching and/or bruxing in response to cervical pain occurring as a result of the cervical whiplash.

I have had the opportunity to see numerous intraoral orthotic appliance designs. The appliances were used for the treatment of TMD and/or MMH related symptoms and dysfunction. Many clinicians relate the success of splint therapy to breaking patterns of occlusal contact and deprogramming the musculature[242,243] that may be compensating for occlusal irregularities.[249] The design of the appliance should fit individual patient needs with full knowledge of the effects it may have on the TMJs, muscles, and teeth (Ch. 6). To be added to this list are the potential effects the appliance may have on the cervical spine. Splint designs should consider not only the occlusion effecting the UPPM and trajectory of jaw closure (Ch. 6)[262] but also that cervical spine dynamics affects the UPPM and trajectory of jaw closure. From the cervical spine perspective, an appliance that has the features listed below will minimize deleterious effects on the cervical spine yet maintain a therapeutic profile for the treatment of TMD and/or MMH. The appliance features listed below follow similar features mentioned in Chapter 6.

1. Full coverage to allow even contact simultaneously during closure
2. Maxillary coverage preferred though mandibular coverage may be required
3. Hard acrylic
4. Thin
5. Anterior portion of the splint provides immediate posterior disclusion in excursive movements

6. Shallow inclines leading into the centric stops still providing the features stated in #5

7. Avoid aggressive centric relation techniques

8. Appliance should ideally be balanced in more than one head posture (i.e., neutral and then extension or with patient reclining in dental chair)

Summary

Patients experiencing pain and/or dysfunction in the cervical spine may not be able to accommodate to mandibular changes as influenced by an intraoral orthotic appliance. An intraoral orthotic appliance may actually be a stimulus to the patient's symptoms in the presence of altered cervical spine dynamics. A healthy cervical spine is a more forgiving cervical spine when mandibular positioning and mobility is sufficiently influenced by the design and chairside balancing of the intraoral orthotic appliance. Comprehensive management of TMD and/or MMH will include cervical spine management. Dr. Mohl states: [197] "It therefore seems reasonable to consider that at least some of the dysfunctional problems involving the masticatory system could be in some way related to the adaptive requirements imposed by chronic or acute postural demands." The multifactorial etiology and pathophysiology of TMD and masticatory muscle hyperactivity is well accepted today. Cervical spine involvement may indirectly influence this complex topic. In select individuals, however, the cervical spine may be the primary feature contributing to pain and dysfunction.

DIAGNOSING "CERVICAL SPINE INVOLVEMENT"

The Diagnostic Dilemma

Previous sections discussed the cervical spine involvement as a source of neck, shoulder, upper extremity, and cephalic symptoms. The clinical implications of cervical spine involvement influencing mandibular position and movement have also been discussed. This section will discuss the criteria needed to diagnose the cervical spine condition that has, thus far, been referred to as cervical spine involvement.

Medical diagnoses that implicate cervical spine involvement as a patient's source of symptoms include such diagnoses as "neck pain," "cervical sprain," "cervical disc disease," "cervical osteoarthrosis," "thoracic outlet syndrome," "myofascial pain syndrome," "cervical fibromyalgia," and "radiculopathy." Such diagnoses may often rely on only anecdotal experience or general informed judgement gathered from the history and physical examination.[263] Yet for other diagnoses, the use of expensive paraclinical procedures including radiographic, electrodiagnostic, and laboratory procedures may be required.

Ideally, the diagnosis should indicate the source of the patient's symptoms and should provide an insight into the treatment(s) required to resolve the patient's problem. The musculoskeletal diagnosis should be easily assessible by clinical tests and measures to determine effectiveness of treatment. The goal for the majority of all spinal pain patients is return to pain-free functional activity. The extent to which the treatment and the projected outcome/prognosis of treatment is influenced by the diagnosis emphasizes the importance of the diagnosis.[264]

Considering the emphasis placed on the diagnosis, hopefully the diagnosis will be correct. However, treatment, outcome of treatments, and prognosis of spinal disorders (lumbar, thoracic, and cervical), may seldom be based upon the previously described diagnostic scenarios. The following facts illustrate the problems and dilemmas of arriving at a medical diagnosis for spinal pain.

1. Radiographs, a common procedure used to diagnose spinal conditions,[265] may provide little, if any, insight into the source of the patient's symptoms.[266–268] Abnormal structural pathologic findings, including disc herniations, have been found in spines of asymptomatic patients.[269–272] Epidemiological studies show that the prevalence of most abnormalities seen in plain radiographs of subjects with spinal pain is similar to those abnormalities seen in subjects that never had spinal pain.[266,267,269,270]

2. New technology involving radiographs, electrodiagnostic, and laboratory procedures has not altered the overall incidence, morbidity, cost, or disability related to spinal pain disorders.[276] With the unnecessary cost and exposure to radiation yielding no additional information regarding etiology and prognosis of spinal pain,[273,274] some authors propose a selective use of radiographs in spinal pain patients.[275–277]

3. The diagnosis is unknown in 90 percent of spinal patients.[278,279] The vast majority of diagnoses that incriminate a particular tissue source are difficult to identify, because the physical signs and symptoms often have little correlation.[87] It is difficult to establish a correlation between tissue source with signs and symptoms because the degrees of dysfunction do not warrant the removal of tissues to be studied.[87]

4. Terminology and nosology of diagnosis currently used for spinal disorders are neither standardized nor validated.[87] The diagnosis thus becomes the fundamental source of error from which the clinician may formulate a treatment plan that may be done for an incorrect diagnosis.[280,281]

5. The ability of a physical therapist to evaluate the effects of physical therapy intervention for a medical diagnosis is hampered for reasons previously mentioned.[280,281] Physical therapy interventions cannot be shown to be effective for any diagnosis of a spinal condition unless there is a clear statement of the condition.[280,281] These are some of the reasons why there are contradictory findings in the literature and in rehabilitative therapy regarding criteria for evaluating the effectiveness of treatment.[87]

The literature continues to be deficient in scientifically admissible studies pertaining to the evaluation, treatment and prognosis in spinal diagnoses.[87]

Scientific studies need to provide better understanding of how to arrive at meaningful diagnoses for spinal conditions. With advanced diagnostic accuracy, more realistic insight as to the prognosis of returning the patient back to a functional and quality life style might be derived.[280,282]

Complexity of the spinal anatomy, physiology, neurophysiology, and the pain phenomenons are some of the inherent features of spinal pain that make it difficult to arrive at a diagnosis.[87,270,279] In an extensive review of the literature in 1987, the Quebec Task Force on Spinal Disorders concluded that of the numerous acute or chronic spinal complaints, *nonspecific* ailments of the lumbar, dorsal and cervical regions, with or without radiation of pain comprise the vast majority of problems for which the patient seeks help.[87] *Nonspecific* implies a nondiseased condition, meaning that no underlying disease can be established. The clinician should be alert to the possibility of disease or an unrelated musculoskeletal condition that can mimic a nonspecific ailment of the spine.[283] If the clinician is ever in doubt, a referral to the appropriate medical and or dental professional is in order.

Given the vast problems of diagnosing nonspecific complaints, the Task Force found it necessary to propose its own classification of spinal disorders.[87] This classification system was not based on radiological, physiopathological, or mechanistic entities, since they remain too vague in most cases. The Task Force proposed a classification based on simple clinical criteria (signs and symptoms) that represent the majority of cases seen in clinical practice. The Task Force proposed a classification called "Activity-Related Spinal Disorders" for patients having nonspecific complaints. The classification of activity related spinal disorders was divided into 11 categories.[87] (Table 11-3) The following is a summary of each category:

Categories 1–3. Based only on localization of pain (history)
Category 4. Based on the results of the clinical examination
Categories 5–7. Based on the result of paraclinical investigations
Categories 8–10. Based on response to treatment
Category 11. Based on conditions seldom seen or of little importance

The reader is strongly encouraged to read the full report of the Quebec Task Force on Spinal Disorders to appreciate the complexity of all factors (i.e., evaluation, diagnosis, treatment and prognosis) relating to spinal disorders with an initial literature review of 7,000 articles.[87] The report lists the 769 references used by the Task Force in reaching their conclusions.

A growing consensus among clinicians and researchers dealing with nonspecific spinal pain agrees that a new widely acceptable diagnostic classification is needed.[269,284–288] Inspired in part by the Quebec Task Force publication, research and clinical testing of various nonspecific classification systems, in which patients are primarily classified according to signs and symptoms, has been pursued in the medical and physical therapy professions.[268,280,283–286,289–291] Classifying/diagnosing patients according to signs and symptoms should provide a direct treatment plan and a better understanding of treatment outcomes.[289,292,293] Physical therapists would share in the domain of diagnosing/

Table 11-3. Classification of Activity-Related Spinal Disorders

Classification	Symptoms	Duration of Symptoms From Onset	Working Status at Time of Evaluation
1	Pain without radiation	a (<7 days)	
2	Pain + radiation to extremity, proximally	b (7 days–7 weeks)	W (working)
3	Pain + radiation to extremity, distally[a]	c (>7 weeks)	I (idle)
4	Pain + radiation to upper/lower limb neurologic signs		
5	Presumptive compression of a spinal nerve root on a simple roentgenogram (i.e., spinal instability or frature)		
6	Compression of a spinal nerve root confirmed by Specific imaging techniques (ie, computerized axial tomography, myelography, or magnetic resonance imaging) Other diagnostic techniques (e.g., electromyography, venography)		
	Spinal stenosis		
7	Postsurgical status, 1–6 months after intervention		
8	Postsurgical status, >6 months after intervention		
9	9.1 Asymptomatic		
	9.2 Symptomatic		W (working)
10	Chronic pain syndrome		I (idle)
11	Other diagnoses		

[a] Not applicable to the thoracic segment.
[b] (From Spitzer et al.,[87] with permission.)

classifying patients according to signs and symptoms that identify the condition. A diagnosis based upon signs and symptoms would be the focus of the physical therapist's treatment and reassessment of the patient's condition during, immediately following and prior to subsequent treatments.[288,289] Diagnosis by a physical therapist has been defined by Sahrmann:[294]

> Diagnosis is the term that names the primary dysfunction toward which the physical therapist directs treatment. The dysfunction is identified by the physical therapist based on information obtained from the history, signs, symptoms, examination, and tests the therapist performs or requests.

Studies on the clinical efficacy of classifying patients with nonspecific complaints based upon signs and symptoms have largely addressed the lumbar spine. Therefore, the following classification for nonspecific ailments of the cervical spine is only a proposal. This classification is based upon the author's present clinical impression of nonspecific complaints of the cervical spine. As clinical research pertaining to classifying nonspecific activity related disorders of the cervical spine is expanded, both the name and criteria used in the history and physical examination will be modified.

The proposed classification and categories for nonspecific complaints of the cervical spine are:

Classification: Movement Dysfunction of the Cervical Spine (MDCS)

Category 1. Neck symptom(s) (central) without radiation.
Category 2. Neck symptom(s) and
  a. Radiation, but not into extremity
  b. Radiation into upper extremity
Category 3. Neck symptom(s) + radiation cephalic
Category 4. Patient perception of a limitation in mobility of the neck
Category 5. Patient perception of a limitation in mobility of the neck along with either Categories 1, 2 or 3

Jette states,[288] "the purpose of having a physical therapist establish a diagnosis is to name and communicate the primary impairment, disability, or handicap toward which the clinician directs his or her treatment within that professional's appropriate scope of practice." A physical therapy diagnosis should not be used to reflect ownership of the condition.[288] The following is an overview of the pertinent history and physical examination needed to arrive at the diagnosis of MDCS.

History

The patient's response to the following questions will direct the clinician towards suspecting MDCS. The series of questions will establish a base line as to how the patient subjectively and functionally is responding to treatments offered for MDCS. Short-term and long-term goals will begin to be formulated during the history and will be determined after the physical examination is completed. Further "testing" may be needed to determine more specifics of impairment and functional limitation. The following questions are not meant to be an exhaustive outline of a detailed medical and/or clinical history.

1. What is your primary complaint(s)?

This question should document the chief complaint, the area of the symptoms, and the description of the symptoms. Patient will be asked if the previous features of their symptoms changed since they first become aware of their symptom(s).

Primary Symptoms can consist of any one or combination of:
Headaches
Facial
Jaw
Neck
Shoulder
Proximal or distal upper extremity symptoms

Secondary Symptoms can consist of any one or combination of:
Dizziness
Eye (pressure behind the eyes, eyes sensitive to light, difficulty in focusing
Ear (subjective hearing loss, fullness, ringing)
Throat (difficulty in swallowing, soreness that does not turn into a sore throat)

Insight as to how the cervical spine can be a source of secondary symptoms has been explained in the section Cervical Spine as a Source of Cephalic Symptoms.

Secondary complaints in the absence of "primary complaints" may suggest that the patient does not have MDCS. Secondary complaint(s) needs to occur in conjunction with a "primary complaint(s)" in order to suggest that the secondary complaints are originating from MDCS, although there are exceptions to this. Bell states[295] that the primary pain may be modulated and inhibited until it is not consciously felt by the patient, leaving the secondary referred pain as his complaint. When this occurs, the therapist finds himself with the task of locating the "silent" primary pain that is the source of the complaint.[295] If a secondary complaint(s) is verbalized as the patient's only complaint(s) with no "primary complaint" expressed by the patient, the clinician will have to rely upon the objectives of the physical examination to suggest that the secondary complaint(s) is stemming from MDCS. If the objectives of the physical examination are not achieved, such secondary complaints expressed as primary complaints may not be related to MDCS and a referral to the appropriate health professional is in order.

The clinician must take note that primary complaints such as headache, jaw, and facial symptoms can occur without other symptoms. In other words, the patient may complain only of jaw symptoms with the source stemming from the silent cervical spine. Thus the importance of establishing a differential diagnosis is emphasized. If the TMJ and associated muscles of mastication are not suspected as a source of the patient's symptoms, then the clinician should investigate the cervical spine.

2. What do you believe caused your symptoms?

Any one or combination of the following are possible responses from the patient that should increase the clinician's suspicion that MDCS is present:

Physical trauma (i.e., MVA, fall, blow to the head and neck)
  Patients who received a direct trauma involving the cervical spine usually take longer to recover and can continue to have symptoms for as long as 15 years.[2]
Occupational trauma (i.e., change in the physical working environment; travelling, lifting, reaching, etc.)
Emotional trauma (family or work related)
Recreational trauma (weekend athlete)
Insidious onset (detailed questioning will often indicate that an insidious onset is actually related to one or a combination of the conditions listed above)

3. When did you first notice the appearance of your symptoms?

Less than 7 days
7 days to 7 weeks
More than 7 weeks

According to the Quebec Task Force,[87] acute pain is restricted to 7 days duration, subacute is defined as lasting from 7 days to 7 weeks, and chronic is defined as lasting more than 7 weeks in duration. The Task Force recognizes that the outlook for recovery grows more ominous as time elapses, emphasizing the need to accurately diagnosis and begin appropriate treatments.[87] The Task Force suggests that symptoms that persist past the seventh week after onset (or treatment) require consultation with a specialist. However, the Task Force indicates even in the case of a patient whose symptoms have lasted 6 months, symptoms can still be treated without significant psychologic components.[87] Clinically, MDCS would best be treated within the first 7 weeks. However, MDCS can be managed well into the chronic stages based upon the skill level of the clinician. Variables as discussed in Chapter 13 may also need to be investigated.

4. Describe the intensity, frequency and duration of your symptom(s)

Intensity. Intensity can be graded on the visual analogue scale of 0 to 10.[296] MDCS can have an intensity anywhere from 1 to 10, most common between a 2 to 8.

Frequency. Frequency associated with MDCS can vary from daily to once a month. The less frequently a person experiences symptoms, the longer the patient will need to be followed to determine if treatments have any effect on symptomatic outcome.

Duration. Duration for MDCS can range from an intermittent "fleeting" symptom to a constant symptom that varies only in intensity. A fleeting primary or secondary symptom usually occurs in the presence of another primary symptom(s). As an example, "my jolting head pain" or "ringing in my ears" lasts for only a few seconds, "but my neck pain is constant." The patient may go on to say that the fleeting pain is noticed when the neck pain intensity increases.

This line of questioning, if appropriate, can be done for each primary and or secondary complaint. Some patients may be able to categorize the intensity, frequency, or duration of their symptoms in relation to morning, afternoon, and evening patterns. Asking the patient if symptom(s) are better, worse or no different since onset will provide an idea of the stage the patient is in at this time.

5. What increases, reproduces or decreases your symptoms?

A patient experiencing MDCS often will identify some form of movement and/or positioning of their neck as increasing, reproducing, or decreasing their symptoms. The clinician will recall the silent pain phenomenon explained earlier. If the patient has difficulty in answering this question, the clinician can ask lead questions such as:

Are your symptoms affected by movement or activities involving your head, neck, shoulders, or arms?

Are your symptoms affected by how you hold your head, neck, shoulders, or arms?

Are your symptoms affected by work-related, family-related or self-induced stress situations?

Do you have trouble in getting to sleep, or staying asleep, or are your symptoms present first thing in the morning? Do you find that you have to support your neck a certain way at night in order to get to sleep?

6. What can you not do since you have been experiencing your symptom(s)?

This line of questioning will determine how MDCS is effecting the patient's ability to function. Question the patient about functional activities both at work and at home, sleeping patterns, and recreational activities. If function is not affected then inquire about how their symptoms interfere with their quality of life (i.e., "I do not like going out," "I do not like being sociable or being with my spouse." Still other patients will state they can still do everything but are in pain while doing the activity.

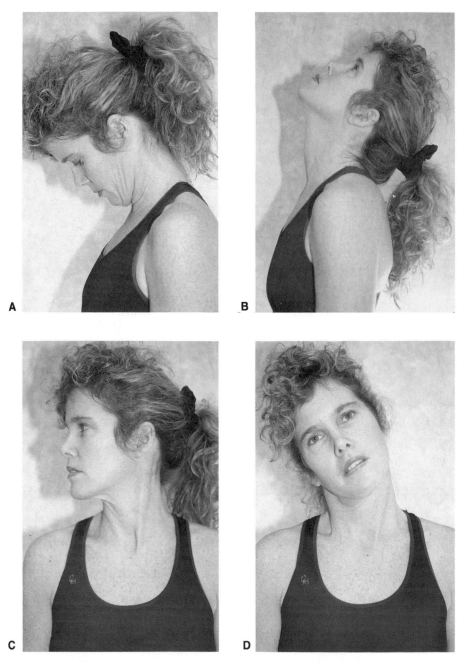

Fig. 11-7. Active movements in the cardinal planes of motion (**A**) Flexion. (**B**) Extension. (**C**) Rotation (right). (**D**) Side Bending (right).

Physical Examination

The physical examination will consist of the following three objectives. Any two of the three objectives along with the pertinent history questions previously covered will help in arriving at the diagnosis of Movement Dysfunction of the Cervical Spine.

Objective I

The patient's symptom(s) is either reproduced, increased or decreased (effected) by either or both (1) active movement(s) performed by the patient; (2) manual procedure(s) performed by the clinician.

Active Movement(s) Performed by the Patient.   Active movements would include the cardinal plane movements of flexion, extension, rotation, and side bending (Fig. 11-7). Combined active movements of diagonal extension, right or left, and diagonal flexion, right or left, may be necessary to effect the patient's symptoms (Fig. 11-8). During and immediately following the active movements, the patient will be asked if the symptoms were affected by any of the active movements.

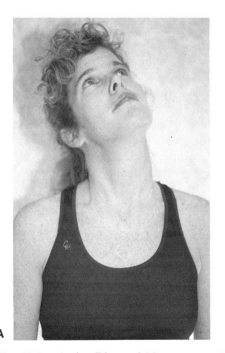 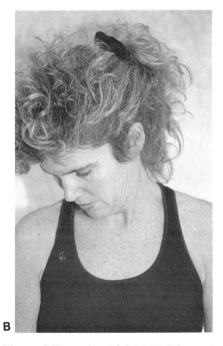

A   **B**

Fig. 11-8.   Active Diagonal Movements. **(A)** Diagonal Extension (right). **(B)** Diagonal Flexion (right).

Manual Procedure(s) Performed by the Clinician. (The specifics as to the manual procedures will be discussed in Objective III.) Active or manual procedures may not affect the patient's symptom(s) all the time. Tissue "irritability" often determines whether or not a patient's symptoms will be affected with active and or manual procedures. Tissue irritability is defined as the clinician's observation as to the ease in which the patient expresses either verbally ("that hurts") or nonverbally (protective posturing) nociceptive activity caused by mechanical or chemical irritation of the involved tissue(s) in response to the active and or manual procedures.

Objective II

The active movements and or manual procedure(s) must incriminate an area that is commonly associated with a primary and or secondary symptom(s).

Active Movements. Active movements of the cervical spine would involve the cervical spine tissues (facet joints and nerve roots) and associated tissues (muscles and peripheral nerves). The clinician may want to stabilize the shoulders of the patient during cervical spine active movements, to ensure that active movements are occurring in the cervical spine area and not the thoracic area.

The clinician should record active range of motion (AROM) performed in the cardinal planes. If AROM is limited by MDCS then treatment of MDCS may result in symptomatic improvement. The patient's perception of improved mobility as well as an observed improvement in mobility by the clinician may also result from the treatment of MDCS.

Recording AROM provides objective data for the examination. The clinician is referred to Youdas and co-workers[297] for comparative analysis of three methods for reliability of measurements for active cervical range of motion.

Clinicians should avoid using previously reported singular values as estimates of normal cervical AROM for both genders and across all ages.[298] In a study involving 337 healthy subjects ages 11 to 97, Youdas and co-workers[298] concluded that AROM had a significant relationship to age and gender. Females usually have more AROM than males[298] and for each 10-year change in age, both females and males lose approximately 5 degrees of neck extension AROM and 3 degrees of AROM for the remaining cardinal planes of motion.[298,299] Due to the wide normal variation of active movements (age, gender, build, and habit) the value of AROM lies more in monitoring progress than in diagnosing.[300]

Manual Procedures. Manual procedures of palpation and passive mobility will be directed toward the six areas outlined in Figure 11-9. Empirical evidence indicates that manual procedures in these areas are frequently correlated with the patient's symptoms. Questions pertaining to specifics of hand placement, direction of force, amount of force, duration of force, and palpatory findings

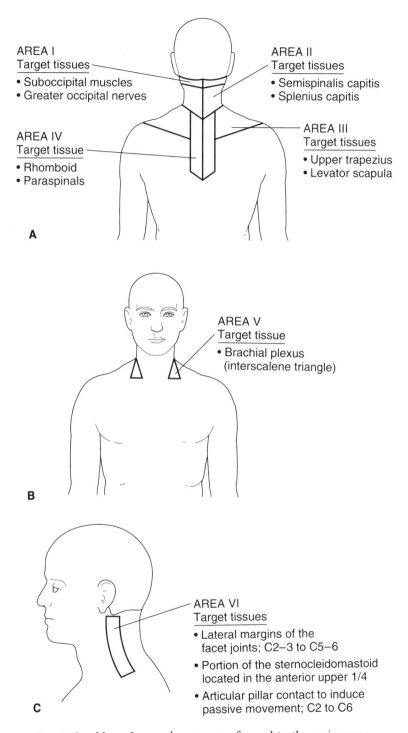

Fig. 11-9. Manual procedures are performed to these six areas.

are beyond the scope of this chapter. Knowledge of anatomy and clinical experience are variables that factor into the skilled application of manual procedures and into the interpretation of the subjective and objective findings.

Objective III

If a manual procedure(s) effects the patient's symptom(s), can the clinician identify altered mobility, position, and or tissue condition in the area(s) being examined?

Target Tissues. A clinical impression of altered mobility (joint, soft tissue), position (osseous positional faults) or tissue condition (increase, decrease of normal muscle, or soft tissue tension) may be determined by the clinician for the targeted tissue(s) in the appropriate area. There are, of course, other tissues that have not been named that are located in these areas. The purpose is not to identify all tissues, but to gather an impression about "key" tissue involvement that will help to arrive at the diagnosis of MDCS.

Area I (Fig. 11-10) Target Tissues
  Suboccipital muscles
  Greater occipital nerve

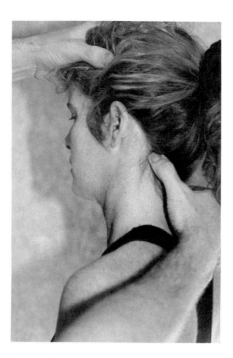

Fig. 11-10.   Area I. Target tissues: suboccipital muscles, greater occipital nerve.

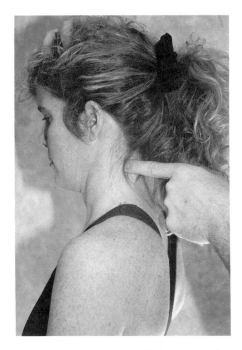

Fig. 11-11.   Area II. Target tissues: semispinalis capitis, splenius capitis.

Area II (Fig. 11-11) Target Tissues
    Semispinalis capitis
    Splenius capitis
Area III (Fig. 11-12) Target Tissues
    Upper trapezius
    Levator scapula
Area IV (Fig. 11-13) Target Tissues
    Rhomboid
    Paraspinals
Area V (Fig. 11-14) Target Tissue
    Brachial plexus (interscaleni triangle)
Area VI Target Tissues
    Lateral margins of the facet joints C2–3 to C5–6 (Fig. 11-15A)
    Portion of the sternocleidomastoid in the anterior upper quarter of area
        VI
    Articular pillar (Fig. 11-1) contact to induce passive movement from C2
        to C6 (Fig. 11-15B)
Areas I–VI (Fig. 11-16)
    Manual traction test.[79] This test is directed to all areas and tissues. It is
    a nonspecific test of the patient's subjective response to a traction force
    applied to the head and neck. Often the patient will report symptoms have

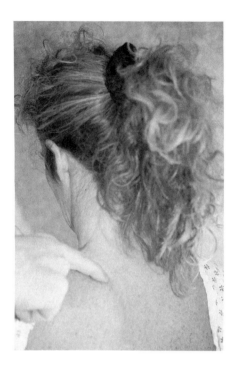

Fig. 11-12.   Area III. Target tissues: upper trapezius, levator scapula.

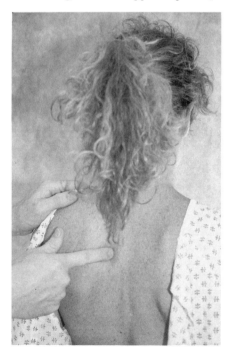

Fig. 11-13.   Area IV. Target tissues: rhomboid, paraspinals.

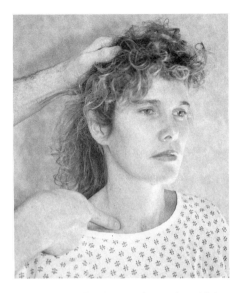

Fig. 11-14. Area V. Target tissue: brachial plexus.

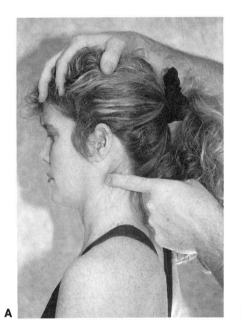
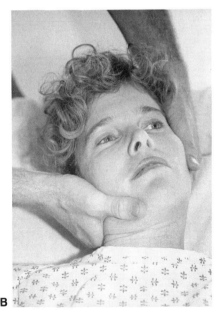

Fig. 11-15. Area VI. Target tissues: (**A**) Lateral margins of the facet joints (C2–3) (a portion of the sternocleidomastoid can be palpated in the anterior upper quarter of area VI). (**B**) C4 articular pillar contact by the right metacarpal phalangeal joint, inducing a passive right side bending motion.

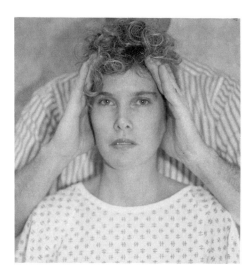

Fig. 11-16. Areas I–VI. Target tissues: a nonspecific passive cephalic traction force applied by the lateral aspect of the thumb of both hands to the mastoid processes.

decreased while the traction is applied. The amount of force is dependent upon the degree of tissue irritability and ability of the patient to relax.

Postural Evaluation. It has long been suggested that faulty posture may be involved in the etiology of spinal pain.[301] In a study of Refshauge and co-workers,[302] 25 subjects with pain in the cervical or trapezius region were age-matched with 25 volunteers. The study failed to show that the size of the cervico-thoracic kyphosis in habitual standing is associated with the presence of pain in the cervical and trapezius area.[302] Griegel-Morris and co-workers[303] looked at postural abnormalities in the thoraco–cervical–shoulder region of 88 healthy volunteers between the ages of 20 to 50 years. The relationship between the severity of postural deviations and the severity and frequency of pain in the thoraco–cervical–shoulder region was not significant.[303] Based upon these studies, ideal postural alignment may need to be redefined. My clinical observations have placed less emphasis on the evaluation of head–neck–shoulder (HNS) posture for the purpose of arriving at the diagnosis of MDCS. This is not to infer that postural instructions are not given to the patient. Patient education about maintaining an upright postural position during standing and sitting postures appears to be extremely therapeutic (Fig. 11-17). With reliability and predictability in question, it appears that an actual "measurement" of posture is not needed in order to diagnose MDCS. What may be more important than static posture is the dynamics of HNS relationship as well as active and passive segmental dynamics. If the patient has good regional and segmental dynamics and is instructed on concepts of good posture, then the HNS relationship obtained by the patient may be considered normal.

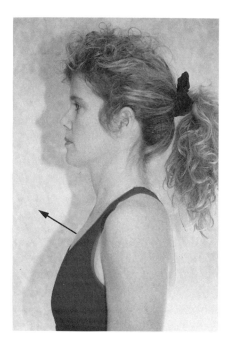

Fig. 11-17. An upright postural relationship of the HNS. Shown also is a line extending up and out from the chest to assist in the awareness of an upright postural position.

Comments on the Three Objectives of the Physical Examination

Additional objectives, areas, and tissues can be included in this form of an examination. For now, I find that if the above objectives are addressed, this will be sufficient to either include or exclude the diagnosis of MDCS. This form of examining is most reliable, valid, predictive, and teachable when combined with sound clinical reasoning. Clinical reasoning is here defined as the cognitive process or thinking used in the evaluation and management of a patient.[304,305] Clinical reasoning is the essential bridge between a history and physical examination and knowing the answer. I do not want to lead the reader to believe that all aspects of reliability, validity, and predictive value of the proposed physical examination have been worked out and documented, for they have not. It is recommended that the clinician read the "Standards for Tests and Measurements in Physical Therapy Practice," developed by a task force of the Committee on Research (1987) by the American Physical Therapy Association.[306] As a profession we need to achieve quality of our tests and measurements, ". . . not only among ourselves and our medical colleagues, but also, more relevantly, among those who must render decisions about our services and livelihood." (S Wolf)[306]. "Clinical practice cannot wait and testing will usually have to proceed; however, physical therapists should be aware of and should acknowledge the limitations of the measurements they are using."[306]

Special Findings of the Physical Examination

Special findings of the physical examination may modify the approach to treatment for MDCS. Manual therapy is a significant portion of the treatment approach. Manual therapy involves a wide spectrum of procedures that are aimed at specific objectives. Contraindications to manual therapy are all relative depending on the special findings of the individual patient and the clinician's skill level. The following special findings will influence the clinician's choice of manual therapy procedures.

Cervical Spondylosis

Cervical spondylosis is a condition involving degeneration[83] and is identified by radiographs. Patients with minimal degenerative changes as seen on x-rays can tolerate manual therapy to the cervical spine. Patients with severe degenerative changes may also benefit from manual therapy depending on which techniques are chosen and how they are delivered.

Standardization of radiographic interpretation for cervical spondylosis is needed so that both the medical and physical therapy professions will know what is meant by minimal, moderate, and severe spondylotic changes. Studies have shown the need to elaborate, validate, and standardize the criteria to improve on the reliability of interpreting plain radiographs[307] and CT scans.[269,307,308] Correlating degenerative changes with history and other physical findings of the examination for the symptomatic patient may provide insight into symptomatic and functional outcomes of physical therapy treatment for MDCS.

Radiculopathy

Upon examination, no finding by itself will validate the presence of radiculopathy. Radiculopathy will require a combination of the following findings on examination:

Neurologic Examination.   Positive for incriminating a specific nerve root based upon muscle, reflex, and cutaneous testing. See neurologic examination section below for additional discussion.

Radiographic Findings of Cervical Spondylosis.   The more severe the degenerative changes on x-rays, the more potential for stenosis of the intervertebral foramina resulting in radiculopathy.

Repeated Active or Passive Diagonal Extension Patterns. Extension of the cervical spine causes a statistically significant decrease in the intervertebral foramina diameter when compared to the intervertebral foramina diameter in a neutral cervical spine position.[309] Combining sagittal extension and ipsilateral rotation (diagonal extension—Fig. 11-8A), causes the most foraminal encroachment at C5, C6, and C7.[309] Diagonal extension patterns may be useful for eliciting pain as a provocative procedures for radiculopathy.[309]

Reproduction of neck symptoms with or without radiation into the shoulder and or upper extremity during diagonal extension patterns requires cautious interpretation. Reproduction of symptoms can be attributed to tissues (muscle, facet joint, peripheral nerve), other than nerve root irritation/compression. Pain in the arm is only a symptom and other tests need to be performed to confirm direct nervous tissue irritation. Reflex mechanisms causing referred symptoms are believed to be more common than mechanical nerve lesions.[310] Even in the presence of a known radiculopathy, I find that a majority of patients can do quite well with manual therapy to the cervical spine.

Upper Limb Tension Tests. The upper limb tension test (ULTT) has been termed the straight leg raise of the arm.[311] The relevant anatomy and biomechanics of the ULTT have been the focus of recent attention.[311-316] The ULTT can be used to test the mobility of cervical nerve roots and peripheral nerve mobility.[312] This procedure combines shoulder depression, shoulder abduction, extension, lateral rotation, forearm supination and elbow extension, and wrist/finger extension.[312] The major cervical nerve roots affected by the above procedure are C5 and C6,[314,315] which are also the main nerve roots involved with radiculopathy.[75] The absence, reproduction or increase in the patient's neck or upper extremity symptoms during or following the completion of the ULTT may help to determine the presence of neural tissue entrapment (central or peripheral). The clinician will need to do a differential examination of the glenohumeral, elbow, and wrist joints and their associated tissues so as to clear other sources of shoulder and upper extremity symptoms.

In summary, correlation of the neurologic assessment, radiographic findings of cervical spondylosis, diagonal extension patterns, and the patient's response to the ULTT will assist the clinician to conclude whether or not radiculopathy is present. If present, the clinician may need to modify certain manual therapy techniques. If the patient does not respond to the proposed management discussed in the next section, and uncertainty about the presence of radiculopathy persists, then additional radiographic and/or electrodiagnostic tests may need to be performed by the physician (Ch. 12).

Neurologic Assessment

A screening neurological examination is performed to assess for sensory, motor or reflex deficits (Ch. 12).

Sensory Testing. Sensory testing for signs and symptoms of nerve root involvement would be indicated in the presence of parasthesia in the dermatomal distribution of the nerve root (i.e., medial and lateral aspect of the upper arm—C5, thumb—C6, middle finger—C7, and ring and little fingers—C8 and T1).[4] Similarly, myotomal pain radiation in the nerve root distribution to distal muscles (C5–6 to the proximal shoulder muscle group, C7 to the triceps and pectoralis major, and C8–T1 to the distal hand intrinsics) may be factored into the clinician's reasoning.[4] Hypoalgesia may be a more valid index of nerve root involvement than hyperalgesia, which is thought to be only a reflection of severity of pain.[317,318]

Muscle Testing. Muscle testing can involve a number of false positives. The therapist's ability to determine the patient's ability to contract maximally in the presence of pain will factor into the clinician's interpretation of a manual muscle test. Research has demonstrated that muscle weakness may be due to pain inhibition that may be abolished by local anaesthetic.[319,320] Saal and Saal[321] found no statistically significant difference in outcome in low back patients with neurologic weakness or with extruded discs from the total study population. They found that the presence of muscle weakness does not adversely affect the outcome of nonoperative treatment, and should not be used as overwhelming evidence that surgery is needed.[321] Radiculopathy can be treated very successfully with aggressive nonoperative care.

Reflexes. Diminished reflexes as with muscle weakness have been shown to be abolished by local anaesthetic.[319,320] The clinician will be alert to false positives during this form of neurologic assessment.

Summary. Composite findings of radiographs and radiculopathy testing may suggest the deferral of manual therapy. Otherwise, I recommend commencing with manual therapy in the treatment of MDCS even in the presence of minimal to moderate neurologic findings, with the understanding that neurologic signs and symptoms will be reassessed prior to and following each treatment session.

Dizziness

As discussed earlier, dizziness can result from peripheral or central disorders. Ischemic dizziness that is caused by the extrinsic factor of vertebral artery involvement will need to be acknowledged before manual therapy is administered to the cervical spine. The vertebral artery test, though described different ways, would classically involve combining active or passive cervical spine rotation and extension.[322,323] The test position should be held for no less than 10 seconds so as to recognize any latent response. The patient's eyes should be observed for nystagmus and the patient should report any symptoms of dizziness. Aspinall[148] suggests a building block approach to clinical testing that should reduce the risk to the vertebral artery. According to Aspinall, testing procedures are performed first in the sitting position, then in the lying position.[148] Positioning for the vertebral artery tests in the upper and lower cervical spine would then be performed individually for each position previously mentioned.[148] A vertebral artery test that is positive will be considered a strict contraindication for manual therapy, especially if significant cervical spondylitic changes are present on x-rays and the patient reports dizziness with certain neck positions (e.g., looking up). If a vertebral artery test is positive, with no prior history of dizziness and normal x-rays, then manual therapy may be only a relative contraindication in the hands of a skilled clinician. Questions arise about the specificity of this testing, as other tissues in the cervical spine can cause dizziness (i.e., reflex vertigo). As discussed in the section on Ischemic Vertigo, symptoms either associated or not associated with dizziness such as diplopia, drop attacks, dysarthria, and/or dysphagia are a strict contraindication to manual therapy or any physical therapy management until the etiology of such symptoms are investigated.

Upper Cervical Instability

The presence of upper cervical instability is usually suspected by history of trauma and rheumatoid arthritides.[324] Instability is confirmed by various radiographic views and or upper cervical ligament integrity testing.[325,326] However, clinicians should be skeptical when interpreting findings from ligamentous testing in the cervical spine because the reliability and validity of these tests have not been established in a clinical setting. The reader is referred to the references for additional information on upper cervical ligament integrity testing.[326,327]

MANAGEMENT OF MOVEMENT DYSFUNCTION OF THE CERVICAL SPINE

The natural history of nonspecific spinal disorders is that they usually improve spontaneously with time.[87,328,329] This known progression towards resolution has been used by doctors to support the advice of bed rest and the use of anti-inflammatories, analgesics and muscle relaxants.[330] Although there is a tendency for spinal pain to improve with time, Roland and Morris[328] concluded that up to one-quarter of patients report increasing disability during the first week after presentation, and one-quarter also report increasing disability during the subsequent 3 weeks. Given that 10 to 20 percent of patients who have a nonspecific spinal disorder do not follow the natural history of spontaneous recovery, a large number of patients continue to require treatment.[331,332] This smaller group of patients is growing and accounts for up to 85 percent of the total cost of spinal pain.[331,333] This group of symptomatic patients may progress from a simple neck pain problem to a chronic neck pain problem that becomes costly. Marbach et al.[334] speculated that because chronic facial pain patients have a larger number of consultations and that most consultations result in no treatment or referral, chronic facial pain patients must resort to an emphasis on the sensory aspect of their complaints to obtain attention from health care providers.

Until criteria are established that will help to identify those patients who will not follow the natural history of resolution from those who do, early physical therapy intervention is suggested for the majority of patients with a nonspecific condition of the cervical spine. Often this may involve only a session on patient education pertaining to posture and activity.[330] Early conservative management can help reduce overall cost and may greatly decrease the chances that acute neck pain will become chronic. Waddell[332] states that "... acute and chronic pain are not only different in time scale but are fundamentally different in kind." The profile of a chronic patient is one of emotional distress, depression, failed treatment, and adoption of a sick role.[332] Early intervention by a physical therapist is strongly recommended to prevent such a catastrophe.

Research that investigates an *approach* using a variety of treatments may be more clinically relevant, as the application of one technique that will remedy the patient's total problem is rare.[335] The following are suggested treatments to be used in an *approach* to the management of an acute or chronic patient with MDCS.

Patient Education

Patient education may be the single most important area in physical therapy management of nonspecific symptoms. The first obstacle in patient education is overcoming the patient's fear, anxiety, misconception, and advice from friends about the meaning of their symptoms. Acknowledging that their feelings and confusion are real and normal may provide a level of comfort for the patient. In an essay by Norman Cousins, it is stated:[336]

> Somewhere in our early education we become addicted to the notion that pain means sickness. We fail to learn that pain is the body's way of informing the mind that we are doing something wrong, not necessarily that something is wrong.

Patients may also perceive "something to be wrong" not only from their symptoms but also from their diagnosis. A diagnosis may actually enhance the feelings of fear and anxiety, which in turn may intensify symptoms and lead the patient to believe that a cure is not available. For example, the diagnosis of "cervical arthritis" or "degenerative disc disease" may create an image of having to learn to live with pain. The diagnosis of "disc herniation" may influence some patients to believe the only cure for their symptoms is surgery. Patients need to be informed that unless there is explicit clinical criteria, their symptoms may originate from tissues other than the disc, which can be treated conservatively. Only in selected patients have surgical procedures of discectomy or fusion demonstrated reduced pain and neurologic deficit.[273] Often, the results of surgically treated patients are less satisfactory than those of conservatively treated patients.[337] In a blinded controlled study of low back surgery, a follow-up at 4 and 10 years showed that patients who had undergone surgery were no better than those who had not.[338] Parry[339] has noted a general belief among specialists that surgery for lumbar pain syndromes has been widely overprescribed. By inference, the same concerns must be raised about cervical spinal surgery.[340] In a follow-up of nonsurgical patients the value of an educational program for potential surgery patients was demonstrated.[341] Education provided the patient with tools to make informed decisions as well as to motivate them to continue their home program and set new goals. In patients who avoided surgery, education provided the opportunity to increase activity without fear of increased pathology.[341]

Health professionals should be careful about the "label" they give the patient considering that the precise diagnoses in the majority of spinal pain patients are unknown.[87,342] Patients' interpretations of the meaning of their diagnosis along with the misconceptions associated with spinal pain suggest a great deal of patient education is needed. Patients should be told that the primary tissues that will be addressed with physical therapy are muscle and joint. Symptoms originating from nervous tissue (peripheral and central) and discogenic involvement will be helped indirectly by addressing the muscle and joint conditions. Patients need to know their symptoms may be managed by addressing the muscle and joint involvement regardless of the degenerative/discogenic involvement. Exceptions to this will be based upon the special objective findings previously covered.

Once the meaning of the diagnosis is understood by the patient, their role in the treatment process is explained to them. Improvement of symptoms and functional limitations is assisted by the patient's active participation in a treatment program. Focusing the patient's attention on ways to reduce and control abnormal stress on the cervical spine is important as unnecessary stress on the pathologic or normal cervical spine and surrounding tissues can exacerbate symptoms.[343] These stresses may occur nocturnally and diurnally. Patient awareness will be directed to sleeping and upright postures, cervical collars, and a specific and/or general exercise program.

Sleeping Postures

Primary and secondary symptoms may interfere with the patient's ability to sleep, stay asleep, or the symptoms may be present upon awakening in the morning. Nocturnal parafunctional activities often have been attributed to causing or aggravating headaches and jaw, and neck symptoms. Treatment for nocturnal parafunction has focused on the use of an intraocclusal appliance.

What should not be overlooked in controlling nocturnal symptoms is proper support to the cervical spine. The cervical spine may not only be a source of the patient's symptoms, but also a possible cause of nocturnal parafunction, as discussed earlier in this chapter. Patient education regarding tongue-up, teeth apart, breathing, and swallowing (as covered in Ch. 7) may carry over into the night to minimize parafunction.

Sleeping positions should be supine and/or sidelying; stomach sleeping will usually exacerbate the patient's symptoms. In the supine or sidelying position, a cervical pillow will be used. The physical therapist may choose from among several cervical pillows. I have observed that pillows that are softer, with a larger diameter, are usually more therapeutic.

Supine Sleeping Posture

A cervical pillow is placed under the patient's neck. Depending upon the patient's anterior to posterior chest position and/or forward head posturing, a regular thin pillow may be placed under the cervical pillow, extending just under the patient's shoulders. (Fig. 11-18) The regular thin pillow may eventually be removed to allow the patient to be in a neutral head posture. However, the forward posturing of some patient heads may be normal; therefore, the regular pillow may always remain under the cervical pillow. Patients who have a long neck may lay with their head slightly in extension over the cervical pillow. If this is observed, a regular thin pillow should be placed under the cranium, which will support the head in a neutral position to the neck in combination with the cervical pillow.

Patients who regularly awaken with upper extremity symptoms secondary to a peripheral or central entrapment may need to have a pillow placed under their involved arm(s) while sleeping. Shoulder girdle depression and traction

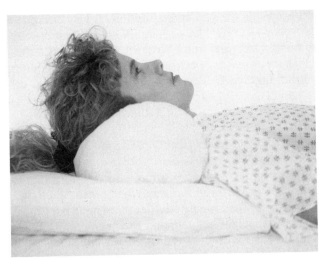

Fig. 11-18. Cervical pillow used in the supine sleeping posture.

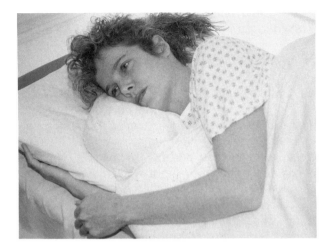

Fig. 11-19. Cervical pillow used in the sidelying sleeping posture.

through the extended arm are means of tensioning the brachial plexus and cervical nerve roots.[344] Elevating the involved arm will lessen tension of the neural tissue in the areas of potential peripheral and/or central entrapments. Placing several pillows under the patient's knees will complete the instructions in the supine sleeping posture.

Sidelying Sleeping Posture

Patients will be told to sleep on their uninvolved side. The cervical pillow will be placed under the cervical spine. (Fig. 11-19) Depending on the width of the patient's shoulders, a regular thin pillow will be placed under the cervical pillow. Depending on the length of the cervical spine, another regular thin pillow will be positioned behind the cervical pillow to support the head. A pillow or two should be placed under the top arm so as to decrease neural tissue tension. A pillow or two between the knees will complete the instructions in the sidelying sleeping posture.

Difficulty in these positions may be due to cervical restrictions that are advanced and cannot accommodate to the supported neck position. If such a situation occurs, manual therapy to the cervical spine for several treatment sessions should be offered first, followed by the use of the cervical pillow.

Upright Postures

Upright postures will focus on the relationship between the (HNS) areas. HNS postures can vary in the sagittal, horizontal and transverse planes. As discussed earlier, several studies showed no correlation between neck–shoulder–thoracic posture and symptoms.[302,303] This does not decrease the importance of educating the patient on postural concepts. Sedentary habits, poorly equipped work sites that result in prolonged positioning in poor postural alignment, and lack of postural awareness may be responsible for poor posture.[303] Tendencies to "yield to gravity" may become more pronounced with age.[345]

The easiest and most effective way for me to quickly educate the patient on the awareness of avoiding poor posture is instructing the patient on "chest up." The patient will visualize a string extending from their upper chest. (Fig. 11-17) The patient will be told to follow the string with their chest. By visualizing the string and the resulting chest position, the patient should be able to avoid a slumped HNS posture during the majority of activity carried out in the upright posture.

Avoiding the poor HNS posture in the sitting position is more difficult for the patient. Static sitting tends to allow gravity to force the patient away from an upright posture. The physical therapist will need to educate the patient about proper chair support and perhaps offer one of the various low back pillow supports that are available. (Fig. 11-20) Supporting the lumbar spine helps to avoid a poor HNS posture. Depending on the patient's work environment and job description, instructing the patient in the use of a pillow or two under their

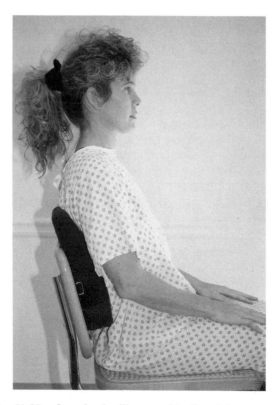

Fig. 11-20.   Low back pillow used in the sitting posture.

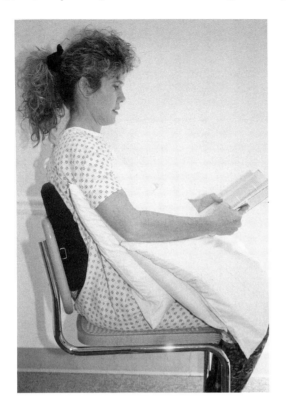

Fig. 11-21.   Low back pillow and pillows under the arms used in the sitting posture.

arms will reduce the tractional force of the arms and shoulders on the neck. Elevating the arms will also decrease neural tissue tension. If pillows under the arms are not practical at work, the pillows can be placed under the arms at home while reading, watching television, etc. (Fig. 11-21) The patient will be told not to watch television or read in bed.

Manual Therapy

Manual therapy consisting of palpation, passive mobility testing, and manual traction was incorporated into the physical examination to assist in the diagnosis of MDCS. Manual therapy will now be discussed as a treatment tool to help in managing the symptoms and dysfunction associated with MDCS.

Manual therapy may consist of hands-on repetitive oscillations, steady stretch or high velocity thrusts of joints, or the application of various forms of soft tissue massage, muscle stretching, or shortening.[346] The potential therapeutic value in manual therapy evolves around the mechanical, neurologic, neurophysiologic and psychological effects of manual therapy.[346-353]

A comprehensive understanding of clinical and scientific viewpoints on manual therapy from clinicians and researchers can be obtained from the references.[346–353]

Clinical discussions pertaining to the cause and effect of mechanical, neurologic, and neurophysiologic involvement of a tissue, the identification of a tissue, and optimal techniques or treatments are diversified.[354] Grieve[355] describes the present state of manual therapy:

> We continue to sound as though we know so much, when we know comparatively little. It might be a good thing to admit this. We make much of clinical science, enthusiastically referring to this or that part of the massive mountain of literature which best serves our particular interest.... Much of what we do is simply what has been proven on the clinical shop floor to be effective in getting our patients better—we do not always know why.[355]

Therapeutic outcome resulting from the use of manual therapy does not necessarily mean that the tissue(s) causing the patient's symptoms have been identified.[356] The spine is a multisegmental system in which tissues work together and potentially fail together through either insidious or traumatic onsets. Singular tissue involvement is the exception rather than the rule. Clinical reasoning used to incriminate a tissue must be kept in proper perspective since the evaluation tools and manual procedures used by physical therapists have not been shown to be completely reliable and valid.[284,306] Steps have and continue to be taken to document the efficacy of the evaluation and treatment using manual therapy. DiFabio[356] in a review of the literature, identified 14 studies that were judged to be valid demonstrations of the efficacy of manual therapy in the treatment of patients who have somatic pain syndromes. DiFabio concluded there was clear evidence to justify the use of manual therapy in the treatment of patients who have back pain.[356] Recently a study has documented that a trained manual therapist is as objective and sensitive as controlled diagnostic blocks in identifying cervical facet joint dysfunction.[45]

Clinicians treat patients on a day-to-day basis and are looking for new directions in improving functional outcomes in patient care. More than we care to acknowledge, clinicians often treat by recalling what worked best for one patient or group of patients and applying that treatment approach to a current patient of similar history and physical findings. Guidelines in research should consider these clinical observations.

In an article by Shepard et al.,[357] entitled *"Alternative Approaches to Research in Physical Therapy: Positivism and Phenomenology,"* two philosophical approaches to research in physical therapy were discussed.[357] This article attempted to detail the subtle philosophical issues of quantitative (positivism) and qualitative (phenomenology) research methods in a comprehensive way. Justice to the contents of this article cannot be done in a few paragraphs. A brief definition of these two different philosophical perspectives is appropriate because they may assist the clinician's ability to formulate and research clinical observations.

The philosophical orientation of positivism is associated with empiricism.[357] The article of Shepard and co-workers quoted Polit and Hungler[358] defining positivism as:

> ... the process whereby evidence rooted in objective reality and gathered directly or indirectly through the human senses is used as a basis for generating knowledge.

Examples of empirical evidence include heart rate, leg length discrepancy, and stride length. Cause and effect relationships are best researched through the positivistic perspective.[357]

Phenomenology tries to understand social phenomena or human activity from the viewpoint of the person being studied.[357] Reality is believed to be socially constructed by the individual, and thus multiple realities exist, not a finite number of objective truths.[357] In defining multiple realities, Sheppard and co-workers quoted Merriam as saying:

> The world is not an objective thing out there but a function of personal interaction and perception. It is a highly subjective phenomenon in need of interpreting rather than measuring. Beliefs rather than facts form the basis of perception.[359]

In a commentary to Shepard et al., Mattingly states:

> Often it is not enough to fix the "body" of the patient. Therapists are also asking the client to become an active participant in therapy, to practice exercises at home, to "buy on" to the goals of therapy. They may even set goals collaboratively, trying to individualize treatment to meet the needs and lifestyles of their clients. Phenomenological approaches have much to offer health practices, especially those such as physical therapy, whenever it matters not only what a patient's physical dysfunctions are but how those dysfunctions affect the patient's life. Put differently, phenomenological research is essential whenever the health professional must address the patient's 'illness experience'."[360] "... If treatment is 'treating a life,' so to speak, and not just a body, then it is important to do research that illuminates the phenomenological aspects of treatment...."[360]

In order to document if manual therapy is better than doing nothing at all, both philosophical approaches to research in physical therapy will need to be addressed. *A classification system that offers consistency to an approach in treatment would be insignificant in manual therapy unless the physical therapist had the ability to modify the approach based upon the individual needs of the patient.* What follows is one of multiple manual therapy treatment approaches. Manual therapy by itself, without involving the other forms of management that have and will be discussed, will not be very effective. I have favored the following manual therapy approach for some time.

Three-Dimensional Movement Techniques

The identification/isolation of a spinal tissue is difficult if not impossible to achieve. Even if the tissue can be identified, it is difficult to know if the treatment is specific to the named tissue. This often leads to a major obstacle in deciding where to begin with a manual therapy approach. The inability to identify and name the tissue(s) does not imply that manual therapy cannot be specific to the dysfunction (restrictions) of a tissue(s) that is causing the patient's symptoms. The naming of a specific tissue (i.e., right upper trapezius muscle, left C2–3 facet joint, right GON or right C5 nerve root) for the majority of patients experiencing MDCS is often not necessary unless a positivistic perspective is strongly suggested from the history and physical examination.

The *initial* approach taken by this author is to use techniques that address *restrictions in movement patterns* of the cervical spine. The techniques are referred to as "three-dimensional movement techniques." Three-dimensional movement techniques are used when there is active and/or passive restrictions contributing to the patient's symptoms and dysfunction. The goal of three-dimensional movement techniques is to improve upon *passive functional movement patterns* that may result in the improvement of *symptoms and active functional movement patterns*.

Before applying three-dimensional movement techniques or other manual therapy techniques, the following criteria is needed: (1) MDCS is present, identified by the history and physical examination; and (2) Acknowledge the presence of "special findings" that may modify the three-dimensional movement techniques.

The three-dimensional movement techniques involve any one or combination of *rotational, diagonal*, and *spiral* movement patterns. To detail hand placement, direction of movement, speed of movement, amount of stretch, duration of stretch, etc., is not the intent of this text. The reader is referred to the photographs in Figure 11-22 to obtain a general idea of the movement patterns created with these techniques. The application of these techniques and others by a skilled therapist will allow for the identification and treatment of specific or general restrictions of the tissue(s). During the application of the three-dimensional movement techniques, a continuum of treatment and reassessment occurs. The application of three-dimensional movement techniques may be all that is needed with some patients to manage symptoms and dysfunction associated with MDCS. For other patients these techniques will facilitate the application of other appropriate manual or medical (i.e., injections) techniques that are directed towards a named tissue or to a specific or general restriction that was not resolved with three-dimensional movement techniques.

Fig. 11-22. (**A–H**) Three-dimensional movement techniques involving any one or combination of *rotational, diagonal* and *spiral* movement patterns. (**A**) Upper arc. (**B**) Lower arc. (**C**) Melt. (*Figure continues.*)

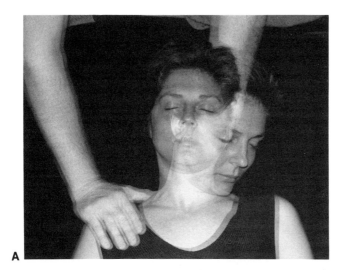

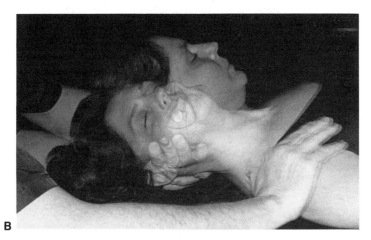

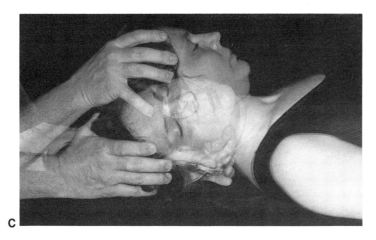

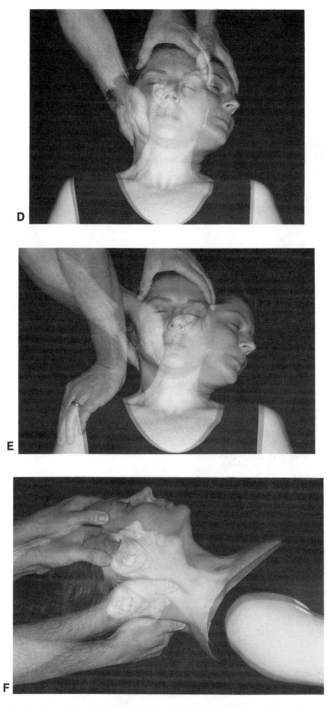

Fig. 11-22. (*Continued*) (**D**) Melt with thumb. (**E**) Melt with thumb cross over arm. (**F**) Bilateral lift. (*Figure continues.*)

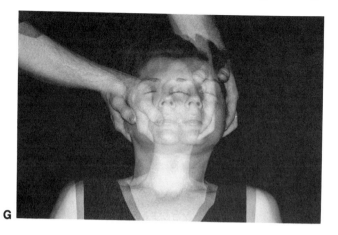

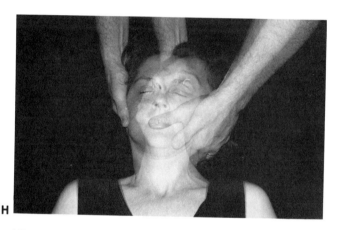

Fig. 11-22. (*Continued*). (**G**) Lateral arc. (**H**) Gap. The names indicate the movement patterns through which the cervical spine is moved. These photographs are not intended to detail hand placement, direction of movement, speed of movement, amount of stretch, or duration of stretch. The application of these techniques by a skilled therapist will allow for the identification and treatment of specific or general restrictions of the tissue(s). During the application of the three-dimensional movement techniques, a continuum of treatment and reassessment occurs.

Traction

Traction is often indicated when radiculopathy is suspected. The objective of traction is to separate the posterior intervertebral space in the presence of a compressed or irritated nerve root. When possible, manual therapy should be rendered over several treatment sessions before offering traction. Manual therapy will help to prepare the patient for traction by decreasing muscle and soft tissue tone and by improving the mobility of facet joints.

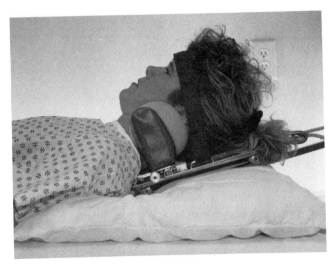

Fig. 11-23. Patient set up for the application of mechnical traction. Note the thin pillow positioned under the patient's shoulders and traction unit. Extra foam may be placed under the mastoid processes for the patient whose tissues are sensitive in this area and/or who is receiving a higher poundaged pull.

Traction can be applied through a variety of different cervical/head harnesses using weight or mechanical machinery. Mechanical traction using a head halter as shown in Figure 11-23 is my preferred way to ensure that a force of traction is occurring in the cervical spine. If the patient is set up correctly, minimal forces from the traction unit would arrive at the mandible and thus the TMJ. In my view, any home traction units or head halters other than that in Fig. 11-23 may not achieve the objectives of traction.

Colachis and Strohm[361,362] found that a traction force of 30 lbs for a duration of only 7 seconds can separate the cervical intervertebral space with the amount of separation increasing with flexion. Wong and co-workers found that traction either in the horizontal neck position or flexed to 30 degrees provided significant separation of the intervertebral space from C3–4 to C6–7 measured posteriorly and anteriorly.[363] Posterior intervertebral separation for all levels was best in the horizontal head position. The traction force used was 13.5 kg (approximately 30 lbs) for a duration of 8 seconds followed by unloading for 6 seconds alternately for a period of 20 minutes.[363] Traction was preceded by application of a heat pack. Clinically, a force of 20 to 25 lbs for a duration of 30 seconds and unloading for less than 5 secs for 15 minutes is therapeutic.

Cervical Collars

Cervical collars are seldom required in the treatment of MDCS, except in known traumatic injury. The most common traumatic injury is usually associated with a whiplash.[364] Cervical whiplash represents a collection of symptoms following injury to the neck, usually hyperextension/flexion occurring as a result of a rear-end accident.[365] The pathology of whiplash is poorly understood and described because the forces involved vary from incident to incident and fresh post-mortem cervical spines are not readily available for study.[364,366] Other than the apparent soft tissue and joint injury, Twomey[77] and Osti[367] describe "rim lesions" that may result from a whiplash injury. A rim lesion is best described as clefts in the cartilage plates and annulus fibrosus.[77,89] The clefts are in the peripheral part of the disc, near the vertebral rim and usually parallel with the end-plate.[77] Rim lesions principally involve the avascular cartilage plate, but have been observed to extend into the outer annulus, which contains nerves and blood vessels, and into the bony end-plate which is highly vascular.[77,89,368] Patients experiencing a significant whiplash injury may need to be supported with a collar. Twomey and Taylor state[77]; "It is essential that there be an early period of immobilization of the neck to allow for resolution of effusion and to ensure that bleeding into the damage areas ceases." However, when using a cervical collar, the importance of early mobility cannot be overlooked so as to avoid secondary problems associated with immobility. Patients who have become dependent upon the collar present with additional clinical concern. Questions as to how long the neck should be immobilized are largely an individual matter between patient and attending clinician. Collars should be designed and worn with the narrow section in front of the neck so that cervical hyperextension is avoided.[369]

Exercise

The passive application of modalities and manual therapy do not replace the need for a specific and general exercise program in the prophylaxis and treatment of nonspecific spinal disorders. Application of modalities and manual therapy procedures may often need to precede the initiation of an exercise program in order to decrease symptoms and increase passive and active mobility.

It is very clear that disuse has harmful affects on skeletal health.[370] Twomey indicates that bone and muscle both respond positively to exercise and adversely to disuse.[46] There is an increasing body of evidence supporting the value of regular exercise in preserving skeletal health.[46] Shepard[371] and Menard and Stanish,[372] indicate that the reduction in muscle mass that occurs with increasing age is due to disuse and can be substantially reversed by a program of activity. Pardini[373] has demonstrated that most elderly Americans can show up to 50 percent improvement in muscle strength after a relatively short exercise program. Aniansson and others[374] show that it is possible to increase muscle strength, endurance, and hypertrophy into old age. Aloia et al.[375] reported a significant increase in total body calcium in postmenopausal women who exercised regularly for 1 year, in contrast with a decline in total body calcium in a matched sedentary group. These findings were later supported by the work of Smith et al.[376]

Strength, endurance, and flexibility are important but without coordination and proper recruitment of motion, spinal symptoms may still occur or reoccur. Irregular movement patterns with or without poor posture may contribute to repetitive microtrauma of cervical structures, including muscles, facet joints and nervous tissue.[377,378] Poor movement patterns contribute to habitual overuse of isolated motion segments while they minimize normal movement at others.[379] Patients experiencing pain originating from MDCS will require a comprehensive exercise program. Exercise programs will need to be individualized and consistent with personal goals.

SUMMARY

Muscles, facet joints, peripheral nerves, and nerve roots can cause neck, shoulder, and upper extremity symptoms. Each of these can prove to be a major source of cephalic symptoms, mimicking symptoms believed to be originating from a temporomandibular disorder and or from a masticatory muscle disorder. Cervical spine involvement needs to be acknowledged in patients who receive dental intervention such as equilibration, intraoral appliance, orthodontics, or orthognathic/joint surgical procedures. Dental intervention may need to come during or after the management of the cervical spine involvement.

The dilemma surrounding the inability to diagnose nonspecific spinal complaints is very real. Although it is preferable for a diagnosis/classification of a nonspecific spinal condition to be based on a unitary principle (i.e., anatomical [bone spur], pathologic [disc degeneration], or etiologic [cervical sprain], this is not always possible.[87] A diagnosis rarely exists as a pure entity explaining the patient's condition.[87] Caution therefore should be taken when the clinician, patient, and third party payers place too much emphasis on the medical diagnosis for a nonspecific condition of the spine.

Treatment strategies for nonspecific lumbar complaints based upon signs and symptoms are currently being developed. I propose a classification for nonspecific disorders of the cervical spine referred to as "Movement Dysfunction of the Cervical Spine." The pertinent history and criteria of physical examination that are needed to derive at the diagnosis of "Movement Dysfunction of the Cervical Spine" is outlined.

Management of movement dysfunction of the cervical spine begins with patient education to resolve the myths surrounding a specific condition and diagnosis. Patient education regarding proper sleeping and upright postures is vital so as to avoid further unnecessary stress to the cervical spine and associated structures. The therapeutic value of manual therapy, supported as needed with modalities, will decrease symptoms and improve function. Traction would be indicated when radiculopathy is present. Establishing a specific and/or general exercise program for individual patients of all ages will promote a more functional and independent quality of life.

ACKNOWLEDGMENT

I would like to thank Carolyn Law, M.P.T., for her invaluable assistance with manuscript preparation.

REFERENCES

1. Kelsey JL: Epidemiology of Musculoskeletal Disorders. p. 146. Oxford University Press, New York, 1982
2. Gore D, Susan B, Gardner G et al: Neck pain: a long-term follow-up of 205 patients. Spine 12:1, 1987
3. Accident Facts—1980 Edition. Chicago, National Safety Council, 1980
4. LaBan M: "Whiplash": its evaluation and treatment. p. 293. In: Saal J (ed): Physical Medicine and Rehabilitation: Neck and Back Pain: State of the Art Reviews, V. 4, No 2, Hanley & Belfus, Philadelphia, 1990
5. Insurance Bureau of Canada: Fact Book. p. 20. 15th Ed. Toronto, Canada, 1987
6. Ameis A: Cervical whiplash: consideration in the rehabilitation of cervical myofascial injury. Can Fam Phys 32:1871, 1986
7. Hodson SP, Grundy M: Whiplash injuries: their long-term prognosis and the relationship to compensation. Neuro-Orthop 7:88, 1989
8. Dvorak J, Valach L, Schmid S: Cervical spine injuries in Switzerland. Manual Med 4:7, 1989
9. Quarrier N: Performing arts medicine: the musical athlete. JOSPT, 17:90, 1993
10. Holmstrom E, Lindell J, Moritz: Low back and neck/shoulder pain in construction workers: occupational workload and psychosocial risk factors. Part 2: relationship to neck and shoulder pain. Spine 17:672, 1992
11. Hagberg M, Wegman D: Prevelance rates and odds ratios of shoulder-neck diseases in different occupational groups. Br J Ind Med 44:602, 1987
12. Leino P: Symptoms of stress predict musculoskeletal disorders. J Epidemiol Community Health 43:293, 1989
13. Linton S: Risk factors for neck and back pain in a working population in Sweden. Work and Stress 4:41, 1990
14. U.S. Department of Health and Human Services, Public Health Service, Center for Disease Control, National Institute for Occupational Safety and Health, HETA 89-299-2230 U.S. West Communications, July 1992
15. Rundcrantz B, Johnsson B, Mortiz U: Pain and discomfort in the musculoskeletal system among dentist. Swed Dent J 15:219, 1991
16. Goldenberg DL: Fibromyalgia syndrome: An emerging but controversial condition. JAMA 2783, 1987
17. Friction J: Myofascial pain syndrome, Neuro Clin 7:413, 1989
18. Awad E: Interstitial myofibrositis: hypothesis of mechanism. Arch Phys Med Rehabil 54:449, 1973
19. Thompson J: Subspecialty clinics: physical medicine and rehabilitation, Mayo Clin Pro 65:1237, 1990
20. Yunnus M, Kalyan-Raman U, Kalyan-Raman K: Primary fibromyalgia syndrome and myofascial pain syndrome: Clinical features and muscle pathology, Arch Phys Med Rehabil 69:451, 1988
21. Travell J, Simons D: Myofascial pain and dysfunction, the trigger point manual. New York: Williams & Wilkins, New York, 1983
22. Travell JG: On myofascial pain. J Clin Orthod 23:468, 1989
23. Bogduk N: Headaches and the cervical spine (editorial). Cephalalgia 4:7, 1984
24. Simons D: Muscular pain syndromes. Adv Pain Res Ther 17:1, 1990
25. Bennett R: Myofascial pain syndromes and the fibromyalgia syndrome: a comparative analysis. Adv Pain Res Ther 17:43, 1990
26. Campbell S: Regional myofascial pain syndromes. Rheum Clin North Am 15:31, 1989

27. Simons D: Myofascial pain syndromes: where are we? where are we going? Arch Phys Med Rehabil 69:207, 1988

28. Thompson J: Tension myalgia as a diagnosis at the Mayo Clinic and its relationship to fibrositis, fibromyalgia and myofascial pain syndrome. Mayo Clin Proc 65:1237, 1990

29. Yunas M, Masi A, Calabro J et al: Primary fibromyalgia (fibrositis): clinical study of 50 patients with matched normal controls. Semin Arthritis Rheum 11:151, 1981

30. Bennett R: Fibrositis: Does it exist and can it be treated? J Musculoskel Med, 57, 1984

31. Bennett R: Fibromyalgia. JAMA, 257:2802, 1987

32. Wolfe F: Fibrositis, fibromyalgia, and musculoskeletal disease: the current status of the fibrositis syndrome. Arch Phys Med Rehabil, 69:527, 1988

33. Hubbard D, Gregory B: Myofascial trigger points show spontaneous needle EMG activity. Spine 18:1803, 1993

34. Kent B: Anatomy of the trunk. Phys Ther, 1974

35. Hayashi K, Yabuki T: Origins of the uncus and of Von Luschka's joint in the cervical spine. J Bone Joint Surg, 67A:788, 1985

36. Carrera G, Williams A: Current concepts in evaluation of the lumbar facet joints. CRC Crit Rev Diagn Imaging 21:85, 1984

37. Mooney R: The facet syndrome. Clin Orthop 115:149, 1976

38. Dory A: Arthrography of the lumbar facet joints. Radiology 140:23, 1981

39. Leyshon A, Kirwan E, Parry C: Electrical studies in diagnosis of compression of the lumbar root. J Bone Joint Surg 36:71, 1981

40. Wyke BD: Neurology of the cervical spinal joints. Physiotherapy 65:72, 1979

41. Wyke BD, Polacek P: Articular neurology: the present position. J Bone Joint Surg 7B:401, 1975

42. Bogduk N, Marsland A: The cervical zygapophyseal joints as a source of neck pain. Spine 13:610, 1988

43. Dwyer A, Aprill C, Bogduk N: Cervical zygapophyseal joint pain patterns I: a study in normal volunteers. Spine 15:453, 1990

44. Aprill C, Dwyer A, Bogduk N: Cervical zygapophyseal joint pain patterns II: A clinical evaluation. Spine 15:458, 1990

45. Jull G, Bodguk N, Marsland A: The accuracy of manual diagnosis for cervical zygapophyseal joint pain syndrome. Med J Aus 148:223, 1988

46. Twomey L: A rationale for the treatment of back pain and joint pain by manual therapy. Phys Ther 72:885, 1992

47. Mercer S: The menisci of the cervical synovial joints. p. 109. Proceedings from the Fourth Biennial Conference of Manipulative Therapist Association of Australia, Brisbane, May 22–25, 1985

48. Bogduk N, Engel R: The menisci of the lumbar zygapophyseal joints: a review of their anatomy and clinical significance. Spine 9:454, 1984

49. Kos J, Wolfe J: Les menisques intervertebraux et leur role possible dans les blocages vertebraux. Ann Med Phys 15:203, 1972

50. Engel R, Bogduk N: The menisci of the lumbar zygapophyseal joints. J Anat 135: 795, 1982

51. Kos J, Wolf J: Die "Menisci" der Zwischenwirbelgelenke und ihre mogliche rolle lei Wirbelblockierung. Manuelle Medizine, 10:105, 1979

52. Yu S, Sether L, Haughton V: Facet joint menisci of the cervical spine: correlative MR imaging and cryomicrotomy study. Radiology 164:79, 1987

53. Lewin T, Moffett B, Viidik A: The morphology of the lumbar or synovial intervertebral joints. Acta Morphol Neerl-Scand 4:299, 1962

54. Lewit K: The contribution of clinical observation to neurobiological mechanisms in manipulative therapy. p 3. In Korr I (ed): The Neurobiologic Mechanism In Manipulative Therapy. Plenum Press, New York, 1978
55. Droz-Georget JH: High-velocity thrust and pathophysiology of segmental dysfunction. In Idczak RM (ed): Aspects of Manipulative Therapy. Proceedings of a Multidisciplinary International Conference on Manipulative Therapy. Melbourne, August 1979
56. Kopell H, Thompson W: Peripheral Entrapment Neuropathies. Williams & Wilkins, Baltimore, Maryland, 1963
57. Pratt N: Neurovascular entrapment in the regions of the shoulder and posterior triangle of the neck. Phys Ther 66:1894, 1986
58. Riddel D, Smith B: Thoracic and vascular aspects of thoracic outlet syndrome. Clin Orthop 207:31, 1986
59. Cuetter A, Bartoszek D: The thoracic outlet syndrome: controversies, overdiagnosis, overtreatment, and recommendations for management. Musc and Nerve, 410, 1989
60. Sunderland S: Traumatized nerves, roots and ganglia: musculoskeletal factors and neuropathological consequences. Editor Korr I. In Korr I (ed): The Neurobiologic Mechanisms in Manipulative Therapy. Plenum Press, New York, 1978
61. Sunderland S: Nerves and Nerve Injuries, 2nd Ed. Churchill Livingstone, New York, 1979
62. Schaumburg H, Spencer P: Pathology of spinal root compression. p 141. In Goldstein M (ed): The Research Status of Spinal Manipulative Therapy, U.S. Department of Health, Education, and Welfare. NINCDS Monograph No. 15, DHEW Publication No (NIH) 76-998, Feb 2–4, 1975
63. Seddon H: Three types of nerve injuries and repair. In Microsurgery Workshop Symposium. CV Mosby, St Louis, 1975
64. Bogduk N: The clinical anatomy of the cervical dorsal rami. Spine 7:319, 1982
65. Cox C, Cocks G: Occipital neuralgia. J Med Assoc State Ala 48:23, 1979
66. Hunter C, Mayfield F: Role of the upper cervical roots in the production of pain in the head. Am J Surg 78:743, 1949
67. Saadah H, Taylor F: Sustained headache syndrome associated with tender occipital nerve zones. Headache 27:201, 1987
68. Jansen J, Markakis E, Rama B, Hildebrandt J: Hemicranial attacks or permanent hemicrania—a sequel of upper cervical root compression. Cephalalgia 9:123, 1989
69. Perelson N: Occipital nerve tenderness: a sign of headache. South Med J 40:653, 1947
70. Bovim G, Bonamico L, Fredriksen T et al: Topographic variations in the peripheral course of the Greater Occipital Nerve; autopsy study with clinical correlations: Spine 16:475, 1991
71. Sjaastad O, Fredriksen T, Stolt-Nielsen A: Cervicogenic headache, C2 rhizopathy, and occipital neuralgia: a connection? Cephalalgia 6:189, 1986
72. Hildebrandt J, Jansen J: Vascular compression of the C2 and C3 roots—yet another cause of chronic intermittent henicrania? Cephalalgia 4:168, 1984
73. Rosenberg W, Swearingen B, Poletti C. Contralateral trigeminal dysaesthesias associated with second cervical nerve compression: a case report. Cephalalgia 10: 259, 1990
74. Sunderland S: Anatomical perivertebral influences on the intervertebral foramen. p. 129 In: The Research Status of Spinal Manipulative Therapy. U.S. Department of Health, Education, and Welfare. NINCDS Monograph No. 15, DHEW Publication No (NIH) 76-998, Feb 2–4, 1975

75. Dillin W, Booth R, Cuckler J et al: Cervical Radiolopathy. A review. Spine 11: 988, 1986
76. Mixter W, Barr J: Rupture of the intervertebral disc with involvement of the spinal canal. N Engl J Med 211:210, 1934
77. Twomey L, Taylor J: The whiplash syndrome: pathology and physical treatment. J Man Manipul Ther 1(1):26, 1993
78. Taylor J: Growth and Development of Human Intervertebral Disc. PhD Thesis, University of Edinburgh, 1973
79. Kramer J: Intervertebral disc lesions: Causes, Diagnosis, Treatment and Prophylaxis. Georg Thieme Verlag, Stuttgart, 1981
80. Bowden R: Cervical spondylosis. Proceedings of the Royal Society of Medicine, 59:62, 1966
81. Twomey L, Taylor J: Joints of the middle and lower cervical spine: age changes and pathology. In Jones H, Jones M, Milde M (eds): Sixth Biennial Conference Proceedings, Manipulative Therapists Association of Australia, Adelaide, South Australia, 1989
82. Lawrence J: Disc degeneration: its frequency and relationship to symptoms. Ann Rheum Dis 28:121, 1969
83. Parke W: Correlative anatomy of cervical spondylotic myelopathy. Spine 13:831, 1988
84. Friedenberg ZB, Edeiken J, Spencer HN et al: Degenerative changes in the cervical spine. J Bone Joint Surg 41A:61, 1959
85. Juntura E, Raininko R, Videman T et al: Evaluation of cervical disc degeneration with ultralow field MRI and Discography. Spine 14:616, 1989
86. Brain L, Wilkinson M: Cervical Spondylosis and other disorders of the cervical spine. WB Saunders, Philadelphia, 1967
87. Spitzer WO, LeBlance F, Dupuis M: Scientific approach to the asessment and management of activity-related spinal disorders: a monograph for clinicians. Report of the Quebec Task Force on Spinal Disorders. Spine 12(suppl 7):51, 1987
88. Mendel T, Wink C, Zimny M: Neural elements in human cervical intervertebral disc. Spine 17:132, 1992
89. Taylor J, Twomey L: Acute injuries to cervical joints. Spine 18:1115, 1993
90. Bogduk N: Cervical causes of headache and dizziness. p. 289. In Grieve G (ed): Modern Manual Therapy. Churchill Livingstone, Edinburgh, 1986
91. Everett N: Functional Neuroanatomy 6th ed, Lea & Febiger, Philadelphia, 1972
92. Kerr F: Mechanism, diagnosis and management of some cranial and facial pain syndromes. Surg Clin N Am 43:951, 1963
93. Kerr F, Olafson R: Trigeminal and cervical volleys. Arch Neurol 5:171, 1961
94. Kerr F: A mechanism to account for frontal headache in cases of posterior fossa tumors. J Neurosurg 18:605, 1961
95. Kerr F: Structural relation of the trigeminal spinal tract to upper cervical roots and the solitary nucleus in the cat. Exp Neurol 4:134, 1961
96. Cyriax J: Rheumatic Headache. Br Med J 2:1367, 1938
97. Campbell D, Parsons C: Referred head pain and its concomitants. J of Nervous and Mental Diseases 99:544, 1944
98. Feinstein B, Langton J, Jameson R et al: Experiments on referred pain from deep somatic tissues. J Bone Joint Surg 36A:981, 1954
99. Bogduk N, Marsland A: C3 Headaches. Paper presented at the International Meeting on Pain and Regional Anaesthesia. Australasian Pain Society, Perth, February, 1983

100. Bogduk N, Corrigan B, Schneider G et al: Cervical headache. Med J Australia 143:202, 1985
101. McNeill C (ed): Temporomandibular Disorders: Guidelines for classification, assessment, and management. The American Academy of Orofacial Pain. Quintessence Pub. Co., 1993
102. Ad Hoc Committee on the Classification of Headache. JAMA 179:717, 1962
103. Classification and Diagnostic Criteria for Headache Disorders, Cranial Neuralgias and Facial Pain. First Ed. International Headache Society. Cephalagia 8(suppl 7): 1988
104. Edmeads J: The cervical spine and headache. Neurology 38:1874, 1988
105. Barré JA: Le syndrome sympathique posterior. Rev Neurol (Paris) 33:248, 1926
106. Bartschi-Rochiax W. Headache of cervical origin. p. 192. In Vinken PJ, Bruyn GW (eds): Handbook of Clinical Neurology. Vol 5. Headache and cranial neuralgias. North Holland Publ Co., Amsterdam, 1968
107. Sjaastad O, Saunte C, Hovdahl H et al: "Cervicogenic" headache. An hypothesis. Cephalalgia 3:249, 1983
108. Pfaffenrath V, Dandekar R, Pollmann W: Cervicogenic headache—the clinical picture, radiological findings and hypotheses on its pathophysiology. Headache, 27:495, 1987
109. Fredriksen T, Hovdal H: "Cervicogenic headache": clinical manifestation. Cephalalgia 7:147, 1987
110. Pfaffenrath V, Dandekar R, Mayer E et al: Cervicogenic headache: Results of computor-based measurements of cervical spine mobility in 15 patients. Cephalalgia 8:45, 1988
111. Fredriksen T, Wysocka-Bakowska M, Bogucki A et al: Cervicogenic headache—pupillometric findings. Cephalalgia 8:93, 1988
112. Fredriksen T: Cervicogenic headache: the forehead sweating pattern. Cephalalgia 8:203, 1988
113. Sjaastad O, Fredriksen T, Sand T et al: Unilaterality of headache in classic migraine. Cephalalgia 9:71, 1989
114. Fredriksen T, Fougner R, Tangerud A et al: Cervicogenic headache. Radiological investigations concering head/neck. Cephalalgia 9:139, 1989
115. Jaeger B: Are "cervicogenic" headaches due to myofacial pain and cervical spine dysfunction? Cephalalgia 9:157, 1989
116. Farina S, Granella F, Malferrari et al: Headache and cervical spine disorders: Classification and treatment with transcutaneous nerve stimulation. Headache 26: 431, 1986
117. Ziegler DK, Hassanein R, Hassanein K: Headache syndromes suggested by factors analysis of symptom variable on a headache prone population. J Chronic Dis 25: 353, 1972
118. Rose F: Headache: definition and classification. p. 1. In Rose F (ed): Handbook of Clinical Neurology. Vol 4 (48): Headache, Elsevier, NY, 1986
119. Appenzeller O: Pathogenesis of vascular headache of the migrainous type: The role of impaired central inhibition. Headache 15:177, 1975
120. Rose F, Capildeo R: Migraine: definition and classification. Cephalalgia 3:225, 1983
121. Walters E: The epidemiological enigma of migraine. Int J Epidemiol 2:189, 1973
122. Bakal D, Kaganov J: Muscle contraction and migraine headache: Psychophysiologic comparison. Headache 17:208, 1977
123. Olesen J: Some clinical features of the acute migraine attack. An analysis of 750 patients. Headache 18:268, 1978

124. Kaganov J, Bakal D, Dunn B: The differential contribution of muscle contraction and migraine symptoms to problem headache in the general population. Headache 157, 1981

125. Carlsson J, Fahlcrantz A, Augustinsson L: Muscle tenderness in tension headache treated with acupuncture or physiotherapy. Cephalalgia 10:131, 1990

126. Sjaastad O: Cluster headache. p. 217. In Vinken PJ, Bruyn G, Klawans H, Rose F (eds): Handbook of Clinical Neurology. Vol. 4. Elsevier, Amsterdam, 1981

127. Jensen O, Nielsen F, Vosmar L: An open study comparing manual therapy with the use of cold packs in the treatment of post-traumatic headache. Cephalalgia 10: 242, 1990

128. Jensen O, Justesen T, Nielsen F et al: Functional radiographic examination of the cervical spine in patients with post-traumatic headache. Cephalalgia 10:295, 1990

129. Frykholm: Clinical picture. p. 5. In Hirsch, Zotterman (eds): Cervical Pain. Pergamon Press, Oxford, 1971

130. Smith D: Dizziness, a clinical perspective. Neurol Clin 8:199, 1990

131. Adams R, Victor M: Principles of Neurology. 3rd Ed. McGraw-Hill, New York, 1985

132. Brown J: A systemic approach to the dizzy patient. Neurol Clin 8:209, 1990

133. Uemura T, Suzuki J, Hozawa J: Neuro-otological examination with special reference to equilibrium function tests. Baltimore: University Park Press, 1977

134. Troost B: Dizziness and vertigo in vertebrobasilar disease. Part I. Stroke 11:301, 1980

135. Troost B: Dizziness and vertigo in vertebrobasilar disease. Part II. Stroke 11:413, 1980

136. Herdman S: Treatment of benign paroxysmal positional vertigo. Phys Ther 70: 381, 1990

137. Herr R, Zun L, Mathews J: A directed approach to the dizzy patient. Ann Emerg Med 18:664, 1989

138. Baloh R, Honrubia V, Jacobson K: Benign positional vertigo: clinical and oculographic features in 240 cases. Neurology 37:371, 1987

139. Schuknecht H: Cupulolithiasis. Arch Otolaryngol. 90:765, 1969

140. Hall S, Ruby R, McClure J: The mechanisms of benign paroxysmal vertigo. J Otolaryngol 8:151, 1979

141. Brandt T, Daroff R: Physical therapy for benign paroxysmal positional vertigo. Arch Otolaryngol 106:484, 1980

142. Shumway-Cook A, Horak F: Rehabilitation strategies for patients with vestibular deficits. Neurol Clin 8:441, 1990

143. Shumway-Cook A, Horak F: Assessing the influence of sensory interaction on balance. Phys Ther 66:1548, 1986

144. Fisher C: Vertigo in cerebrovascular disease. Arch Otolaryngol 85:529, 1967

145. De Jong J, Bles W: Cervical dizziness and ataxia. p. 185. In Bles W, Brandt T (eds): Disorders of Posture and Gait. Elsevier, Amsterdam, 1986

146. Coman W: Dizziness related to ENT conditions. In Grieve G (ed): Modern Manual Therapy of the Vertebral Column. Churchill Livingstone, Edinburgh, 1986

147. Hutchison M: An investigation of pre-manipulative dizziness testing. In Jones H, Jones M, Milde M (eds): Sixth Biennal Conference Proceedings. Manipulative Therapists Association of Australia. Adelaide, South Australia, 1989

148. Aspinall W: Clinical testing for cervical mechanical disorders which produce ischemic vertigo. JOSPT 11:5, 1989

149. Grant R: Dizziness testing and manipulation of the cervical spine. p. 111. In Grant

R (ed): Physical Therapy of the Cervical and Thoracic Spine. Clinics in Physical Therapy. Vol 17. Churchill Livingstone, New York, 1988

150. McCouch G, Deering I, Ling T: Location of receptors for tonic neck reflexs. J Neurophysiol 14:191, 1951
151. Abrahams V: The physiology of neck muscles; their role in head movement and maintenance of posture. Can J Physiol Pharmacol 55:332, 1977
152. Goodwin GM, McCloskey DI, Matthews PBC: The persistence of appreciable kinesthesia after paralysing joint afferents but preserving muscle afferents. Brain Res 37:326, 1972
153. Manzoni D, Pompeiano O, Stampacchia G: Tonic cervical influences on posture and reflex movements. Arch Ital Biol 117:81, 1979
154. Wyke B: Articular neurology—a review. Physiotherapy 58:94, 1972
155. Cohen L: Role of eye and neck proprioceptive mechanisms in body orientation and motor coordination. J Neurophysiol 24:1, 1961
156. Igarashi M, Watanabe T, Maxian P: Role of neck proprioceptors for the maintenence of dynamic bodily equilibrium in the squirrel monkey. Laryngoscope 79:1713, 1969
157. Cope S, Ryan GMS: Cervical and otolith vertigo. J Laryng 73:113, 1959
158. Gray LP: Extralabyrinthine vertigo due to cervical muscle lesions. J Laryng 70: 352, 1956
159. Weeks VD, Travell J: Postural vertigo due to trigger areas in the sternocleido-mastoid muscle. J Pediat 47:315, 1955
160. De Jong PTVM, De Jong JMBV, Cohen B, Jongkees LBW: Ataxia and nystagmus induced by injection of local anesthetics in the neck. Ann Neurol I:240, 1977
161. Hinoki M: Vertigo due to whiplash injury: A neurotological approach. Acta Oto-laryngol (Stockh). (suppl 419):9, 1985
162. Barlow D, Freedman W: Cervico-ocular reflex in the normal adult. Acta Otolar-yngol (Stockh) 89:487, 1980
163. Kobayashi Y, Yagi T, Kamio T: Cervico-vestibular interaction in eye movements. Auris-Nasus-Larynx (Tokyo) 13:87, 1986
164. Carlsson J, Rosenhall U: Oclumotor disturbances in patients with tension head-ache treated with acupuncture or physiotherapy: Cephalalgia 10:122, 1990
165. Preiskel HW: Some observations on the postural position of the mandible. J Pros Dent 15:625, 1965
166. Kazis H, Kazis AJ: Complete mouth rehabilitation. Henry Kimpton, London, 1956
167. Thompson JR: The rest position of the mandible and its significance to dental science. Am Dent Assoc 33:151, 1946
168. Beyron HL: Characteristics of functionally optimal occlusion and principles of occlusal rehabilitation. J Am Dent Assoc 48:648, 1954
169. Atwood DA: A review of the fundamentals on rest position and vertical dimension. Internat Dent J 9:6, 1959
170. Murpy WM: Rest position of the mandible. J Pros Dent 17:329, 1967
171. Rugh JD, Drago CJ: Vertical dimension: A study of clinical rest position and jaw muscle activity. J Pros Dent 45:670, 1981
172. Garnick J, Ramfjord SP: Rest position. An electromyographic and clinical inves-tigation. J Pros Dent 12:895, 1962
173. Kawamura Y, Fujimoto J: Some physiologic considerations on measuring rest position of the mandible. Med J Osaka Univ 8:247, 1957
174. Wessberg GA, Epker BN, Elliott AC: Comparison of mandibular rest positions induced by phonetics, transcutaneous electrical stimulation, and masticatory elec-tromyography. J Pros Dent 49:100,1983

175. Lund J, Widmer C: An evaluation of the use of surface electromyography in the diagnosis, documentation, and treatment of dental patients. J Craniomand Disord Facial Oral Pain. 3:125, 1989
176. Krajicek DD, Jones PM, Radzyminski SF et al: Clinical and electromyographic study of mandibular rest position. J Pros Dent 11:826, 1961
177. Turrell AJ: Clinical assessment of vertical dimension. J Prosthet Dent 28:238, 1972
178. Weinberg LA: Vertical dimension: a research and clinial analysis. J Prosthet Dent 47:290, 1982
179. Fieldman S, Leupold RJ, Staling LM: Rest vertical dimension determined by electromyography with biofeedback as compared to conventional methods. J Pros Dent 84:216, 1978
180. George JP, Boone ME: A clinical study of rest position using the kinesiograph and myomonitor. J Prosthet Dent 41:456, 1979
181. Basler FL, Douglas JR, Moulton RS: Cephalometric analysis of the vertical dimension of occlusion. J Pros Dent 11:831, 1961
182. Yemm R: Irrelevent muscle activity: D Pract 19:51, 1968
183. Atwood DA: A cephalometric study of the clinical rest position of the mandible. Part I: the variability of the clinical rest position following the removal of occlusal contacts. J Pros Dent 6:504, 1956
184. Carlsson GE, Ericson S: Postural face height in full denture wearers. A longitudinal x-ray cephalometric study. Acta Odontol Scand 25:145, 1967
185. Landa JS: Integration of structure and function of the temporomandibular joint. N York J Dent 24:290, 1954
186. Hackney J, Bade D, Clawson A: Relationship between forward head posture and diagnosed internal derangement of the temporomandibular joint. J Orofacial Pain 7:386, 1993
187. Shock P: Current concepts of the aging process. JAMA 175:108, 1961
188. Kiernander B: Discussion on postural re-education—a critical examination of methods. Proc R Soc Med Section of Physical Medicine 49:667, 1956
189. Igarashi M, Watanabe T, Maxian P: Role of neck propriocepters for the maintenence of dynamic bodily equilibrium in the squirrel monkey. Laryngoscope 79:1713, 1969
190. Manzoni D, Pompeiano O, Stampacchia G: Tonic cervical influences on posture and reflex movements. Arch Ital Biol 117:81, 1979
191. Fukuda T: Studies on human dynamic postures from the viewpoint of postural reflexes. Acta Otolaryng (Stockholm), Suppl. 161:1, 1961
192. Bizzi E. Polit A, Morasso P: Mechanisms underlying achievement of final head posture. J Neurophysiol 39:435, 1976
193. Gibbs C: The continuous regulation of skilled response by kinaesthetic feedback. Brit J Psychol 45:24, 1954
194. Eccles J, Sabah N, Schmidt R et al: Modes of operation of the cerebellum in the dynamic loop control of movement. Brain Res 41:73, 1972
195. Tinbergen N: Ethology and stress diseases. Science 185:20, 1974
196. Tinbergen N: Functional ethology and the human sciences. Proc R Soc Lond (Ser B) 182:385, 1972
197. Mohl DM: The role of head posture in mandibular function. p. 97: In Solberg WK, Clark GT (eds): Abnormal Jaw Mechanics Diagnosis and Treatment. Quintessence Publishing, Chicago, 1984
198. Posselt U: Studies on the mobility of the human mandible. Acta Ondontol Scand 10:1, 1952

199. Brill N, Lammie GA, Osborne J et al: Mandibular positions and mandibular movements. Br Dent J 106:391, 1959

200. Dombrady L: Investigation into the transient instability of the rest position. J Pros Dent 16:479, 1966

201. Basmajian JV: Muscles alive. Their functions revealed by electromyography. 2nd Ed. Williams & Wilkins, Baltimore, 1967

202. Granit R: The Basis of Motor Control. Academic Press, New York, 1970

203. Yemm R: The mandibular rest position: the roles of tissue elasticity and muscle activity. J the DASA, January 1975

204. Carlsoo S: An electromyographic study of the activity of certain suprahyoid muscles, and of reciprocal innervation of the mandible. Acta Anatomica, 26:81, 1956

205. Mohamed SE, Christensen LV: Mandibular reference positions. J Oral Rehab 12: 355, 1985

206. Darling DW, Kraus SL, Glasheen-Wray MB: Relationship of head posture and the rest position of the mandible. J Prosthet Dent 52:111, 1984

207. Wyke BD: Neuromuscular mechanisms influencing mandibular posture: a neurologist's review of current concepts. J Dent 2:111, 1972

208. Guyton AC: Textbook of Medical Physiology. 4th Ed. WB Saunders, Philadelphia, 1971

209. Goodgold J, Eberstein A: Electrodiagnosis of neuromuscular diseases. Williams & Wilkins, Baltimore, 1972

210. Bratzlavsky M, Vander Eecken H: Postural reflexes in cranial muscles in man. Acta Neurol Belg 77:5, 1977

211. Magnus R: Some results of studies in the physiology of posture. Lancet 2:531, 1926

212. Magnus R: Korperstellung, pp. XIII, 740, Berlin, 1924, Julius Springer, Animal Posture, Croonian Lecture, Proc. Roy. Soc., Series B., Vol 98, No B 690, pp 339–353

213. Magnus R, DeKleijn A: Die Abhangigkeit des Tonus der Extremitatenmuskeln von der Kopfstellung. Pflug Arch. Ges. Physiol., 145:455, 1912

214. McCouch G, Deering I, Ling T: Location of recepters for tonic neck reflexes. J Neurophys 14:191, 1951

215. Funakoshi M, Amano N: Effects of the tonic neck reflex on the jaw muscles of the rat. J Dent Res 52:668, 1973

216. Sumino R, Nozaki S, Katoh M: Trigemino-neck reflex. p 81. In Kawamura Y, Dubner R: Oral-Facial Sensory and motor functions. Quintessence, Tokyo, 1981

217. Funakoshi M, Fujita N, Takehana S: Relations between occlusal interference and jaw muscle activities in response to changes in head position. Journal Dent Res 55:684, 1976

218. Forsberg C-M, Hellsing E, Linder-Aronson S et al: EMG activity in neck and masticatory muscles in relation to extension and flexion of the head. Eur J Orthodon 7:177, 1985

219. Mohl N: Head posture and its role in occlusion. New York State J. 42:17, 1976

220. McClean LF: Gravitational influences on the afferent and efferent components of mandibular reflexes. PhD dissertation, Thomas Jefferson University of Philadelphia, 1973

221. Lund P, Nishiyama T, Moller E: Postural activity in the muscles of mastication with the subject upright, inclined, and supine. Scand J Dent Res 78:417, 1970

222. Watt DM: Gnathosonics—a study of sounds produced by the masticatory mechanism. J Pros Dent 16:73, 1966

223. Eberle WR: A study of centric relation as recorded in a supine position. J Am Dent Assoc 42:15, 1951

224. McLean LW, Brenman HS, Friedman MGF: Effects of changing body position on dental occlusion. J Dent Res 52:1041, 1973

225. Brenman HS, Amsterdam M: Postural effects on occlusion. Dent Prog 4:43, 1963

226. Goldstein DF, Kraus SL, Williams WB, et al: Influence of cervical posture on mandibular movement. J Prosthet Dent 52:421, 1984

227. Ramfjord SPM, Ash MM Jr: Occlusion. 2nd Ed. WB Saunders, Philadelphia, 1971

228. Carlsson GE, Ingervall B, Gulumser K: Effect of increasing vertical dimension on the masticatory system in subjects with natural teeth. J Prosth Dent 41:284, 1979

229. Rivera-Morales WC, Mohl N: Relationship of occlusal vertical dimension to the health of the masticatory system. J Prosthet Dent 65:647, 1991

230. Halbert R: Electromyographic study of head position. J Can Dent Assoc 24:11, 1958

231. Davis PL: Electromyographic study of superficial neck muscles in mandibular function. J Dent Res 58:537, 1979

232. Green JD, Groot GD, Sutin J: Trigemino-bulbar reflex pathways. Am J Physiol 189:384, 1957

233. Manni E, Palmier G, Marini R et al: Trigeminal influences on extensor muscles of the neck. Exp Neurol 47:330, 1975

234. Sumino R, Nozaki S: Trigemino-neck reflex: Its peripheral and central organization. In Anderson DJ, Matthews B (eds): Pain in the Trigeminal Region. Elsevier/North-Holland Biomedical Press, 1977

235. Manns A, Miralles R, Guerrero F: The changes in electric activity of the postural muscles of the mandible upon varying the vertical dimension. J Pros Dent 45:438, 1981

236. Daly PD, Preston CB, Evans WG: Postural response of the head to bite opening in adult males. Am J Orthod 82:157, 1982

237. Vig PS, Showfety KJ, Phillips C: Experimental manipulation of head posture. Am J Orthod 77:258, 1980

238. Root GR, Kraus SL, Razook SJ et al: Effect of an intraoral appliance on head and neck posture. J Prosth Dent 58:90, 1987

239. Salonen M, Raustia A, Huggare J: Head and cervical spine posture in complete denture wearers. J Craniomandib Pract 11:30, 1993

240. Williamson E: The interrelationship of internal derangements of the temporomandibular joint, headache, vertigo, and tinnitus: a survey of 25 patients. J Craniomandib Pract 8:301, 1990

241. Seligman D, Pullinger A: The role of intercuspal occlusal relationships in temporomandibular disorders: a review. J Craniomandib Dis Fac Oral Pain 5:96, 1991

242. Naeije M, Hansson T: Short-term effect of stabilization appliance on masticatory activity in myogenous craniomandibular disorder patients. J Craniomandib Dis Fac Oral Pain 5:245, 1991

243. Wilkinson T, Hansson T, McNeil C et al: A comparison of the success of 24-hour occlusal splint therapy versus nocturnal occlusal splint therapy in reducing craniomandibular disorders. J Craniomandib Dis Fac Oral Pain 6:64, 1992

244. Seligman D, Pullinger A: The functional occlusal relationships in temporomandibular disorders: a review. J Craniomandib Dis Fac Oral Pain 5:265, 1991

245. Seligman D, Pullinger A: Association of occlusal variables among refined TM patient diagnostic groups. J Craniomandib Dis Fac Oral Pain 3:227, 1989

246. Lipp M: Temporomandibular symptoms and occlusion: a review of the literature and the concept. NY State J Dent 56:58, 1990
247. Carlsson GE, Droukas BC: Dental occlusion and the health of the masticatory system. J Craniomand Pract 2:141, 1984
248. Kirveskari P, Alanen P, Jamsa T: Association between craniomandibular disorders and occlusal interferences. J Prosthet Dent 62:66, 1989
249. Nielsen I, McNeill C, Danzig W et al: Adaptation of craniofacial muscles in subjects with craniomandibular disorders. Am J Orthod Dentofac Orthop 97:20, 1990
250. Nomenclature Committee of the Academy of Denture Prosthetics: Glossary of prosthodontic terms, 5 Ed. J Prosthet Dent 58:713, 1987
251. Krough-Poulsen WB, Olssen A: Management of the occlusion of the teeth. p 236. In Schwartz L, Chayes CM (eds): Facial Pain and Mandibular Dysfunction. WB Saunders Co., Philadelphia, 1968
252. Pruzansky S: The application of electromyography to dental research. J Am Dent Assn 44:49, 1952
253. Jarabak JR: An electromyographic analysis of muscular and temporomandibular joint disturbances due to imbalances in occlusion. Angle Orthodont 26:170, 1956
254. Perry HT: Functional electromyography of the temporal and masseter muscles in Class II, Division I malocclusion and excellent occlusion. Angle Orthodont 26:49, 1955
255. Karlsson S, Cho S-A, Carlsson G: Changes in mandibular masticatory movements after insertion of nonworking-side interference. J Craniomand Disord Facial Oral Pain 6:177, 1992
256. Dawson PE: Evaluation, Diagnosis and Treatment of Occlusal Problems. p. 49. Baltimore: CL Mosby, Baltimore, 1989
257. Rugh J, Ohrbach R: Occlusal parafunction. p. 249. In Mohl ND, Zarb GA, Carlsson GE, Rugh JD (eds): A Textbook of Occlusion. Quintessence, Chicago, 1988
258. Kronn E: The incidence of TMJ dysfunction in patients who have suffered a cervical whiplash injury following a traffic accident. J Orofac Pain 7:209, 1993
259. Braun B, DiGiovanna A, Schiffman E et al: A cross-sectional study of temporomandibular joint dysfunction in post-cervical trauma patients. J of Craniomandib Disord Facial Oral Pain 6:24, 1992
260. Pullinger AG, Seligman DA: Trauma history in diagnostic groups of temporomandibular disorders. Oral Surg Oral Med Oral Pathol 71:529, 1991
261. Howard R, Benedict J, Raddin J et al: Assessing neck extension-flexion as a basis for temporomandibular joint dysfunction. J Oral Maxillofac Surg 49:1210, 1991
262. Maruyama T, Nishio K, Kotani M, Miyauchi S: The effect of changing the maxillomandibular relationship by a bite plane on the habitual mandibular opening and closing movement. J Oral Rehab 11:455, 1984
263. Begg C: Statistical Methods In Medical Diagnosis. CRC Critical Reviews in Medical Informatics, 1(1):1, 1986/1988
264. Kassirer J, Pauker S: Should diagnostic testing be regulated? New Engl J Med 299:947, 1978
265. Koch H, Gagnon R: Office visits involving x-rays. p. 79. National Ambulatory medical care survey: United States 1977. Advance Data from Vital and Health Statistics, No. 53, DHEW Publication, PHS, 1979
266. Boden S, Davis D, Dina T et al: Abnormal magnetic resonance scans of the lumbar spine in asymptomatic subjects. J Bone Joint Surg 72A:403, 1990
267. Deyo R: Plain roentgenography for low back pain: Finding needles in a haystack. Arch Inter Med 149:27, 1989

268. Coste J, Paolaggi J, Spira A: Classification of nonspecific low back pain. II. Clinical Diversity of organic forms. Spine 17:1038, 1992

269. Wiesel S, Tsourmas N, Feffer H et al: A study of computer-assisted tomography. I. The incidence of positive CT-scans in an asymptomatic group of patients. Spine 9:949, 1984

270. Torgerson W, Dotter W: Comparative roentgenographic study of the asymptomatic and symptomatic lumbar spine abstracted. J Bone Joint Surg 58A:850, 1976

271. Teresi L, Lufkin R, Reicher M et al: Asymptomatic degenerative disk disease and spondylosis of the cervical spine. MR Imaging. Radiology 83, 1987

272. Jackson R, Cain J, Jacobs R et al: The neuroradiographic diagnosis of lumbar herniated nucleus pulposus: II. Spine 14, 1989

273. Haldeman S: Failure of the pathology model to predict back pain: Presidential Address, North American Spine Society. Spine 1990; 15:718, 1990

274. Miles K, Maimaris C, Finlay D et al: The incidence and prognostic significance of radiological abnormalities in soft tissue injuries to the cervical spine. Skeletal Radiol 17:493, 1988

275. Deyo R, Diehl A: Lumbar spine films in primary care: Current use and effect of selective ordering criteria. J Gen Intern Med 1:20, 1986

276. Liang M, Komaroff A: Roentgenograms in primary care patients with acute low-back pain: a cost-effectiveness analysis. Arch Intern Med 142:1108, 1982

277. Scavone J, Latshaw R, Rohrer G: Use of lumbar spine films: Statistical evaluation at a university teaching hospital. JAMA 426:1105, 1981

278. Nachemson A: Advances in low-back pain. Clin Orthop 200:266, 1985

279. Spratt K, Lehmann T, Weinstein J et al: A new approach to the low-back physical examination. Spine 15:96, 1990

280. Guccione A: Physical therapy diagnosis and the relationship between impairments and function. Phys Ther 71:499, 1991

281. Binkley J, Finch E, Hall J et al: Diagnostic classification of patients with low back pain: report on a survey of physical therapy experts. Phys Ther 73:138, 1993

282. Jette A: Using health-related quality of life measures in physical therapy outcomes research. Phys Ther 73:528, 1993

283. Boissonnault WG: Examination in Physical Therapy Practice—Screening for medical disease. Churchill Livingstone, New York, 1991

284. DeRosa C, Porterfield J: A physical therapy model for the treatment of low back pain. Phys Ther 72:261, 1992

285. Coste J, Paolaggi J, Spira A: Classification of nonspecific low back pain. I. Psychological involvement in low back pain. Spine 17:1028, 1992

286. Delitto A, Cibulka M, Erhard R et al: Evidence for use of an extension-mobilization category in acute low back syndrome: A prescriptive validation pilot study. Phys Ther 73:216, 1993

287. Diagnosis in Physical Therapy. A roundtable discussion. Delitto A, Guccione A, Jette A, Sahrmann S, Moderator Magistro C. In PT Magazine, 58, 1993

288. Jette A: Diagnosis and classification by physical therapists: A special communication. Phys Ther 69:967, 1989

289. Dekker J, van Baar M, Curfs E et al: Diagnosis and treatment in physical therapy: an investigation of their relationship. Phys Ther 73:568, 1993

290. Riddle D, Rothstein J: Intertester reliability of McKenzie's classifications of the syndrome types present in patients with low back pain. Spine 18:1333, 1993

291. Khalil T, Asfour S, Martinez L et al: Stretching in the rehabilitation of low-back pain patients. Spine 17:311, 1992

292. Sikorski J: A rationalized approach to physiology for low-back pain. Spine 10: 571, 1985
293. McKenzie R: The Lumbar Spine: Mechanical Diagnosis and Therapy. Spinal Publications, Waikanae, New Zealand, 1981
294. Sahrmann S: Diagnosis by the physical therapist—a prerequisite for treatment. A special communication. Phys Ther 68:1703, 1988
295. Bell W: Orofacial Pains; Differential Diagnosis. 2nd Ed. p. 56. Year Book Medical Pub, Chicago, 1980
296. Tait R, Pollard C, Margolis R et al: The pain disability index: psychometric and validity data. Arch Phys Med Rehabil 68:438, 1987
297. Youdas J, Carey J, Garrett T: Reliability of measurements of cervical spine range of motion—comparison of three methods. Phys Ther 71:98, 1991
298. Youdas J, Garrett T, Suman V et al: Normal range of motion of the cervical spine: An initial goniometric study. Phys Ther 72:770, 1992
299. Dvorak J, Antinnes J, Panjabi M et al: Age and gender related normal motion of the cervical spine. Spine 17:5393, 1992
300. Burn L, Paterson J: Musculoskeletal Medicine. The Spine. p. 152. Kluwer Academic Publishers, Boston, 1990
301. Kendall H, Kendall F, Boynton D: Posture and Pain. Williams & Wilkins, Baltimore, 1952
302. Refshauge K, Bolst L, Goodsell: The relationship between cervicothoracic posture and the presence of pain. Proceedings from the International Federation of Orthopaedic Manipulative Therapists, Vail, Colorado June 1–5, 1992
303. Griegel-Morris P, Larson K, Mueller-Klaus K et al: Incidence of common postural abnormalities in the cervical, shoulder, and thoracic regions and their association with pain in two age groups of healthy subjects. Phys Ther 72:425, 1992
304. Hayes K: The effect of awareness of measurement error on physical therapists' confidence in their decisions. Phys Ther 72:515, 1992
305. Wolf S: Clinical Decision Making in Physical Therapy. FA Davis Company, Philadelphia, 1985
306. Standards for tests and measurements in physical therapy practice. Task Force members, Rothstein J, Campbell S, Echternach J, et al. Phys Ther 71:589, 1991
307. Coste J, Paolaggi J, Spira A: Reliability of interpretation of plain lumbar spine radiographs in benign, mechanical low-back pain. Spine 16:426, 1991
308. Deyo R, McNiesh L, Cone R: Observer variability in interpretation of lumbar spine radiographs. Arthritis Rheum 28:1066, 1985
309. Yoo J, Zou D, Edwards W et al: Effect of cervical spine motion on the neuroforaminal dimensions of human cervical spine. Spine 17:1131, 1992
310. Lewit K: The contribution of clinical observation to neurobiological mechanisms in manipulative therapy. In Korr I (ed): The Neurobiologic Mechanisms in Manipulative Therapy. Plenum Press, New York, 1978
311. Kenneally M, Rubenach H, Elvey R: The upper limb tension test: The SLR test of the arm: In Grant R (ed): Physical Therapy of the cervical and thoracic spine. Clinics in Physical Therapy 17. Churchill Livingstone, New York, 1988
312. Elvey R: Brachial plexus tension tests and the pathoanatomical origin of arm pain. p. 105. In Idczak R (ed): Aspects of Manipulative Therapy, Lincoln Institute of Health Sciences, 1980
313. Breig A: Adverse Mechanical Tension in the Central Nervous System. John Wiley and sons, New York, 1978

314. Butler D, Gifford L: The concept of adverse mechanical tension in the nervous system. Part 1: testing for "Dural Tension." Physiotherapy 75:622, 1989
315. Butler D, Gifford L: The concept of adverse Mechanical tension in the nervous system. Part 2: Examination and Treatment. Physiotherapy 75:629, 1989
316. Elvey R: Treatment of arm pain associated with abnormal brachial plexus tension. Austr J Physiother 32:225, 1986
317. Whitty C, Willison R: Some aspects of referred pain. Lancet ii:226, 1958
318. Lewis T, Kellegren J: Observations relating to referred pain, visceromotor reflexes and other associated phenomena. Clin Sci 4:47, 1939
319. Mooney V, Robertson J: "The Facet Syndrome." Clin Orthop 115:149, 1976
320. Leyshon A, Kirwan E, Parry C: Electrical studies in diagnosis of compression of the lumbar root. J Bone Joint Surg 36B:71, 1981
321. Saal J, Saal J: Nonoperative treatment of herniated lumbar intervertebral disc with radiculopathy, an outcome study. Spine 14:431, 1989
322. Hutchison M: An investigation of premanipulative testing. p. 104. Proc of 6th Bienn. Conf MTAA, Adelaide, Australia, 1989
323. Powell V: An investigation of testing procedures for vertebrobasilar insufficiency. Aust J Physiother 36:31, 1990
324. Yochum T, Rowe L: Arthritides of the upper cervical complex. p. 22. In Idczak R (ed): Aspects of Manipulative Therapy. Proceedings of a Multidisciplinary International Conference on Manipulative Therapy, Melbourne, Aug 1979, Lincoln Institute of Health Sciences, 1980
325. Pettman E: Stress testing the anatomy. Proceedings from the International Federation of Orthopaedic Manipulative Therapists. Vail, Colorado, June 1–5, 1992
326. Paris SV: S3 Course Notes. p. 78. Institute of Graduate Physical Therapy, Inc. St. Augustine, Florida, 1992
327. Aspinall Wendy: Clinical testing for the craniovertebral hypermobility syndrome. JOSPT 12:47, 1990
328. Roland M, Morris R: A study of the natural history of low back pain. Spine 8: 145, 1983
329. Waddell G: A new clinical model for the treatment of low back pain. Spine 12: 632, 1987
330. Nachemson A: A critical look at the treatment for low back pain. Scand J Rehab Med 11:143, 1979
331. Benn R, Wood P: Pain in the back: an attempt to estimate the size of the problem. Rheumatol Rehabil 14:121, 1975
332. Berquist-Ullman M, Larsson U: Acute low back pain in industry. Acta Orthop Scand 170(suppl):1, 1977
333. Andersson G, Pope M, Frymoyer J: Epidemiology. p. 101. In Pope M, Frymoyer J, Andersson G (eds): Occupational Low Back Pain. Praeger, New York, 1984
334. Marbach et al: Psychother Psychocom 39:47, 1983
335. Farrell J, Twomey L: Acute low back pain, comparison of two conservative treatment approaches. Med J Aust 1:160, 1982
336. Cousins N: A nation of hypochondriacs. p. 88. Time, June 18, 1990
337. Greenough C, Fraser R: Assessment of outcome in patients with low-back pain. Spine 17:36, 1992
338. Weber H: Lumbar disc herniation: a controlled prospective study with ten years of observation. Spine 8:131, 1983
339. Parry W: The failed back. p. 341. In Wall PD, Melzack (eds): Textbook of Pain. Edited by PD Wall and Melzack. Churchill Livingstone, New York, 1989

340. Wetzel F: Chronic Benign Cervical Pain Syndromes. Surgical Considerations. Spine 17(suppl):S367, 1992

341. McCoy C, Selby D, Henderson R et al: Patients avoiding surgery; pathology and one-year life status follow-up. Spine 16(suppl)S198, 1991

342. Nelson M (ed): Low back pain and industrial and social disablement. Proceedings of symposium. London: Back Pain Association, 1983

343. McKenzie R: The Lumbar Spine: Mechanical Diagnosis and Therapy. Spinal Publications, Waikanae, New Zealand, 1981

344. Cooper D, Jenkins R, Bready L et al: The prevention of injuries of the brachial plexus secondary to malposition of the patient during surgery. Clin Orthop 228: 33, 1988

345. Russek AS: Diagnosis and treatment of scapulocostal syndrome. JAMA 150:25, 1982

346. Zusman M: Spinal manipulative therapy: review of some proposed mechanisms, and a new hypothesis. Austr J Physiother 32:89, 1986

347. Korr (ed): The Neurobiologic Mechanisms in Manipulative Therapy. Plenum, New York, 1978

348. Idczak R (ed): Aspects of manipulative therapy. Proceedings of a Multidisciplinary International Conference on Manipulative Therapy, Melbourne, Aug 1979, Lincoln Institute of Health Sciences, 1980

349. Burn L, Paterson J (eds): Musculoskeletal Medicine. Kluwer Academic Publishers, Boston, 1990

350. Rothstein J (ed): Manual Therapy: Special Issue. Phys Ther 72:(12), 1992

351. Goldstein M (ed): The Research Status of Spinal Manipulative Therapy. U.S. Department of Health, Education, and Welfare. DHEW Publication No. (NIH) 76-998. NINCDS Monograph No. 15, 1975

352. Zusman M, Edwards B, Donaghy: Investigation of a proposed mechanism for the relief of spinal pain with passive joint movement. J Manual Med 4:58, 1989

353. Manipulative Physiotherapists Association of Australia, 7th Biennial Conference. Nov 27–30, 1991, Blue Mountains, New South Wales. Manipulative Physiotherapists Association, Australia, North Fitzroy Victoria, Australia.

354. Bogduk N: A scientific approach to cervical diagnosis. p. 151. Proceedings from the Fourth Biennial Conference of the Manipulative Therapist Association of Australia, Brisbane, May 22–25, 1985

355. Grieve G (ed): Modern Manual Therapy of Vertebral Column. Churchill Livingstone, New York, 1986

356. Di Fabio R: Efficacy of manual therapy. In Rothstein J (ed): Manual Therapy: Special Issue. Phys Ther 72:853, 1992

357. Shepard K, Jensen G, Schmoll B et al: Alternative approaches to research in physical therapy: positivism and phenomenology. Phys Ther 73:88, 1993

358. Polit D, Hungler B: Nursing Research: Principles and Methods. 4th Ed. JB Lippincott, Philadelphia, 1991

359. Merriam S: Case study research in education: a qualitative approach. Jossey-Bass, San Francisco, 1988

360. Mattingly C: Commentary on Shepard K, Jensen G, Schmoll B et al: Alternative approaches to research in physical therapy: positivism and phenomenology. Phys Ther 73:98, 1993

361. Colachis S, Strohm B: Radiographic studies of cervical spine motion in normal subjections, flexion and hyperextension. Arch Phys Med Rehabil 46:753, 1965

362. Colachis S, Strohm B: Relationship of time to varied traction force with constant angle of pull. Arch Phys Med Rehabil 47:353, 1966

363. Wong A, Leong C, Chen C: The traction angle and cervical intervertebral separation. Spine 17:136, 1992

364. Twomey LT, Taylor JR: Damage to the cervical disc and facet joints following severe trauma. p. 25. In: Manipulative Physiotherapists Association of Australia, 7th Biennial Conference. Blue Mountains, New South Wales, Nov. 27–30, 1991, Manipulative Physiotherapists Association Australia, North Fitzroy Victoria, Australia, 1991

365. Pearce J: Whiplash injury: a reappraisal. J Neurol Neurosurg Psy 52:1329, 1989

366. Davis S, Teresi L, Bradley W et al: MRI Findings in cervical spine hyperextension injuries. p. 170. Proceedings of the 41st Annual Meeting of the Royal Australian College of Radiologists, 1990

367. Osti O, Vernon-Roberts B, Fraser R: Anulus Tears and intervertebral disc degeneration: an experimental study using an animal model. Spine 15:762, 1990

368. Taylor J, Twomey L: The development of the human intervertebral disc. p. 39. In Ghosh P (ed): The Biology of the Intervertebral Disc. Vol. 1. CRC Press, Boca Raton, 1988

369. Foreman S, Croft A: Whiplash injuries; The Cervical Acceleration/Deceleration Syndrome. Williams & Wilkins, Baltimore, 1988

370. St Pierre D, Gardiner P: The effect of immobilisation and exercise on muscle function: a review. Physiother Canada 39:24, 1987

371. Shepard R: Management of exercise in the elderly. Applied Sports Sciences 9: 109, 1984

372. Menard D, Stanish W: The aging athlete. Am J Sports Med 17:187, 1991

373. Pardini A: Exercise, vitality and aging. Aging 344:19, 1984

374. Aniansson A, Grimby G, Rundgren A et al: Physical training in old men. Age Ageing 9:186, 1980

375. Aloia J, Cohn S, Cane R et al. Prevention of bone loss by exercise. J Clin Endocrinol Metab 43:992, 1978

376. Smith E, Reddin N, Smith P: Physical activity and calcium modalities for bone mineral increase in aged women. Med Sci Sports Exerc. 13:60, 1981

377. Gustavsen R: Training Therapy: Prophylaxis and Rehabilitation. New York, Thieme, 1985

378. Saal JS: Flexibility training. Physical medicine and rehabilitation: state of the art reviews 1:537, 1987. Philadelphia, Hanley & Belfus, Inc.

379. Sweeney T, Prentice C, Saal J et al: Cervicothoracic Muscular Stabilization Techniques. In: Saal J (guest ed) Physical Medicine and Rehabilitation: State of the Art Reviews. Vol 4, No 2, June 1990. p 335–359, Philadelphia, Hanley & Belfus, Inc.

380. Jansen J, Spoerri O: Atypical frontoorbital pain and headache due to compression of upper cervical roots. p. 14. In Pfaffenrath V, Lundberg P-O, Sjaasdad O (eds): Updating in Headache. Springer, Berlin, 1985

12 | Medical Management of the Cervical Spine

Jonathan P. Lester
Robert E. Windsor
Susan J. Dreyer

A thorough understanding of cervical spinal disorders is important for any practitioner involved in the treatment of TMD. Cervical spine pathology often coexists with TMD in the patient with head and neck symptoms. Furthermore, cervical spinal disorders may become symptomatic if altered cervical biomechanics are used to control TMD-related pain or dysfunction.[1] Cervicogenic head, neck, and upper extremity pain may be secondary to cervical spondylotic disease or nondegenerative dysfunction of innervated cervical structures. Identification of the cause of the symptoms can be achieved through a comprehensive evaluation including physical examination, imaging studies, electrodiagnostic studies, and selective spinal injections. Multidisciplinary treatment programs using physical, medical, and surgical therapies can provide symptomatic relief in most cases.

EPIDEMIOLOGY OF NECK PAIN

Neck and related shoulder pain are common musculoskeletal disorders found in industrialized societies. Although epidemiologic studies vary considerably, most have found that the prevalence of significant neck or shoulder pain is approximately 10 to 20 percent and slightly more common in women.[2] Risk factors for development of neck and shoulder pain include increasing age, stress, frequent material handling,and frequent work above shoulder level.[3]

CERVICAL SPINAL DISORDERS

Degeneration of cervical spinal structures occurs to some extent in all individuals, and it is impossible to say with certainty that a symptomatic lesion of the cervical spine is related or not related to this degenerative process. However, for the sake of the following discussion, disorders of the cervical spine will be divided into those that are directly related to the degenerative process and those that are thought to be caused by mechanical or physiologic dysfunction of nondegenerative cervical spinal structures. One must realize that this is an academic distinction and that in the clinical setting the etiology of a symptom complex may be multifactorial.

Cervical Spondylosis

Cervical spondylosis denotes a series of progressive and well-defined biochemical and morphologic degenerative changes involving the cervical intervertebral discs, vertebral bodies, zygapophyseal (facet) joints, and supporting ligamentous structures.[4] These changes occur progressively in most individuals after the second decade of life and represent the natural aging process of the cervical spine. In some individuals, cervical spondylotic changes are related to the clinical presence of pain or neurologic dysfunction. What determines whether these changes will become pathologic in any particular individual and to what extent specific symptom complexes can be attributed to certain morphologic changes is still not fully understood.

The spondylotic process begins with biochemical changes within the nucleus of the intervertebral disc. Loss of high-molecular-weight mucoproteins decreases the water-binding capacity of the nuclear material and leads to progressive desiccation of nuclear matrix.[4] At the same time, nuclear collagen content increases, producing a stiff, fibrotic, and granular nucleus. Such changes cause the disc to become less efficient at converting axial compression forces to radial tension forces. Because the disc cannot disperse axial forces in the radial direction, the disc annulus is exposed to greater compression forces, leading to increased wear and fibrillation of the collagen fibers comprising the disc annulus. Progressive fibrillation of annular fibers leads to annulus failure, which manifests as disc bulging and loss of disc height. Disc degeneration also results in the loss of segmental lordosis and may allow an increase in segmental motion.[5] The resultant changes in disc morphology and mechanical function stimulate a bony and ligamentous response that may include the development of anterior vertebral body traction spurs, posterior vertebral body osteophytes and bony bar formation, osteophytosis of the posterolateral uncovertebral joints of Luschka, and thickening of the ligamentum flavum. Also, the facet joints may undergo degenerative changes including thinning of articular cartilage, sclerosis, and reactive bone formation. Bony and soft tissue changes resulting from the degenerative process are most prevalent at the C5–6 level (followed in frequency by the C6–7 and C4–5 levels) and may result in narrowing of the central spinal canal and neuroforamina, leading to impingement of neurologic structures.[6-8]

Cervical Disc Protrusion

Cervical spondylosis may become clinically pronounced when nuclear matrix protrudes (herniates) into or through the disc annulus. Disc protrusion may occur acutely with strain or trauma to the cervical spine or chronically without trauma. As the disc annulus fibers suffer progressive fibrillation and weaken, they develop macroscopic radial and circumferential fissures that allow peripheral migration of nuclear material. As the nuclear material approaches the outer annular fibers, the annulus may bulge out (contained disc protrusion) or defects in the annulus and posterior longitudinal ligament (PLL) may allow the nuclear material to escape beyond the disc margin (disc extrusion). Disc protrusion is most frequent in the late fourth or early fifth decade of life, before nuclear desiccation and fibrosis, and affects women slightly more than men.[7] Risk factors for cervical disc protrusion include smoking, frequent recreational diving into water, and frequent heavy lifting. Disc protrusion may be anterior, posterior, posterolateral, or intraforaminal. Intraforaminal and posterolateral protrusions are most common and may produce radiculopathy (pain, sensory disturbance, muscle weakness, and reflex changes in the distribution of a single nerve root) by mechanical compression of the exiting nerve root or dorsal root ganglion.[9] Also, research on lumbar discs has shown that nuclear material contains highly inflammatory substances that may chemically insult the neural elements.[10] Anterior and posterior protrusions are less common, as they are prevented by the anterior longitudinal ligaments and PLLs, which reinforce the annulus in these locations.[11] Posterior protrusions may produce myelopathy (sensory disturbance, weakness, spasticity, and hyperreflexia below the level of the protrusion) caused by compromise of the cervical spinal cord, but symptomatic disc lesions causing myelopathy are usually accompanied by coexistent compromise from bony narrowing of the spinal canal.[4] Disc protrusions can present with neck pain and stiffness, radicular pain, or referred pain to the scapular region.

Cervical Internal Disc Disruption

The cervical intervertebral disc may also be a cause of neck and arm pain without the development of a significant protrusion. Painful disc derangement may develop if acute injury or chronic fatigue creates annular defects, allowing peripheral migration of inflammatory nuclear material to the innervated outer third of the annulus. Crock[12] has termed this condition of painful disorganization of internal disc architecture *internal disc disruption* (IDD). IDD may exist without the disc exhibiting significant disc bulging or focal protrusion on imaging studies. Work by Cloward[13] in the 1950s using cervical discography helped to identify the presence of this condition, as well as to characterize the cervical, brachial, and scapular pain referral patterns of these discogenic lesions (Fig. 12-1).

Cervical Spondylotic Radiculopathy and Myelopathy

Cervical radiculopathy and myelopathy may also be produced by chronic progressive spatial encroachment on the cervical spinal cord and nerve roots or their vascular supply by the bony and ligamentous spondylotic changes previously described. Cervical spondylotic radiculopathy and myelopathy (CSM) most commonly present insidiously in the sixth and seventh decades of life but may become acutely symptomatic after cervical trauma. Clinical signs and symptoms are usually but not always determined by the relative degree of compromise to the central spinal canal and neuroforamina and may present as monoradiculopathy, polyradiculopathy, myelopathy, or combined myeloradiculopathy. Motor findings may be a mixed picture of upper and lower motor neuron deficits but usually include lower motor neuron signs (weakness, atrophy, fasciculations, and hyporeflexia) at the level or levels of spinal stenosis and upper motor neuron signs (weakness, spasticity, and hyperreflexia) below the level of stenosis.[4] Sensory findings also depend on the site of compromise. Disruption of ascending spinothalamic tracts of the cervical spinal cord leads to loss of contralateral pain and temperature sensation, and compromise to the

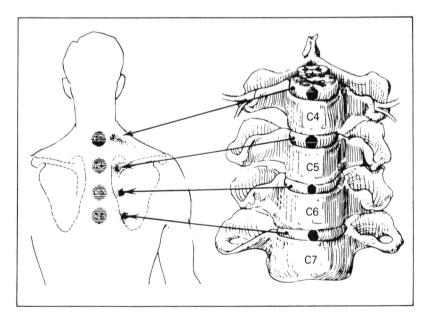

Fig. 12-1. Discogenic pain referred from the anterior surface of the lower cervical discs (From Cloward,[13] with permission.)

posterior columns may cause loss of position and vibration sensory input. Compromise to the dorsal root ganglion or existing nerve root will cause loss of sensation in a dermatomal distribution.[14] Compromise to the cervical spinal cord may also lead to bowel, bladder, and sexual dysfunction (urinary incontinence, fecal incontinence, or impotence). The presentation of CSM may be painless, may include local neck pain and stiffness, or may produce referred arm pain if radicular compromise is part of the underlying pathology.

Although cervical spondylosis occurs to some degree in all individuals, many never experience symptoms. Clinical expression of CSM is thought to be intimately related to the diameter of the cervical spinal canal. Most authors agree that the critical midsagittal diameter for the development of CSM is 12 to 13 mm (the normal diameter between C3 and C7 is 17 to 18 mm).[5,15] Therefore, individuals with initial spinal canal diameters at the lower end of the normal spectrum are predisposed to develop CSM, and those with more generous canal diameters may never develop symptoms despite extensive spondylotic disease. Other factors thought to play a role in the development of CSM include spinal canal shape, degree of soft tissue changes (e.g., ligamentum flavum hypertrophy), and associated vascular compromise.

Also, positional changes of the cervical spine alter the shape and volume of the spinal canal and may affect the degree of symptomatic compromise to cervical neurologic structures. Relative cervical canal stenosis may become absolute stenosis when the cervical spine is extended. In extension, there is posterior bulging of the disc annulus and unfolding of the ligamentum flavum, which decrease the sagittal diameter of the spinal canal and axial compression of the cervical spinal cord, which causes an increase in the cross-sectional area of the cord.[16] Hence, a sudden deceleration–hyperextension injury to the cervical spine as might occur in a "whiplash"-type injury, or prolonged cervical extension from poor sitting posture or sleeping on one's stomach, might contribute to the acute or chronic onset of CSM. Alternatively, anterior cord compression may occur during flexion when the cervical spinal cord is stretched over osteophytes protruding from the posterior vertebral body.

The natural history of CSM is often characterized by the insidious onset of mild or moderate symptoms that remain stable or progress slowly or in a stuttering fashion, often leading to long periods of nonprogressive disability.[17] Acute onset of CSM followed by rapid progressive deterioration of neurologic function is uncommon in the absence of trauma. Conservative care may help control symptoms in mild to moderate cases in which pain is the predominant symptom and significant neurologic compromise is absent but does not appear to be helpful in severe cases in which profound neurologic compromise exists or to affect the ultimate outcome. One must be careful to exclude other causes of neurologic dysfunction such as multiple sclerosis, motor neuron disease (amyotropic lateral sclerosis), low-pressure hydrocephalus, spinal cord tumor, cervical syrinx, or intracranial pathology.[14]

Cervical spondylosis may also lead to bony encroachment on other cervical structures, producing a diverse group of symptoms in addition to pain and neurologic dysfunction.[14] Anterior disc protrusion or anterior traction osteophytes may compromise esophageal function and cause dysphagia.[18] Osteophytosis of the facet or posterolateral uncovertebral joints may cause vertebral artery insufficiency and produce dizziness or the feeling of unsteadiness with cervical rotation. However, direct vascular compression alone rarely produces clinical symptoms unless there is underlying atherosclerotic disease. Also, pressure on the cervical sympathetic chain from anterior disc protrusion or osteophytes may cause dizziness, diplopia, tinnitus, or the vague feeling of cervical constriction.[14]

Cervicogenic Pain

In addition to compromise of the cervical spine from the spondylotic process, symptom complexes believed to originate in the cervical spine may develop from dysfunction of nondegenerative cervical spinal structures. Head, neck, and upper extremity pain without concomitant neurologic compromise may be caused by degenerative changes, injury, or mechanical dysfunction (postural stress, repetitive overuse, altered biomechanics, or altered proprioceptive or nocioceptive input) of cervical spinal structures. The perivertebral muscles, zygapophyseal joints, intervertebral discs and related ligaments, cervical dura matter, and dorsal root ganglion (DRG) are all highly innervated by the cervical spinal nerves with nociceptive endings and may act as pain-generating structures.[19,20] Pain may be felt locally at the site of cervical pathology or referred to a distant site (head, shoulder, arm). Referred pain may be characterized as either radicular (sharp, lacinating, well localized to a dermatomal region) or sclerotomal (dull, aching, poorly localized over a diffuse nondermatomal region). Pain character may give insight into the source of the pain generator.

Muscles

Cervical prevertebral, paravertebral, and postvertebral musculature may develop localized bands of tight, well-defined, painful fibers termed *trigger points*.[21] Trigger points may develop from acute trauma or strain but most commonly develop from repetitive overuse as occurs with frequent overhead reaching or lifting or chronic postural overuse secondary to an individual maintaining a rounded shoulder posture with accentuated scapular protraction and compensatory cervical hyperlordosis. Trigger points within the pericervical musculature may produce localized pain or referred sclerotomal pain to the head, shoulder, scapula, or upper extremity.[21] These referral patterns are thought to be consistent from one individual to another for a given muscle group. In some cases, trigger point formation is secondary to dysfunction of underlying segmental structures such as the intervertebral disc or facet joint.

Facet Joints

The cervical zygapophyseal joints have become well recognized as a frequent cause of neck pain.[22] Inflammatory or degenerative arthritis, acute sprain as may occur with a deceleration whiplash-type injury, or mechanical dysfunction from postural strain or myofascial restriction may lead to the generation of facet pain. A preliminary study by Dwyer et al[23,24] involving provocative facet joint injections in healthy asymptomatic volunteers and analgesic injection in symptomatic patients has led to the characterization of facet joint pain referral patterns (Fig. 12-2). Further studies involving both normal and symptomatic patients may be needed to refine and confirm this work.

Dura Matter

The cervical dura matter investing the cervical spinal cord and exiting nerve roots are also richly innervated and may generate pain. Mechanical compression from osteophytes or chemical irritation from exudative inflammatory substances originating in the intervertebral disc or zygapophyseal joint may stimulate the dura to produce nociceptive input in the absence of symptomatic neural element compromise.[25]

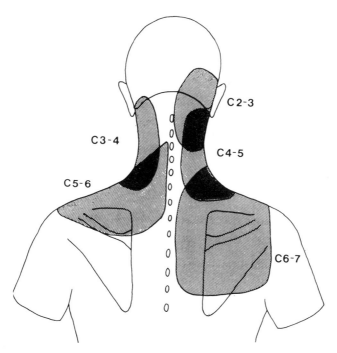

Fig. 12-2. Composite map of the distribution of pain from cervical zygapophyseal joint injections. (From Dwyer,[23] with permission).

Cervicogenic Headache

Head and facial pain may also be secondary to cervical spinal disorders. Afferent sensory pathways from the trigeminal nucleus and upper cervical spinal nerves (C1, C2, and C3) converge in the brain stem, and nociceptive input from the upper cervical spine may be perceived as originating from the trigeminal fields (face) or cutaneous distribution of the C2 and C3 dermatomes (occiput and upper posterior cervical region).[26] Common sources of cervicogenic headache may include the perivertebral and suboccipital muscles, the atlanto-occipital joint, atlantoaxial joint, transverse ligament, alar ligament, C2–3 and C3–4 zygapophyseal joints, and C2–3 intervertebral disc.[26]

Entrapment Syndromes

Peripheral entrapment of neurologic structures originating in the cervical spine may occur and cause head, neck, or upper extremity symptoms. The most well-described of these disorders includes occipital neuralgia and thoracic outlet syndrome. However, an appropriate discussion of the pathophysiology of these disorders and their management is beyond the scope of this chapter, and the reader is referred to alternative references for additional information.[27,28]

EVALUATION

Determining the nature and severity of cervical spinal disorders requires a comprehensive evaluation including a detailed history and physical examination, appropriate imaging studies, electrodiagnostic evaluation, and occasionally selective anesthetic blockade of suspected pain-producing structures. Great care and restraint must be taken when attributing clinical symptom complexes to abnormalities found on imaging studies, as these modalities have become extremely sensitive at defining morphologic changes that may or may not play a role in the clinical symptom complex. To be clinically relevant, imaging abnormalities resulting either from trauma or the degenerative spondylotic process should correlate with subjective complaints, objective physical findings, electrodiagnostic findings, and response to selective anesthetic blockade of appropriate structures. Furthermore, a normal neurologic examination and normal cervical spinal morphology on imaging studies do not rule out the possible presence of a symptomatic cervical spinal disorder from nondegenerative or traumatic pathology. One cannot completely exclude the presence of a painful nondegenerative spinal lesion without performing a thorough manual examination of the cervical spine or performing selective anesthetic blockade of potential pain-producing structures.

History

Obtaining a brief focused history may provide significant insight into the nature of a symptomatic cervical spinal disorder. Acute onset of radicular pain suggests nerve root compromise from soft disc protrusion, whereas insidious development of radicular symptoms suggests spondylotic compromise. Subacute or insidious development of poorly localized pain in the cervical or scapular region may indicate myofascial, facet, or discogenic pain secondary to spondylotic disease or postural overuse. A history of night pain or constitutional symptoms (fever, chills, night sweats, or unexplained weight loss) should alert the clinician to possible tumor or spinal infection. Neck pain in association with pain, swelling, or deformity of the small joints of the hands or feet should suggest the possibility of inflammatory arthritis.

Physical Examination

Physical examination of the cervical spine and related structures should include an orthopaedic assessment, neurologic evaluation, and manual examination. The orthopaedic examination should evaluate cervical motion looking for restrictions or pain during flexion, extension, sidebending, or rotation. Spurling's maneuver, in which the neck is extended, sidebent, and rotated to produce foraminal narrowing, may elicit or intensify radicular symptoms.[29,30]

A screening neurologic examination is performed to assess for motor, sensory, or reflex deficits. A basic motor examination should survey the upper and lower extremity musculature for atrophy or weakness in a peripheral nerve, myotomal, or regional distribution. I usually evaluate the deltoid (C5, C6), biceps (C5, C6), triceps (C7, C8), pronator teres (C6, C7), wrist flexors (C6) and extensors (C7), interossei (C8, T1), abductor pollicis brevis (C8, T1), abductor digiti quinti (C8, T1), hip flexors (L2, L3, L4), quadriceps (L4), ankle dorsiflexors (L5), extensor hallucis longis (L5), and ankle plantar flexors (S1) as an initial screen. Sensory testing should include the C4 through T1 dermatomes, and any deficits in the upper extremity should prompt additional evaluation of the median, ulnar, and radial nerve distributions to discriminate between a radicular pattern of sensory loss and a peripheral nerve pattern.[29,30] Any complaints of sensory deficit involving the chest or lower extremities require a comprehensive sensory examination to search for regional sensory loss or the presence of a myelopathic sensory level. Reflex testing should include evaluation of the biceps, triceps, brachioradialis, knee, and ankle jerks to assess for radiculopathic (decreased or absent reflex) or myelopathic (increased reflex) changes.[29,30] Additional myelopathic reflexes including Hoffman (finger jerks with rapid flexion of the distal interphalangeal joints of the hands) and Babinski (upgoing toes with plantar stimulation) should be checked.[30] Any neurologic deficits found on examination should be compared to determine a common site of compromise such as cervical spinal cord, cervical nerve root, or peripheral nerve.

The comprehensive evaluation of the cervical region also requires a screening manual examination to assess for segmental pain, facet joint dysfunction, or myofascial pain. Segmental examination involves palpation and stress of the cervical spinous processes and may allow one to elicit symptoms and localize the site of pathology to one or two contiguous spinal segments.[31,32] Palpation of the cervical facets may reveal tenderness over symptomatic joints. More experienced examiners may also palpate for soft tissue changes over pathologic facet joints or assess for restrictions in facet joint motion.[31,32] Finally, careful palpation of the cervical and scapular musculature may reveal symptomatic trigger points or changes in tone or flexibility that result from postural overuse.[21,32,33]

Imaging Studies

Radiographs of the cervical spine are indicated in all cases of trauma, suspected tumor, or spinal infection and in the patient with neurologic deficits. Although radiographic findings of spondylotic changes are no more common in symptomatic than asymptomatic patients,[34] positive findings that correlate to deficits on neurologic testing or dysfunction on manual examination in a symptomatic patient may give important information regarding the etiology of the symptom-producing lesion and the degree of compromise from bony structures. Young patients without a history of trauma, constitutional symptoms, or radicular pain or findings of neurologic deficit on examination may not require initial radiologic surgery.

Standard Radiographs

Standard plain films include an anteroposterior (AP), lateral, right and left oblique, open-mouth, and lateral flexion and extension views. The lateral view provides the greatest degree of information. Spondylotic changes may be identified including disc space narrowing, anterior and posterior osteophytes, endplate sclerosis, and facet joint sclerosis or telescopic subluxation.[35] One may also assess cervical lordosis and segmental alignment. Segmental kyphosis may be secondary to a degenerative intervertebral disc or disruption of the PLL. Craniocervical junction abnormalities as a result of congenital dysplasia, os odontoidem, Klippel-Feil anomaly, or inflammatory arthritis may sometimes be identified on the lateral view.[36] Lateral views in flexion and extension give additional information regarding the stability of the cervical and craniocervical articulations. Segmental subluxation of more than 3 mm may indicate disruption of the longitudinal ligament or a severely degenerative disc. Furthermore, separation of the odontoid from the anterior arch of the atlas by more than 2 to 3 mm in adults may indicate fracture of the axis or disruption of the transverse ligament from inflammatory arthritis. The open-mouth view may be used for further assessment of the atlantoaxial articulation. Malalignment of the lateral C1–2 joint line or spread of the lateral masses of C1 beyond the lateral margins of the C2 body may indicate a fracture of C1 (Jefferson fracture). The AP view gives further information regarding cervical alignment and may be useful for evaluation degenerative changes at the posterolateral joints of Luschka. Oblique views demonstrate the patency of the neuroforamina and may show narrowing from bony osteophytes projecting off the joints of Luschka or the medial facet joint margins.

Myelography/Computed Tomography

Cervical myelography may be useful in identifying extradural defects compromising the central spinal canal or proximal nerve root sleeves but cannot always identify the etiology of these defects and has limited use as an isolated imaging modality. However, cervical myelography in concert with thin-slice computed tomography (CT) scanning improves the sensitivity and specificity of these studies. CT scanning after intrathecal contrast injection (CT-myelography) has been the established "gold standard" for evaluating compromise to the cervical dural structures from trauma or spondylotic disease. After identification of abnormal levels on plain myelography, thin-slice CT sections (1.5 to 3.0 mm) can be obtained, and these give excellent spatial resolution of bony and soft tissue structures in the axial plane. Compromise to the dura within the central spinal canal or the root sleeves within the proximal neuroforamina from soft tissue structures (disc protrusion or ligament flavum hypertrophy) or bony osteophytes can be appreciated. Measurements of midsagittal diameter and cross-sectional area can be easily determined.[37] As noted previously, a midsagittal diameter of less than 12 to 13 mm is usually associated with symptomatic cervical myelopathy. Also, a reduction of cervical cross-sectional area to less than 30 percent of normal is correlated with the presence of myelopathic signs.

Complications from myelography may include vertebral artery injury resulting in stroke, death, hemorrhage, or spinal cord trauma from lateral C1–2 puncture. Also, headache or seizures from intrathecal contrast injection or cervical spinal cord injury from hyperextension positioning may occur.[38] These risks have been greatly minimized by use of newer nonionic contrast agents introduced into the thecal space through a lumbar puncture site and by preprocedure screening for patients with severe spondylotic changes or spinal instability that may lead to spinal cord injury from cervical hyperextension.

Plain CT scanning of the cervical spine is useful for surveying the bony architecture and identifying vertebral fractures, congenital stenosis, or frank soft disc protrusion but is relatively insensitive for identifying compromise to dural structures.[39] CT images of the cervicothoracic junction may be compromised by bony artifact from the shoulders.

Thin-slice CT scanning after intravenous contrast injection (CT-IVC) is a useful screening procedure for the evaluation of cervical radiculopathy. Intravenous contrast may allow better visualization of epidural and foraminal soft tissue and vascular structures. Radicular compromise may be identified by displacement of normally enhancing foraminal structures (radicular veins, dura, and dorsal root ganglion) by bone or soft tissue and will be accompanied by passive venous congestion above and below the site of compression. Soft disc protrusion may be identified by an enhancing fibrovascular response to extruded nuclear material.[40] However, risks from CT-IVC may include allergic contrast reaction, and CT-IVC is not commonly performed now that magnetic resonance imaging (MRI) is widely available.

Magnetic Resonance Imaging

Recent advances in MRI make it the modality of choice for studying the cervical spine. MR images are constructed by obtaining signals from the repetitive excitation and relaxation of atomic nuclei within a magnetic field. The relaxation phase is characterized by two main factors, the longitudinal relaxation time (T_1) and the transverse relaxation time (T_2). T_1 and T_2 are intrinsic properties of biologic tissues, and the T_1 and T_2 characteristics of a specific anatomic structure in combination with the density of protons determines the MRI signal.[41] Imaging parameters can be optimized to accentuate the T_1 or T_2 properties of various tissues. T_1 images (short repetition time and short echo time) display a strong signal from fatty tissues and an intermediate signal from tissues high in protein. T_2 images (long repetition time and echo time) display a strong signal intensity from tissues high in water and an intermediate signal from those high in protein. Combining earlier spin echo (SE) T_1 and T_2 acquisitions with newly developed two- and three-dimensional multiplanar gradient recalled (MPGR) images allows one to obtain thin-slice images over a large area with high spatial resolution and excellent soft tissue contrast in orthogonal and oblique planes.[37]

Sagittal T_1 images give excellent anatomic detail and are useful to evaluate for disc space narrowing, disc protrusion, spondylotic vertebral endplate changes, and foraminal narrowing. Axial T_1 images allow good visualization of disc and dural structures in cross section to confirm disc protrusion or compromise to the thecal sac or exiting nerve roots. However, dense sclerotic cortical bone found in many osteophytes does not produce a significant MR signal and the relative contributions of soft tissue and bony elements to compromise of dural structures cannot always be determined by MR images. Sagittal T_2 images provide excellent resolution between disc nucleus, disc annulus, cerebral spinal fluid, and spinal cord elements and have a "myelographic" appearance. T_2 images are very sensitive to loss of nuclear hydration and allow early identification of biochemical and histologic degenerative disc changes (nuclear desiccation, annular fissures, disruption of the posterior nuclear–annular complex) before gross morphologic changes (loss of disc height or disc protrusion). Also, T_2 images may identify signal changes within the spinal cord parenchyma representing edema or malacia secondary to spondylotic compromise.

MPGR images with low flip angle (T_2^*) allow one to obtain T_2-like images in thin sections (1.5 to 3.0 mm) with improved spatial resolution compared with T_2 SE images (Fig. 12-3). Sagittal and axial images are obtained and give excellent visualization of compromise to the dural sac or cervical nerve roots. Also, T_2^* images produce good visualization of foraminal contents and may be supplemented by images constructed in the oblique plane perpendicular to the neuroforamina to clarify subtle pathology. However, T_2^* images are not as sensitive to early desiccative changes of the nucleus as T_2 SE images and may not demonstrate early changes of degenerative disc disease or IDD.

MR may also be performed before and after intravenous injection of gadolinium-DTPA, a paramagnetic contrast agent. Postoperative fibrosis, which appears isointense with other soft tissue structures (protruded disc, ligamentum flavum) on noncontrasted T_1 and T_2 images, will have increased signal intensity after intravenous gadolinium injection. Some centers also obtain cervical sag-

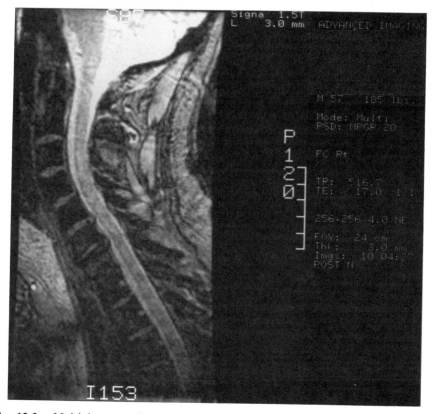

Fig. 12-3. Multiplanar gradient echo sagittal image of the cervical spine showing a moderate protrusion of the C5–6 disc and large protrusion of the C6–7 disc.

ittal MR images in flexed and extended positions to visualize dynamic morphologic changes that may cause cervical spinal cord compromise.

Bone Scan

Bone scanning after intravenous injection of radiolabeled pharmaceutic agents (technetium, gallium) may be a very useful adjuvant imaging modality for the detection of occult spinal lesions such as fractures, malignancy, or spinal infection. Standard bone scanning with radiolabeled technetium is extremely sensitive to vascular changes or reactive bone formation associated with spinal infection, tumor, or metabolic disorders leading to abnormal bone remodeling (Paget disease, hyperparathyroidism).[42] Alternatively, bone scans obtained with gallium are highly selective for disorders such as hematopoietic tumors, sarcomas, and infections. Bone scans may be falsely positive in healed spinal fractures or degenerative conditions and falsely negative in tumors lacking an osteoblastic response, tumors with small nests of cells, or postirradiated tumors. Also, tumors with widespread symmetrically distributed metastatic deposits may appear similar to common degenerative changes.

Choosing the appropriate imaging modality may be a difficult process and may depend on regional availability and costs and preferences of the local orthopaedic or neurosurgical community. CT-myelography offers excellent resolution of bony and soft tissue compromise to the dural elements but requires an invasive procedure and may suffer image degradation from bony artifact at the cervicothoracic junction. MRI is noninvasive, and the combination of SE and MPGR acquisitions allows diagnostic sensitivity that approaches CT-myelography. Also, MRI properties may allow detection of early biochemical and histologic changes within the disc and spinal cord from spondylotic disease that cannot be detected with other imaging formats. However, MR images are very sensitive to motion artifact and may be very difficult to obtain in claustrophobic patients or contraindicated in those with certain ferromagnetic implants (aneurysm clips, cochlear implants, intraoccular foreign bodies, or cardiac pacemakers). Furthermore, older MRI protocols using only SE acquisitions may suffer image degradation from reduced signal-to-noise ratios with thin-slice images and may be less sensitive for intraforaminal pathology than CT-myelography. Plain CT, plain myelography, and CT-IVC are useful imaging modalities but lack the sensitivity of CT-myelography or MRI and have limited indications in the evaluation of cervical spine pathology. Bone scanning with technetium or gallium may be extremely useful as adjuvant imaging modalities when occult cervical spinal lesions are suspected.

Electrodiagnostic Evaluation

Electrodiagnostic evaluation is a minimally invasive method of assessing the functional status of the peripheral and central nervous system (CNS). Unlike the above imaging studies, electrodiagnostic evaluation provides information on the physiologic integrity of the nervous system rather than anatomic morphology. Nerve conduction studies (NCS), electromyography (EMG), and somatosensory-evoked potentials (SEP) may be performed independently or in combination during an electrodiagnostic examination to assess for radiculopathy, cervical spinal cord compromise, peripheral nerve lesions, or neuromuscular disorders. The information gained from electrodiagnostic studies complements the findings on imaging studies and may allow further delineation of symptomatic spondylotic changes and the severity of neurologic compromise from these lesions.

Nerve Conduction Studies

NCSs are used to evaluate the integrity of peripheral sensory and motor pathways. Sensory NCSs involve applying electrical stimulation over a sensory nerve or mixed nerve and recording of the evoked action potential at a standard distance away from the point of stimulation along the course of the nerve. The morphology, latency (time required to travel from the point of stimulation to the recording site), and amplitude of the sensory nerve action potential (SNAP) provides information regarding the function of that nerve. Motor conduction studies are performed in a similar fashion by electrically stimulating a mixed nerve and recording of the evoked compound muscle action potential (CMAP) from a muscle innervated by that nerve. Electrical stimulations at multiple points along the course of the nerve allow calculation of a nerve conduction velocity and identification of a focal entrapment syndrome. NCS of the pathologic nerve is compared with similar conduction studies performed on different nerves within the same extremity, the same nerve in the contralateral extremity, or to normative reference data. Sensory NCSs are not affected in radiculopathy because the site of nerve compromise is proximal to the dorsal root ganglion and stimulation of sensory nerve axons distal to the site of compression results in normal conductions.[43] However, radicular compromise with loss of peripheral motor nerve axons may produce a generalized decrease in the amplitude of the evoked CMAP.

Common sites of upper extremity peripheral entrapment neuropathies that may present with signs and symptoms similar to cervical radiculopathy include compromise to the median nerve in the proximal forearm as it passes through the pronator teres or distally at the carpal tunnel, compromise to the ulnar nerve at the elbow (cubital tunnel) or wrist (Guyon's canal), or compromise to the radial nerve in the proximal forearm as it passes through the supinator.[44] Slowing of the nerve conduction velocity or absolute delays in sensory or motor conduction latencies along the distal segments of multiple nerves may indicate a peripheral polyneuropathy. Peripheral polyneuropathy has many etiologies but may commonly occur secondary to diabetes mellitus, nutritional deficiencies, thyroid dysfunction, or toxic states and may present with pain, sensory disturbance, or weakness similar to cervical radiculopathy.

Although NCSs provide a unique opportunity to assess peripheral nerve function, commonly practiced NCS techniques only allow examination of nerves along their distal course where they are easily accessible to superficial stimulation and recording methods and do not allow evaluation of proximal nerve segments. F-wave analysis is an additional nerve conduction technique that may be performed to assess proximal nerve segments. Unfortunately, F-wave responses are relatively insensitive for detecting monoradicular compromise.

Electromyogram

EMG needle examination represents the single most useful electrodiagnostic technique for assessing radiculopathy. During the EMG examination, a very small specialized needle containing a recording electrode is inserted intramuscularly, and the electrical activity of the muscle is monitored during rest and active contraction. When completely at rest, the muscle should be electrically silent unless the needle is recording from the neuromuscular junction. Spontaneous electrical activity in the form of fibrillation potentials represents the pathologic depolarization of innervated single muscle fibers. The hallmark of active radiculopathy is the finding of spontaneous fibrillation potentials in a myotomal distribution (i.e., multiple muscles with the same root innervation but different peripheral nerve supply). Therefore, EMG examination requires one to survey a variety of muscles innervated by cervical segments above and below the suspected level of compromise and muscles of the same cervical segment innervated by different peripheral nerves. In this manner, one can isolate abnormal findings to a specific cervical root level and exclude peripheral nerve injury. Also, one examines the paraspinal muscles to assess for denervation in the distribution of the posterior rami. When abnormalities are noted in both the ventral and posterior rami distributions, the nerve lesions must be proximal to the level of their division from the nerve trunk, which occurs at the level of the neuroforamina. Assessment of the morphology and recruitment pattern of motor unit action potentials (MUAP) during active muscle contraction adds further diagnostic information. Acute radiculopathy that results in active denervation of peripheral muscle fibers or focal conduction block of motor nerve axons will result in reduced recruitment patterns of normal-appearing MUAPs. Chronic radiculopathy resulting in peripheral denervation and reinnervation from collateral sprouting of surviving axons will result in large-amplitude, polyphasic MUAPs and decreased recruitment patterns. MUAP evaluation also allows detection of myopathy-related MUAP changes. Myopathies may present with weakness and muscular atrophy similar to cervical radiculopathy or myelopathy.

EMG examination provides a simple, minimally invasive, diagnostic test for cervical radiculopathy. In the hands of an experienced electromyographer, EMG examination is very specific and has few false-positive studies. EMG examination may be falsely negative when the radicular compromise is not severe enough to cause axonal loss and peripheral denervation, when there is slow development of root compromise allowing distal reinnervation from collateral sprouting to keep pace with denervation resulting in subtle MUAP changes without findings of active denervation, or when compromise is isolated to the sensory axons.

Evoked Potentials

SEP testing allows evaluation of peripheral and central sensory conduction pathways and may be useful in the diagnosis of cervical radiculopathy or myelopathy.[45–48] After peripheral electrical stimulation of an accessible mixed nerve, segmental sensory nerve, or patch or skin representing a cervical dermatome, evoked potentials may be recorded over the brachial plexus, cervical spine, or scalp overlying the somatosensory cortex. Because of the small amplitude of the potential resulting from a single stimulus compared with background noise, several hundred stimulations are performed repetitively over several minutes and processed to obtain a summated waveform. The latency, amplitude, and morphology of the waveforms are analyzed to assess for focal or absolute conduction delays, loss of amplitude, or significant changes in waveform morphology.

SEPs offer the unique opportunity to assess sensory conduction over proximal peripheral nerve and central pathways and may complement the information gained from NCS and EMG examination. However, SEPs have many practical limitations. First, they require a relaxed patient and meticulous recording techniques to obtain clean, reproducible waveforms. Second, there is large side-to-side and interindividual variability in the waveform amplitudes. Thus, a 50 to 75 percent decrement in waveform amplitude is required to identify an abnormality reliably and discern this from normal variation.[43] Third, conduction delay across a cervical root segment may be small and masked by the normal variability in latency for the entire segment. Fourth, mixed nerve stimulations (median and ulnar), which are the most commonly performed, are carried through multiple root segments and are relatively insensitive to monoradicular compromise. Finally, dermatomal stimulations, which are believed to be most sensitive and specific for single root compromise, are technically demanding and time-consuming to perform and often fail to yield reproducible waveforms that are appropriate for analysis.

Diagnostic Cervical Injections

Identification or confirmation of suspected pain-producing cervical structures can be made by selective anesthetic blockade of the presumed pain-generating tissues. If pain is ablated by anesthetizing a given structure, then that structure is thought to be the source of the patient's pain. Precise diagnostic selective nerve root blocks and cervical facet blocks may be performed under fluoroscopic visualization by experienced physicians in an outpatient radiology setting.

Selective Nerve Root Injection

Selective nerve root blocks are performed by injection of a small amount of long-acting local anesthetic (1 ml of 0.5 percent bupivacaine) into the neuroforamina of a specific root (Fig. 12-4). Shortly after the injection, the patient is re-evaluated for any alteration in pain complaints. In this manner, one or multiple cervical nerve roots may be blocked to delineate the specific nerve root or combination of nerve roots mediating a given patient's pain complex. Selective nerve root injections are most helpful in cases in which there is multilevel radicular pathology or in cases in which radicular pain exists without any obvious source of radicular compromise. One must always consider the possibility of a placebo response in positive responders, and serial blocks may be required to confirm findings.

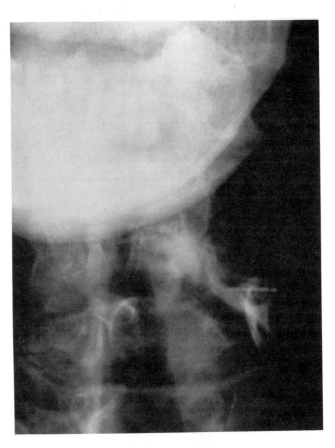

Fig. 12-4. Anteroposterior spot radiograph of the cervical spine showing contrast injection into the neuroforamina before nerve root injection.

Facet Joint Block

The C2–3 through C7–8 zygapophyseal joints may also be anesthetized either through intra-articular injection of local anesthetic (0.5 to 1.0 ml of 0.5 percent bupivacaine) or blockade of the innervation to the joint under investigation (Fig. 12-5). For the C3–4 through C7–8 facet joints, blockade of the medial branches of the posterior primary rami above and below the target joint prevents nocioceptive input from the joint from reaching the brain. For the C2–3 facet joint, blockade of the C3 medial branch and the third occipital nerve provide similar deafferentiation.[49] After facet blockade, subjective pain com-

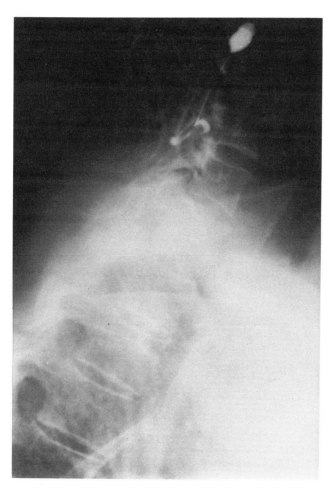

Fig. 12-5. Spot lateral radiograph showing contrast arthrogram of the cervical facet joint before diagnostic or therapeutic injection.

plaints as well as examination for facet tenderness or restricted joint motion are reassessed.

Cervical Discography

The cervical intervertebral disc may also be selectively evaluated as a potential source of neck, shoulder, or arm pain. Cervical discography aids in the identification of a symptomatic disc and in the proper selection of patients who will get successful pain relief with surgical discectomy.[50] Since its introduction in the 1950s, cervical discography has been a relatively controversial procedure but, in my opinion, remains a valuable tool in the evaluation of certain cervical pain syndromes. Cervical discography is indicated in patients with a chronic (greater than 6 months) neck pain unresponsive to comprehensive nonsurgical therapy in which imaging studies and other evaluation methods have been inconclusive in determining a specific source of the pain. Also, cervical discography may be used to restrict or confirm the diagnosis when imaging studies indicate multiple degenerative and potentially painful discs. Cervical discography should be thought of as a presurgical staging tool and should not be performed in an individual who is not thought to be an appropriate operative candidate.

Cervical discography is performed by fluoroscopic-guided placement of a 22-gauge spinal needle into the geometric center of the disc or discs under investigation through the anterolateral approach described by Cloward.[13] After appropriate needle placement, the disc is injected with a small quantity of normal saline, and the pain response of the lightly sedated patient is evaluated for intensity, quality, and location. The response is then graded as being similar or dissimilar to the patient's usual pain complex. Finally, the disc is also injected with a small quantity of nonionic contrast and the internal architecture visualized (Fig. 12-6). Disc levels displaying abnormal internal architecture may also be studied with postdiscography thin-slice CT scans. Great care must be taken when interpreting the pain response to avoid false-positive studies. In our practice, we have found that most all cervical discs examined exhibit some degree of degenerative nuclear morphology and may produce a mild-to-moderate pain response. Therefore, to satisfy the criteria for a positive discogram and to avoid false-positive studies, provocative disc injection must reveal a disc with a significant morphologic derangement and produce moderate-to-severe pain that is familiar both in quality and location to the patient's usual pain complex. When these criteria are satisfied, patients with isolated one- or two-level disc derangements are thought to be good candidates for pain relief with cervical discectomy and anterior interbody fusion.

Although properly performed discography has been shown not to harm the disc,[51] cervical discography has many potential complications. Disc space infection, nerve damage, spinal cord injury, vertebral or carotid artery injury, and laryngeal nerve injury may all occur. However, the potential for these

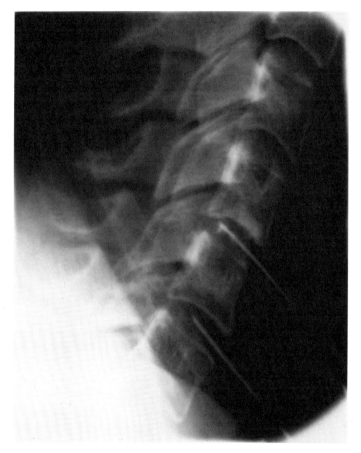

Fig. 12-6.   Spot lateral radiograph demonstrating needle placement before provocative injection of the cervical disc.

complications may be greatly minimized or avoided by meticulous technique and use of perioperative antibiotics.

TREATMENT

Treatment for painful cervical spinal disorders is divided into a pain control phase and a functional restoration phase. Pain control uses medications, physical therapy modalities, manual techniques, and selective spinal injections to provide analgesia, reduce stiffness, and restore normal range of motion (ROM). The patient is then progressed to a program of functional restoration in which strength and flexibility deficits of cervical and upper back musculature are corrected through a program of cervical stabilization exercises.[52] Finally, education and training in optimal cervical biomechanics are taught to allow the patient to prevent or minimize future painful insults to the cervical spine.

Medications

Medications are used in combination with analgesic physical therapy modalities to provide pain control and to reduce inflammation associated with the spinal pathology. Also, medications are used to treat secondary symptoms such as muscle spasm, anxiety, depression, or insomnia that may impede the rehabilitation process.[53] The use of medications for the treatment of TMD and related cervical spinal disorders is discussed further in Chapter 13.

Physical Therapy

Physical therapy reduces pain and facilitates the recovery of normal cervical spine strength, flexibility, posture, and biomechanics. Physical therapy has been found to be most efficacious for our patients when symptoms are due to moderate spondylotic disease or nondegenerative dysfunction of cervical spinal structures. During the pain control phase, therapeutic modalities including hot packs, ice packs, ultrasound, and electrical stimulation are used to alter local blood flow, reduce inflammation, reduce reactive muscle spasm, and provide temporary analgesia.[54] Manual physical therapy techniques include soft tissue mobilization, soft tissue release, and facet and segmental mobilization. These techniques may facilitate removal of local metabolites and remodeling of local connective tissue and may improve segmental motion.[33] Pathologic segments or facet joints may be targeted for more focused therapy. In concert with analgesic therapies, patients are begun on a program of gentle cervical ROM and stretching exercises that are performed in the gym under therapist supervision and then at home on a daily basis. Emphasis is placed on stretching the paraspinal, scalene, levator scapulae, upper trapezius, and pectoralis muscle groups where most individuals suffer from intrinsic or posture-related tightness.

Those individuals with radicular symptoms may also benefit from treatment with cervical traction to provide temporary relief of cervical root compression. If beneficial, patients may be educated in use of a home cervical traction unit. Traction applied by a head halter that pulls under the chin should be avoided in those individuals with concomitant TMD, as this will cause increased compression of the TMJ. Also, patients with cervical instability or spondylotic myelopathy should not undergo mobilization therapies or cervical traction as they may experience worsening of symptoms or risk further neurologic compromise. Therapists that suspect significant spondylotic disease or segmental instability and feel uncomfortable performing mobilization techniques in a patient who has not been evaluated with plain radiographs should alert the referring physician to these concerns so that appropriate radiographs can be obtained or the treatment program altered.

As local and referred pain symptoms are brought under control and cervical motion and biomechanics are improved, the patient is progressed to a program of cervical stabilization exercises. Stabilization exercises are designed to strengthen the supporting cervical, scapular, chest, upper back, and arm musculature and emphasize maintenance of the cervical spine in a neutral position. Neutral cervical posture minimizes forces transmitted across cervical spine segments. By using cervical stabilization techniques throughout all aspects of daily living, an individual may control pain from underlying spondylotic disease or postural overuse of cervical structures and prevent future insults to the cervical spine. Stabilization exercise programs begin with very simple isometric exercises and progress under therapist supervision to incorporate progressive resistance exercises.[52] Additional programs such as McKenzie extension exercises may also be incorporated. Finally, the patient is instructed to continue the exercise program at home or on exercise equipment found in most commercial health clubs.

Monitoring the patient's response to physical therapy provides the physician with important feedback that helps to refine the working diagnosis. As diffuse pain complaints subside, the patient or therapist may be able to localize the pain or dysfunction to a particular segment or facet joint and help target the physician to areas where focal therapeutic interventions such as facet joint injection or selective nerve root blocks may be helpful. Pain that is exacerbated by mobilization suggests segmental instability or underlying internal disc derangement and should prompt the therapist and physician to review the diagnosis and treatment plan.

Therapeutic Spinal Injections

Cervicogenic pain secondary to inflammation of the cervical dura, nerve roots, or facets joints may be relieved or reduced by localized injection of corticosteroid.

Cervical Epidural Steroid Injection

Cervical epidural steroid injection (CESI) may reduce pain and radicular symptoms caused by inflammation of epidural structures or cervical nerve roots. CESI may be performed in an outpatient setting under fluoroscopic guidance. Contrast injection before steroid injection ensures that the corticosteroid is injected into the epidural space and avoids extradural or intravascular injection. However, experienced individuals may elect to perform the procedure without fluoroscopic guidance ("blind injection"). Most investigators report good or excellent long-term results with relief of pain or neurologic symptoms in approximately 40 to 60 percent of patients after injection of 80 mg methylprednisolone (Depo-Medrol).[55-58] In our practice, we routinely inject 18 mg betamethasone (Celestone Soluspan) through the C7–T1 interlaminar space and note best results in patients with acute or subacute (less than 6 months) radicular symptoms. Patients with long-standing symptoms (greater than 1 year), severe bony compromise of radicular structures, or predominantly axial neck pain do not achieve as much relief with CESI. Common side effects from CESI include hiccups, facial flushing, or transient fluid retention. Diabetic or hypertensive individuals may require a reduction in the corticosteroid dose and close monitoring of blood glucose or blood pressure in the early postinjection period. Complications from CESI may include subarachnoid injection, spinal headache, epidural hematoma or abscess, injury to the spinal cord, or nerve damage. Such complications are rare when the CESI is performed by an experienced physician. Repeat injections are only performed on those individuals who experience partial relief of symptoms or when symptoms recur. A poor response to fluoroscopic-guided CESI does not warrant a repeat injection, and routine prescription of a series of injections is discouraged.

Selective Nerve Root Cortisone Injection

Monoradicular compromise that has not responded to CESI may also be treated by selective nerve root injection. In some cases, radicular inflammation and nerve root edema within the neuroforamina, or postoperative changes consisting of epidural scarring or adhesions, may prevent adequate spread of the epidural injectant to the affected nerve root. In these cases, the nerve root may be approached by fluoroscopic-guided injection of corticosteroid into the neuroforamina of the appropriate spinal segment. Contrast injection allows one to confirm spread of the medication along the course of the nerve root. In our practice, 6 to 12 mg Celestone Soluspan is injected during a therapeutic selective nerve root injection and often is combined with 1 ml of 0.5 percent bupivacaine to provide a diagnostic root block. Potential complications include respiratory arrest secondary to epidural or intrasvascular injection with local anesthetic or radicular injury.

Facet Joint Cortisone Injection

Painful inflammatory involvement of the cervical zygapophyseal joints may be treated with intra-articular injection of corticosteroid. Under fluoroscope guidance, the C2–3, through the C6–7 facet joints may be easily entered via a lateral or posterior approach with a 22-gauge spinal needle and the joint infiltrated with a small amount of corticosteroid mixed with either local anesthetic or normal saline.[49,59-61] Intra-articular needle placement is always confirmed by contrast injection. Complications may include respiratory arrest, vertebral artery puncture, intravascular injection, nerve root injury, or epidural injection.

Medial Branch Rhizotomy (Facet Joint Nerve Ablation)

Cervical facet joints with painful, noninflammatory derangements, or facet joints with painful inflammatory lesions unresponsive to intra-articular steroid injections, may be treated by denervation of the appropriate nerve supply. Percutaneous radio frequency denervation of the cervical medial branches is a technically simple outpatient procedure that has been demonstrated to provide successful long-lasting relief of intractable neck pain and occipital headaches of facet origin in approximately 40 to 60 percent of appropriate candidates.[62,63] Selection of facet joints for denervation is made by serial trials of diagnostic reversible medial branch blocks with local anesthetic. Such trials allow proper selection of patients, accurate identification of symptomatic joints, and identification of placebo responders. Also, many patients in our practice receiving diagnostic medial branch blocks report long-lasting pain relief and do not require permanent medial branch nerve ablation. Nerve ablation is achieved by placement of a probe near the target nerve and selective heating of the nerve with a lesion generator (Radionics) until nerve necrosis occurs.[62-64] Probe insertion and placement are performed by the posterior approach described by Bogduk et al.[64] A test stimulation is usually performed before the actual lesion generation to exclude needle placement near the proximal nerve root. Patients with return of their pain after a successful pain-free interval may undergo repeat lesioning. Denervation of the C2–3 facet joint is made by creating lesions in the third occipital nerve as it passes along the lateral margin of the joint and the C3 medial branch as it passes along the waist of the C3 articular pillar. Denervation of the C3–4 through C6–7 joints is performed by lesioning the medial branch above and below the target joint.

Surgery

In cases in which cervical spondylotic disease causes disabling pain or neurologic compromise unresponsive to conservative care, surgical intervention may be necessary. Absolute indications for surgical intervention include moderate-to-severe neurologic compromise or rapidly progressive neurologic compromise. Relative indications include mild stable neurologic compromise or disabling pain originating from a degenerative cervical structure that is amenable to correction with surgical intervention. The goals of surgery may include stabilization or improvement of neurologic deficits or the relief of intractable pain. Unfortunately, there are many types of surgical procedures in practice to treat cervical spondylotic disease, and determining the most optimal surgical approach may be controversial and depends on regional medical opinion and surgeon training or bias. In general, surgical intervention for spondylotic disease can be classified into anterior and posterior procedures. In theory, the approach should be selected based on the pathology. Compression of the cervical nerve roots or spinal cord from posterolateral vertebral osteophytes or posterior vertebral bony bar formation is best treated through an anterior surgical approach, which provides better access for removal of these elements. However, posterior spinal cord compression from a hypertrophic invaginated ligamentum flavum or congenital spinal stenosis from developmental shortening of the pedicles or laminae with a decrease in the midsagittal canal diameter might best be approached from a posterior direction, allowing canal expansion through resection or modification of the ligamentum flavum and lamina.[65] Regardless of the type of procedure performed, most investigators report good or excellent surgical outcomes for spondylotic radiculopathy or myelopathy in approximately 70 to 80 percent of appropriately selected cases.[66–68] However, one must view these results in the light of the fact that in most series the success or failure of the surgical outcome is determined by the surgeon performing the procedure and not by an independent observer. Poorer operative results for CSM are uniformly seen in patients with advanced age, extended symptom duration, multilevel compression, spinal cord atrophy on preoperative imaging studies, and coexisting diabetes mellitus.

Anterior surgical procedures routinely performed for the treatment of spondylotic radiculopathy or myelopathy include anterior cervical discectomy and interbody fusion (ACDF), anterior discectomy without fusion, and anterior vertebrectomy with strut graft fusion. ACDF is believed by most surgeons to be the procedure of choice for spondylotic radiculopathy as it allows excellent exposure to decompress the neuroforamina from posterolateral disc protrusion or bony osteophytes from the joints of Luschka. ACDF is also commonly used to treat one- or two-level spondylotic myelopathy but is believed to be relatively unsatisfactory for treatment of spondylotic myelopathy spanning three or more segments.[66] Complications after ACDF may include injury to the recurrent laryngeal or hypoglossal nerves causing hoarseness or dysphagia; bone graft subluxation or extrusion; hematoma formation at the iliac crest donor graft site; persistent pain or paresthesia at the graft donor site from perioperative injury to the lateral femoral cutaneous nerve (LFCN) or delayed entrapment of the LFCN in postoperative scar formation; and acceleration of spondylotic disease at the adjacent spinal segments above and below the cervical fusion mass. Pseudoarthrosis is also considered a postoperative complication but does not appear to be related to unsuccessful outcome. A final advantage to the use of ACDF is that it may allow subsequent posterior decompression if necessary without the concern for the development of segmental instability.

Anterior discectomy without interbody fusion may also be performed for spondylotic radiculopathy, and the limited data available suggest that results are equivalent to ACDF; however, most investigators do not advocate its use as it does not provide for neuroforaminal distraction and segmental stabilization believed to be necessary for the successful long-term treatment of spondylotic radicular compromise.[66] Anterior discectomy without fusion may be appropriate for individuals with radicular compromise secondary to isolated soft disc protrusion in the absence of spondylotic disease.

Anterior cervical vertebrectomy and strut graft fusion have been advocated for decompression of multilevel spondylotic myelopathy. Autologous iliac crest or fibular bone is used to construct the fusion strut. Complications are similar to those with ACDF, but perioperative morbidity is higher secondary to the greater extent of the operative dissection necessary to gain the appropriate surgical exposure required to perform the procedure.

Posterior decompressive procedures have long been performed for the treatment of cervical spondylotic disease. Posterior laminectomy or laminoplasty is currently advocated for the decompression of multilevel spondylotic myelopathy or spondylotic myelopathy complicated by congenital canal stenosis. Posterior decompression avoids many of the complications seen with ACDF. However, extensive multilevel laminectomies may lead to postoperative kyphotic spinal deformity or segmental instability, further predisposing the cervical spinal cord to compromise from compression over posterior vertebral osteophytes. Furthermore, posterior decompression requires more surgical manipulation of the spinal cord and results in a higher rate of postoperative neurologic injury than anterior procedures. The problem of postoperative deformity or instability may be avoided by performing a laminoplasty in which the laminae are sectioned in the midline or at the lateral margin and the posterior elements "hinged" open.[66] Fusion of the posterior elements in the open-hinged position allows expansion of the cervical spinal canal volume while maintaining intrinsic stability and preventing subsequent deformity.

CONCLUSION

A working knowledge of cervical spinal disorders is necessary to accurately evaluate the patient with head or neck pain in which the differential diagnosis includes cervical spinal disorders in addition to TMD. In such individuals a comprehensive evaluation using historical data, physical examination, imaging and electrodiagnostic studies, and selective spinal injections will allow the practitioner to fully evaluate the extent of symptomatic cervical spinal pathology and to implement appropriate physical, medical, or surgical therapy.

REFERENCES

1. Kraus SL: Cervical Spine influences on the craniomandibular region. In Kraus SL (ed): TMJ Disorders Management of the Craniomandibular Complex. Churchill Livingston, New York, 1988
2. Andersson GB: The epidemiology of spinal disorders. p. 107. In Frymoyer JW (ed): The Adult Spine: Principles and Practice. Vol. 1. Raven Press, New York, 19■■

3. Holmstrom EB, Lindell J, Moritz U: Low back and neck/shoulder pain in construction workers: occupational workload and psychosocial risk factors. Spine 17: 672, 1992

4. Lestini WF, Wiesel SW: The pathogenesis of cervical spondylosis. Clin Orthop 239:69, 1989

5. Parke WW: Correlative anatomy of cervical spondylotic myelopathy. Spine 13:831, 1988

6. Kondo K, Molgaard C, Kurland L, Onofrio B: Protruded intervertebral cervical disc. Minn Med 64:751, 1981

7. Friedenberg ZB, Miller WT: Degenerative disc disesae of the cervical spine. J Bone Joint Surg 45(A):1171, 1963

8. Kelsey JL, Githens PB, Walter SD et al: An epidemiology study of acute prolapsed cervical intervertebral disc. J Bone Joint Surg 66(A):907, 1984

9. Rydevik B, Brown MD, Lundborg G: Pathoanatomy and pathophysiology of nerve root compression. Spine 9:7, 1984

10. Saal JS, Franson RC, Dobrow R et al: High levels of inflammatory phospholipase A_2 activity in lumbar disc herniations. Spine 15:674, 1990

11. Boden SD, Wiesel SW, Laws ER, Rothman RH: Clinical syndromes and physical examination of the cervical spine. p. 41. In: The Aging Spine: The Essentials of Pathophysiology, Diagnosis, and Treatment. WB Saunders, Philadelphia, 1991

12. Crock HV: A reappraisal of intervertebral disc lesions. Med J Aust 1:983, 1970

13. Cloward RB: Cervical discography: a contribution to the etiology and mechanism of neck, shoulder, and arm pain. Ann Surg 150:1052, 1959

14. Clark CR: Cervical spondylotic myelopathy: history and physical findings. Spine 13:847, 1988

15. Bohlman HH, Emery SE: The pathophysiology of cervical spondylosis and myelopathy. Spine 13:844, 1988

16. Panjabi M, White A: Biomechanics of nonacute cervical spinal cord trauma. Spine 13:838, 1988

17. Lees F, Turner JW: Natural history and prognosis of the spinal cord disorder associated with cervical spondylosis. Br Med J 2:1607, 1063

18. Weinshel SS, Maiman DJ, Mueller WM: Dysphagia associated with cervical spine disorders: pathologic relationship? J Spinal Disord 1:312, 1989

19. Bogduk N, Windsor M, Inglis A: The innervation of the cervical intervertebral discs. Spine 13:2, 1988

20. Bogduk N: The clinical anatomy of the cervical dorsal rami. Spine 7:319, 1982

21. Travell JG, Simmons DG: Myofascial Pain and Dysfunction. The Trigger Point Manual. Williams & Wilkins, Baltimore, 1983

22. April C, Bogduk N: The prevalence of cervical zygapophyseal joint pain: a first approximation. Spine 17:744, 1992

23. Dwyer A, Aprill C, Bogduk N: Cervical zygapophyseal joint pain patterns I: a study in normal volunteers. Spine 15:453, 1990

24. Aprill C, Dwyer A, Bogduk N: Cervical zygapophyseal joint pain patterns II: a clinical evaluation. Spine 15:458, 1990

25. Bogduk N: Neck pain: an update. Aust Fam Physician 17:75, 1988

26. Bogduk N: The anatomical basis for cervicogenic headache. J Mainpulative Physiol Ther 15:67, 1992

27. Bogduk N, Marsland: On the concept of third occipital headache. J Neurol Neurosurg Psychiatry 49:775, 1986

28. Sucher BM: Thoracic outlet syndrome—a myofascial variant: part I. Pathology and diagnosis. JOAO 90:686, 1990

29. Magee DJ: Cervical spine. p. 21. In: Orthopedic Physical Assessment. WB Saunders, Philadelphia, 1987
30. Tindall B: Aids to the Examination of the Peripheral Nervous System. WB Saunders, London, 1986
31. Bourdillon JF, Day EA: Detailed examination: the spine. p. 73. In: Spinal Manipulation. 4th Ed. Appleton & Lange, Norwalk, Connecticut, 1988
32. Greenman PE: Principles of Manual Medicine. Williams & Wilkins, Baltimore, 1989
33. Cantu RI, Grodin AJ: Myofascial Manipulation: Theory and Clinical Application. Aspen, Gaithersburg, Maryland, 1992
34. Liang MH, Katz JN, Frymoyer JW: Plain radiographs in evaluating the spine. p. 289. In Frymoyer JW (ed): The Adult Spine. Raven Press, New York, 1991
35. Kramer J, Rivera CA, Kleefield J: Degenerative disorders of the cervical spine. Rheum Dis Clin North Am 17:741, 1991
36. Penning L: Roengenographic evaluation: obtaining and interpreting plain films in cervical spine injury. p. 106. In Sherk HH, Dunn EJ, Eismont FJ et al (eds): The Cervical Spine: The Cervical Spine Research Committee. 2nd Ed. JB Lippincott, Cambridge, Massachusetts, 1989
37. Russell EJ: Cervical disc disease. Radiology 177:313, 1990
38. Robertson HJ, Smith RD: Cervical myelography: survey of modes of practice and major complications. Radiology 174:79, 1990
39. Modic MT, Ross JS, Masaryk TJ: Imaging of degenerative disease of the cervical spine. Clin Orthop 239:109, 1989
40. Jahnke RW, Hart BL: Cervical stenosis, spondylosis, and herniated disc disease. Radiol Clin North Am 29:777, 1991
41. Herzog RJ: Selection of imaging studies for disorders of the lumbar spine. p. 7. In Herring SA (ed): Physical Medicine and Rehabilitation Clinics of North America: Low Back Pain. Vol. 2. WB Saunders, Philadelphia, 1991
42. Ono K, Okada K, Nakashima H, Yamashita K: Roengenographic evaluation: scintigraphy and selective angiography. In Sherk HH, Dunn EJ, Eismont FJ et al. (eds): The Cervical Spine: The Cervical Spine Research Committee. 2nd Ed. JB Lippincott, Cambridge, Massachusetts, 1989
43. Wilbourn AJ, Aminoff MJ: AAEE minimonograph #32: the electrophysiologic examination in patients with radiculopathies. Muscle Nerve 11:1099, 1988
44. Kimura J: Mononeuropathies and entrapment syndromes. p. 495. In: Electrodiagnosis in Diseases of Nerve and Muscle: Principles and Practice. 2nd Ed. FA Davis, Philadelphia, 1989
45. Khan MR, McInnes A, Hughes SP: Electrophysiologic studies in cervical spondylosis. J Spinal Disord 2:163, 1989
46. Heiskari M, Sivola J, Heikkinen ER: Somatosensory evoked potentials in evaluation of decompressive surgery of cervical spondylosis and herniated disc. Ann Clin Res 18:107, 1986
47. Sivola J, Sulg I, Heiskari M: Somatosensory evoked potentials in diagnosis of cervical spondylosis and herniated disc. Electroencephalogr Clin Neurophysiol 52:276, 1981
48. Eisen A, Hoirch M, Moll A: Evaluation of radiculopathies by segmental stimulation and somatosensory evoked potentials. Can J Neurol Sci 10:178, 1983
49. Bogduk N: Back pain: zygapophyseal blocks and epidural steroids. p. 935. In Cousins MJ, Bridenbaugh PO (eds): Neural Blockade In Clinical Anesthesia and Management of Pain. 2nd Ed. JB Lippincott, Philadelphia, 1988
50. Cloward RB: The anterior approach for removal of ruptured cervical discs. J Neurosurg 15:602, 1958

51. Johnson RG: Does discography injure normal discs? Spine 14:424, 1989
52. Sweeney T, Prentice C, Saal J et al: Cervicothoracic muscular stabilization techniques. p. 335. In Saal JA (ed): Physical Medicine State of the Art Reviews: Neck and Back Pain. Vol. 4. Hanley and Belfus, Philadelphia, 1990
53. Robinson JP, Brown PB: Medications in low back pain. p. 97. In Herring (ed): Physical Medicine and Rehabilitation Clinics of North America: Low Back Pain. Vol. 2. WB Saunders, Philadelphia, 1991
54. Basford JR: Physical agents and biofeedback. p. 257. In Delisa JA (ed): Rehabilitation Medicine. JB Lippincott, Philadeplhia, 1988
55. Rowlingson JC, Kirschenbaum LP: Epidural analgesis techniques in the management of cervical pain. Anesth Anal 65:938, 1986
56. Mangar D, Thomas PT: Epidural steroid injections in the treatment of cervical and lumbar pain syndromes. Reg Anesth 16:246, 1991
57. Cicala RS, Thoni K, Angel JJ: Long-term results of cervical epidural steroid injections. Clin J Pain 5:143, 1989
58. Warfield CA, Biber MP, Crews DA, Dwarakanath GK: Epidural steroid injection as a treatment for cervical radiculitis. Clin J Pain 4:201, 1988
59. Dory MA: Arthrography of the cervical facet joints. Radiology 148:379, 1983
60. Hove B, Gyldensted C: Cervical analgesic facet joint arthrography. Neuroradiology 32:456, 1990
61. Wedel DJ, Wilson PR: Cervical facet arthrography. Reg Anesth 16:246, 1991
62. Schaerer JP: Radiofrequency facet rhizotomy in the treatment of chronic neck and low back pain. Int Surg 63:53, 1978
63. Hildebrandt J, Argyrakis A: Percutaneous nerve block of the cervical facet—a relatively new method in the treatment of chronic headache and neck pain: pathological-anatomical studies and clinical practice. Man Med 2:48, 1986
64. Bogduk N, Macintosh J, Marsland A: Technical limitations to the efficacy of radiofrequency neurotomy for spinal pain. Neurosurgery 20:529, 1987
65. White AA, Panjabi MM: Biomechanical considerations in the surgical management of cervical spondylotic myelopathy. Spine 13:856, 1988
66. Herkowitz HN: The surgical management of cervical spondylotic radiculopathy and myelopathy. Clin Orthop 239:94, 1989
67. Saunders RL: Anterior reconstructive procedures in cervical spondylotic myelopathy. Clin Neurosurg 37:682, 1991
68. Whitecloud TS: Anterior surgery for cervical spondylotic myelopathy: Smith-Robinson, Cloward, and vertebrectomy. Spine 13:861, 1988

13 | Psychological and Medical Management of Myofascial Pain

J. David Haddox

The management of pain of TMJ-related disorders is not conceptually different from the management of most chronic nonmalignant pain syndromes. Comprehensive management requires understanding of the biopsychosocial model of illness, as a purely medical-surgical model often proves inadequate to conceptualize and treat these patients. The acceptance of and willingness to work in this model often require paradigm shifts that are substantial and foreign to the general dental, medical, physical therapy, or occupational therapy practitioner. The resistance to this model stems primarily from the insecurity of the practitioner, especially in the realm of the psychosocial aspects of the patient's presentation. To accept this approach, one must enter into areas that are considered "soft" science by many health care providers because of a perceived lack of "objective" evidence of pathology in the psychosocial aspects of a patient's life. Despite this common reluctance, to fully comprehend and therefore manage these disorders, one must begin to look at the person as a complex entity, not simply as a limited range of mandibular motion. Much time and money are often spent trying to elucidate a definite and sole organic cause for a person's complaints, when the problem is just not that easily reducible to a finite, simplistic dysfunction of a joint.

I believe that most patients who are referred to a multidisciplinary pain center with the label "TMJ syndrome" are suffering from myofascial pain involving the primary and accessory muscles of mastication and, in fact, have little, if any, specific joint pathology that can account for their pain. As such, these individuals are all suffering from a *psychosomatic disorder* in the purest sense, that is, a disorder in which a somatic dysfunction (muscle tone, muscle-generated pain) is influenced (enhanced, diminished) by psychological factors that may or may not be derived from the somatic dysfunction. In other words, pre-existing psychological issues may predispose to the development of myofascial pain and may influence how it is perceived by the patient, whereas the presence of myofascial pain, which may occur independently of any psychological stressors, may precipitate the onset of psychological changes in the individual that may, in turn, influence muscle function and the perception of or reaction to nociception derived from the muscles. As used here, the term *psychosomatic* is not meant to imply the representation of intrapsychic conflict as bodily symptoms, which is the classic psychoanalytic definition.

This chapter starts with a brief review of the basics of neurophysiology, progresses into a more "holistic" view of the pain patient, and then discusses some specific interventions and clinical dilemmas. It is hoped by this author that readers will weigh each section of this work equally, for only by doing so will one begin to grasp the complexity of caring for patients who suffer with chronic pain syndromes.

NEUROPHYSIOLOGY OF NOCICEPTION

Understanding the patient suffering from pain begins with a review of what is currently known about the afferent nociceptive system in normal and diseased functioning. This section, despite its title, does not really focus on pain, for that is a very complex concept. Rather, this section strives to explain some salient features of how nociceptive information may be generated, transmitted, and modified to influence the nociceptive substrate on which a painful experience may be based. Although much of this information has shed some light on the management of painful conditions, one must resist the temptation to substantially alter clinical practice or make inappropriate inferences on the basis of this simplistic review.

Four basic processes occur with every painful event. The first is *transduction,* which is the manner in which peripheral stimuli lead to appropriate activity in the primary nociceptive afferent neuron. After the stimulus is transduced, *transmission* occurs along neural pathways from the periphery to the central nervous system (CNS), through a series of relay stations in the CNS and to the thalamocortical connections. *Modulation* can occur anytime after transduction and refers to the influencing of neural traffic to alter its meaning. The final step is *perception* by which the activity in the nervous system produces a subjective awareness of events. This, not surprisingly, is the least well understood of this sequence of events but is dealt with in a later section.

Peripheral Nervous System

The cutaneous nerves are of several types. These can be categorized by fiber diameter or by conduction velocity. Because the anatomic and physiologic properties are interdependent, most individuals refer to the fibers by conduction velocity. There are three major groups by this labeling system: *A fibers,* with conduction velocities in the 12 to 120-m/s range; *B fibers,* conducting in the 3- to 15-m/s range; and *C fibers,* which conduct in the 0.5- to 2-m/s range. Within the first category, subgroupings are A-α, A-β, A-γ, and A-δ, in decreasing order of size and conduction velocity. More information is known about cutaneous afferents than afferents in other tissues, so much of what follows necessarily applies to skin innervation unless otherwise specified.

Nociceptors can be characterized further by their propensity to carry certain types of traffic. The overwhelming majority of A-fiber nociceptors are lightly myelinated A-delta fibers that conduct impulses, on average, at a rate of 15 m/s. These fibers have receptive fields that consist of a cluster of spots, each about 1 mm in diameter, with each fiber covering a total area of about 5 mm². A-fiber nociceptors typically are divided into A-mechanoheat receptors (AMH) and high-threshold mechanoreceptors (HTM). The AMH fibers respond to both noxious heat and noxious mechanical stimulation. The HTMs, as their name implies, respond initially only to noxious mechanical stimuli and not to heat or algesic chemical substances. Both of these fiber types exhibit a phenomenon called *sensitization.* This means that, with repetitive exposure to noxious stimuli, the action potential threshold lowers (i.e., less stimulus energy is required to generate impulses or more impulses are generated from the same stimulus energy). Another interesting phenomenon occurs in regards to the HTM. Although this fiber does not normally respond to noxious heat, repetitive exposure to heat in a noxious range causes this fiber to respond to this mode of stimulation. Interestingly, the HTM's threshold to noxious mechanical stimulation does not change in this experimental paradigm, so the sensitization of this fiber is stimulus modality-specific. Many chemical compounds such as substance P, prostaglandins, histamine, and bradykinin are released from damaged cells or synthesized in an area of injury after tissue trauma and may directly activate or sensitize primary afferents, especially C fibers.

A common clinical example of thermal sensitization is sunburn. While feeling the temperature of a shower with your hand, you adjust the water to a comfortably warm level. When you put your sunburned shoulders under the shower head, however, it feels quite hot, perhaps even painfully hot. Your HTMs, which before thermal sensitization would ignore the warm water, now respond to it as if it were of noxious intensity. This process has significance in the propagation of discharges from injured sites.

Most nerve fibers in the periphery are afferents. Most of these are unmyelinated C fibers. These fibers conduct impulses with a mean conduction velocity of 1 m/s. In practical terms, this means an impulse arising in your great toe takes 1 full second to reach the dorsal horn of your lumbar spinal cord. The bulk of the C fibers are referred to as *C-polymodal nociceptors* (C-PMN), because they respond to a wide variety of noxious stimuli, such as chemical mediators of inflammation, noxious heat, and noxious mechanical stimulation. Their receptive fields are smaller than A fibers and are found in a single area, instead of clusters. C-PMNs are also capable of being sensitized. Excellent research has been performed that correlates the rate of firing of C-PMNs with subjective rating of pain intensity to thermal stimuli.

It is believed that both C-PMNs and A-delta fibers are operant in a noxious event. Empirical evidence, such as a painful stimulus giving rise to two distinct sensations, is part of the basis of this assumption. When a noxious stimulus is applied to an extremity, subjects will often report two distinctly different sensations. The first is almost immediate and is the sharp, well-localized pain. There follows, *after a perceptible pause,* the agonizing, diffuse, often deep and/or burning pain. The first pain is mediated by A-delta fibers and is instantaneous because of their rapid conduction velocity. The second pain is mediated by C fibers and is slower in onset because of their 1-m/s conduction time. The difference in conduction times accounts for the pause between the two sensations.

Further evidence of this thesis can be generated by selective blocking of each fiber type. It is accepted that, in many instances, a dilute local anesthetic solution can somewhat selectively block C fibers. If this is done, one will experience only the initial aspect of a painful experience. A fibers, because of their dependence on vasa nervorum, are much more susceptible to ischemic blockade. If a tourniquet is placed on an extremity for approximately 20 minutes before the onset of a noxious stimulus, then the initial, sharp, well-localized component is not appreciated, but the slow diffuse pain is felt, sometimes in excess of before the tourniquet placement.

A-beta fibers are large and heavily myelinated, conduct impules very rapidly (50 m/s mean), and subserve sensations of touch, pressure, and vibration. In the normal setting, they do not conduct noxious traffic. As is discussed below, they may have an important role in modulation of nociceptive information.

Central Nervous System

As primary afferents travel up the dorsal root, they begin to arrange themselves in a topographic order, with the smaller-diameter afferents congregating on the ventrolateral aspect of the root and entering Lissauer's tract at the dorsolateral edge of the dorsal horn and the large-diameter afferents entering the dorsal columns. The dorsal horn is segregated into Rexed's laminae, with lamina I being most superficial, hence the name *marginal layer.* Lamina II often has a clear gelatinous appearance and is called the *substantia gelatinosa.* Primary afferents tend to terminate on the cells of laminae I and V (A fibers) and lamina II (C fibers).

Several second order neurons in the cord have been characterized. The first of these are the nociceptive-specific (NS) cells of lamina I. These cells receive input from many primary afferents and, therefore, have receptive fields that are much larger than a single primary afferent. They are considered to be high-threshold in that they only respond to noxious stimuli.

A second type of neuron is called the *wide dynamic range neuron* (WDR). These neurons receive input from a variety of primary afferents, including nonnoxious stimuli. Depending on stimulus parameters, these cells are capable of responding in a dynamic manner to a wide variety of stimuli, generally with higher firing rates in response to more intense stimuli.

A third type of cell, called *complex* (CX) by some authors, resides in the deeper laminae and is characterized by complex receptive fields, often including disparate parts of the body and cutaneous as well as deep visceral inputs. Convergence of afferent input is maximal with these cells.

The dorsal horn is a site of modulation of afferent impulses. Via descending opioid-monoamine pathways, afferent impulse transmission may be inhibited by presynaptic interference with the release of substance P, a nociceptive neurotransmitter or by postsynaptic hyperpolarization of second-order nociceptive cells. Large-diameter non-noxious afferent input, such as that carried by A-beta fibers, may also decrease the likelihood of C-fiber traffic being faithfully communicated. This is cited as one of the bases for transcutaneous electrical nerve stimulation (TENS) when used with conventional settings and would logically occur to a degree with massage. Whether other manual therapies specifically activate these fibers is not known.

The dorsal horn is also probably the primary site of the phenomenon of referred pain, which is observed commonly with myofascial pain syndromes. Referred pain describes a perception of pain in one location when, in fact, the nociceptive focus is in another place. Perhaps the most commonly known example of this is arm or jaw pain during a myocardial infarction. In this instance, electrocardiograph (ECG) and muscle enzyme analysis clearly indicate that the pathology is in the myocardium, but often most of or all the pain is perceived as coming from (referred to) the arm. Examination of the arm is not likely to reveal anything significant, although pectoralis muscle trigger points have been described in association with cardiac events.

Some of the central cells are capable of a form of sensitization referred to as *wind-up*. With repetitive stimulation in the noxious range, WDR neurons can undergo plastic changes that enhance their responsiveness to stimuli. Their apparent receptive field can also enlarge considerably, sometimes encompassing an entire extremity, even crossing the midline! This wind-up is at least in part mediated by excitatory amine neurotransmitters, such as glutamate, acting on the NMDA receptor, because NMDA receptor antagonists, such as MK801, can block this phenomenon in laboratory experiments.

Nociceptive impulses reach higher centers primarily via the anterolateral quadrant of the spinal cord. There are many targets, but the main destination appears to be the thalamus. The input to the thalamus shows a somatotopic arrangement as well. The neurons in the medial division of the spinothalamic tract, the so-called paleospinothalamic tract because of its analog in lower vertebrates, terminates predominantly in the intralaminar complex and nucleus submedius. The lateral division, or neospinothalamic tract, terminates in the ventrobasal and posterior nuclei. Most of the cells projecting to the intralaminar complex derive from the deeper laminae of the dorsal horn (CX cells). In contrast, the ventrobasilar projections come from predominantly NS and WDR neurons. The lateral aspects of the thalamus also receive information from the dorsal columns (joint position and mild mechanical stimulation, such as vibration), which can further modulate nociceptive impulses and decrease their impact.

The various thalamic nuclei then project to different areas of the cortex. The medial thalamus, which receives wide-ranging connections, projects to many areas in the cerebral cortex and the limbic system, which is involved in emotion. The lateral (neospinalthalamic tract) thalamic neurons project to the somatosensory cortex. These latter neurons are thought to convey the "sensory" aspects of nociception, whereas the former are believed to influence the affective responses to nociception.

Abnormal Pain Impulses

The preceding information represents a summary of what is known about the behavior of the nervous system in the usual realm of human experience. When significant injury occurs, especially when nerves themselves are injured, abnormal signals may arise that are often vexing to manage. The term *neuropathic pain* is used to distinguish pain arising from tissue injury that is transmitted by the nervous system from that arising from injuries or abnormalities of the nervous system itself. In other words, when the nerves are injured, they have the capability to generate impulses spontaneously. These are often perceived by patients as being uncomfortable in a very unusual way that is beyond the normal pain experience most of us experience.

To further delineate these phenomena, the characteristics of injured nerves have been studied extensively in the experimental setting. To create an injury, one either severs a nerve and caps it, promoting the development of a neuroma or one loosely ligates a nerve and creates a somewhat selective destruction of the myelinated fibers.

In the neuroma model, several differences from the normal setting are noted. First, there is the phenomenon of *spontaneous discharge*. This has been invoked to explain spontaneous pain arising from neuromata in the clinical situation. The second feature is that of *excessively vigorous discharge* in response to innocuous stimuli. This is consistent with some forms of hyperalgesia. The third feature is that of *afterdischarge* (i.e., the continuation of neural discharges long after cessation of the stimulus). This seems to parallel the clinical observation known as hyperpathia.

When one examines the cellular activity in an experimental neuroma, it becomes apparent that injury causes production and transport of receptors down the axon to the neuroma. These receptors include sodium, potassium, and calcium channels and alpha receptors. It has been shown that activation of the alpha receptors by sympathetic stimulation or by the injection of exogenous catecholamines increases the discharge rate. Similarly, blockade of these receptors by phentolamine causes a reduction in event-related firing rates. This explains the efficacy of various sympathetic blockade maneuvers in treating certain types of painful conditions.

In the ligature model, the animals behave as though they have a hyperalgesic paw. They protect the paw and demonstrate reduction of threshold to hot plate–induced paw licking. A depletion of norepinephrine is seen in the paw after the ligature is placed. This model, although not as well characterized as the neuroma model, is being studied to reveal insight into conditions such as reflex sympathetic dystrophy.

Startling new information is emerging about the plasticity of the nervous system. In this context, plasticity refers to the observation that the commonly accepted neural circuitry is not nearly so "hardwired" as was previously thought. In one study, the cutaneous receptive field of a single somatosensory neuron was determined in macaque monkeys. The peripheral nerve supplying the cutaneous area was then severed. Not surprisingly, virtually no cutaneous stimuli in the previous receptive field could induce a response in the somatosensory cortical cell. If, however, the investigators waited a few weeks, before regeneration of the cut nerve could occur, they found that stimulation of areas outside the previously determined receptive field excited the cortical cell. These areas often encompassed large areas of the monkey's body and frequently crossed the midline! Whether this represents the development of new connections or the activation of pre-existing dormant connections remains controversial. However, the inherent plasticity of the CNS, whatever the explanation, is no longer in question. This information has an effect on our understanding of deafferentation pain states, such as spinal cord injuries and traumatic neurectomies, and on the practice of neuroablative procedures for chronic pain syndromes.

APPROACH TO THE CHRONIC PAIN PATIENT

Before beginning the treatment of patients suffering from chronic pain, it is important to understand the distinction between chronic and acute pain. Acute pain is thought to be of value as an alarm or warning of a threat that, if not managed, could endanger the integrity of the organism. Recall that formerly people died from splinters and other minor trauma, largely because of lack of antimicrobial therapy. Therefore, it was probably an evolutionary advantage to experience acute pain to make one vigilant in finding the cause and rectifying it before too much harm was done. Pain frequently results in the inhibition of function of a body part that, in the acute recuperation phase of in injury, may be adaptive. The most common emotional concommitant of an acute pain experience is anxiety. (This is generated by the arousal that the pain causes, the need to know what and how severe the insult is, and the worry about how long the pain and impairment will last.) This is readily observed in the development of children and the way they handle painful experiences. Early on, they will react very vigorously to even minor injuries, because they lack the experience to know that the consequences of these are generally minimal. Often, the main solace a mother supplies is the interpretation of the pain by such statements as "it will be all right" or "it's just a little booboo," which communicate the minimal significance of the event to the child. As the child ages, he or she will normally internalize this information and will begin to react minimally to minor cuts and bumps.

The survival advantage of chronic pain to the organism is unclear to me. It generally serves no useful purpose. The predominant emotional feature of chronic pain is despair. Patients feel rejected or misunderstood by the health care system. They often experience or fear significant losses of esteem, income, roles in society and family, and abilities to engage in pleasurable or rewarding activities. The fear of the unknown with regard to their diagnosis and prognosis often wears on chronic pain-sufferers as well.

The treatment of patients with chronic pain syndromes is a different clinical experience than treating acute postoperative or traumatic pain. In the chronic situation, the affective, behavioral, and cognitive aspects of pain play a greater role in the presentation and in the management philosophy. The preceding section reviewed some principles of how peripheral neural traffic associated with injury or the threat of injury travels to the central cortex. This section focuses, instead, on the processes involved in interacting with patients complaining of chronic pain.

Definitions/Conceptual Model

The International Association for the Study of Pain defines pain as "an unpleasant sensory and emotional experience associated with actual or potential tissue damage or described in terms of such damage." There are four key elements in this definition: (1) pain is *unpleasant,* which is intuitive; (2) it has a *sensory* component, a concept with which most health care providers are very familiar; (3) it also has an *emotional* component, which is present in some degree in every painful situation; and (4) it is an *experience* that is private, totally subjective, and impossible to quantify accurately. I have taken these salient features and presented them graphically in a conceptual model of pain (Fig. 13-1).

By conceptualizing any pain experience on this diagram, one can better understand the patient's suffering. An example is the chronic low back pain patient who has had two laminectomies, neither of which have helped the pain, who has significant complaints of nondermatomal back pain with some radiation into the lower extremities and sleep disturbance, and who has been out of work for 3 months after the last surgery. This person statistically has little neurologic findings and unrevealing electromyography (EMGs) and radiologic studies and probably has muscle pain as a primary nociceptive focus, which would represent point A on Figure 13-2. The behavioral influences, affective factors, and cognitions about the nociceptive input contribute significantly to the experience, however, and elevate the "ABC" axis to a degree that the final position is quite far from the origin (i.e., the patient perceives a great deal of suffering from the pain), represented by point B on Figure 13-2.

Following through with this notion, if you attempt to address this indivi-

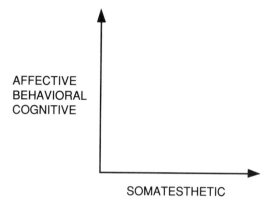

Fig. 13-1. Conceptual model of pain.

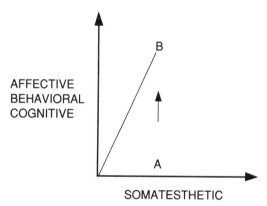

Fig. 13-2. Application of conceptual model in Figure 13-1. See text for explanation.

dual's problem as though it were primarily nociceptive with, perhaps, an epidural injection of local anesthetic and steroid or ultrasound followed by a massage, it is likely that this will be a therapeutic failure, based on inaccurate conceptualization of the problem with incorrect attribution of symptom causality. Remember that low back pain is a symptom or complaint, not a diagnosis. One could argue that if the same patient had been treated with physical therapy and myofascial trigger point injections, the results would have been different, but in most cases that are as advanced as this typical presentation, a transient reduction in nociception is not adequate to bring about a dramatic reduction in the ABC axis because environmental influences often contribute to the maintenance of pain behaviors in the absence of nociception. Likewise, cognitive aspects of the chronic pain experience may become ingrained in the individual's psyche and not resolve with transient decreases in nociception.

Affective/Behavioral/Cognitive Influences

The most common affective concomitants of a pain experience that becomes chronic are depressive in nature. With any given patient, there is always a "chicken and egg" question (i.e., which condition came first). Most typically, when good historical information is available, it is obvious that the affective state is a reaction to prolonged suffering and loss, instead of being a long-standing personality trait of the individual. Although some patients clearly meet DSM-III-R (Diagnostic and Statistical Manual of Mental Disorders, Third Edition, Revised, American Psychiatric Association Press, Washington, DC, 1987) criteria for major depression, most have what I refer to as depressive features (adjustment disorder with depressed mood, to be proper). These individuals have some features that are depressive in nature but usually do not manifest the entire spectrum of a major depression.

Another related emotional state often observed in the chronic pain patient is that of anger. Often these people appear angry at the world. Frequently, they bring anger into the provider–patient relationship, even though it may not be directly related to anything you have done. (If anticipated, this anger can often be addressed therapeutically and not reacted to at face value.) Anger is related to depression in its origin (loss, frustration) and may be a desperate person's attempt to hold onto something to keep from slipping into a depression. Strategies for dealing with anger include acknowledgment of its legitimacy (most chronic pain patients really do have plenty to be angry about), empathy and understanding (knowing that the anger is misdirected and is not actually intended for you), identification ("You know, if that had happened to me, I think I'd be pretty angry, too") and using the "Pillsbury Dough Boy" ploy (nonreactivity to anger, i.e., allowing the patient to "punch" you until he or she just tires out.) Once the anger has dissipated, the patient will often be in a much more approachable position, will form a stronger therapeutic alliance with you, and will tend to be more compliant with your management plan.

Behavior influences can do much to perpetuate suffering in a chronic pain situation. Pain behaviors (limping, grimacing, moaning, symptom amplification, refraining from activity, taking medicine, doctor shopping, etc.) can be, like all behaviors, subject to environmental influences. Most often, reinforcement is forthcoming from the environment in the form of money, privileges, attention, or avoiding of noxious or dangerous situations (work-related hazards or work itself). As part of a comprehensive management plan, these behavioral issues must be addressed in addition to any antinociceptive strategies.

Cognitions, or the way people think about pain, also may need to be a focus of treatment. Some patients react in a cognitive way that tends to heighten their sense of suffering ("I can't take this any longer!" "If this gets any worse, I just know I'll die!"). Others can use cognitions to their benefit ("It's just a tightening sensation; I can handle that"). Cognitive therapies, such as reframing or self-control strategies can be useful components of a treatment plan.

Provider Influences

Common impediments to effective management of patients with chronic pain include attitudes of the provider, simplistic or unimodal approaches, and countertransference.

Attitudes regarding chronic pain patients abound among health care providers, most of which are unfounded or self-fulfilling. Many physicians believe that this group of patients is malingering (i.e., faking symptoms to achieve a conscious gain). Studies have indicated that malingering in this population is rare. Symptom amplification, however, is quite commonly seen in these patients and merely represents another sign of the diagnosis analogous to the alcoholic underestimating daily consumption and to the social/occupational sequelae incurred with alcoholism.

Others believe that chronic pain patients are suffering from neurotic conditions, such as conversion reactions, or the unconscious production of a bodily symptom as a way of symbolizing a repressed emotion. Although this notion is very intriguing to psychoanalysts and does occur, it is clearly not a very likely cause of pain. Most often, this diagnosis is made incorrectly, based on the apparent lack of organic findings (with muscle pain syndromes, such as myofascial pain syndrome and fibromyalgia, being the most commonly missed diagnoses), instead of the presence of positive psychological history and findings that clearly explain the production of a particular symptom.

Drug-seeking behavior is common in chronic pain patients and, in and of itself, represents no particular deviation from the norm. The *reason* for drug seeking is far more important than the existence of it. Most chronic pain patients appear to be seeking drugs, when in reality what they are seeking is relief. Although inappropriate drug use and frank abuse are found in this population, it is far more common to see *drug misuse,* or the inappropriate use of medication caused by lack of understanding or desperation, than *drug abuse,* or the use of agents to change emotional state (achieve a "buzz" or "get high").

Practitioners who approach chronic pain from the antinociceptive focus alone will have some successes but statistically will have many more failures. The carpenter's syndrome ("when all you have is a hammer, all the world looks like a nail") is seen in all health care providers from time to time and frequently represents a great source of frustration for patient, physician, and insurance carrier.

Transference is a term used in psychiatry to describe the approach to a person that is a rehashing of an approach learned in a previous interaction. In essence, patients sometimes react to a physician or other health care provider as they might react to any figure of authority. Such behavior can be frequently traced to the relationship with their father (as a common example). In this instance, the interactional style may be compliance, admiration, fear, mistrust, or noncompliance, to name but a few, and manifests by patients reacting to you (an authority figure) as they had previously acted toward their father (also an authority figure for many people). If this is not recognized as transference, the practitioner may react to the patients' approach at face value and impair the development of a therapeutic relationship. Likewise, we providers also react in "preprogrammed" ways, especially in certain situations. This is, by convention, referred to as *countertransference*. This is defined as a provider's reaction to the transference but is often used in a casual sense to imply any reaction on the part of the practitioner to aspects of the patient's presentation. When you are interviewing a patient and get a knot in your stomach, this most likely represents a countertransference reaction on your part. You should mentally take a step back and try to realize what aspect of the patient you are actually reacting to, as it may change your approach to the patient.

The Four "Whats"

I have found that four pieces of information are useful to ascertain on the first visit with a chronic pain patient. Answering these four questions can give useful information about some of the psychological aspects mentioned previously.

What are your expectations of treatment? This is the most important question of all. If a patient is referred to you for treatment and expects you to "give me a treatment to make all my pain go away," it is likely that this patient will be disappointed. It is imperative to get a good understanding of what the patient believes (or wishes) you can do for them. If the patient has an unrealistic expectation, which, by definition, cannot be met, your treatment is, ipso facto, doomed to fail.

What is the meaning of the pain? By posing this question, one can often get information about what patients perceive is wrong with them and gauge some idea of the impact on their life. The patients' notion of what is wrong is often the beginning of an education to help patients understand what is actually causing their pain and, often more importantly, what is not causing it. By understanding the impact on the patient's life, you can participate in a more effective overall plan that will ultimately improve the outcome of any therapy you initiate. This can include referral to a pain physician or dentist, a physical or occupational therapist, a psychologist, a psychiatrist, or a social worker, who can begin to address some of the relevant issues with the patient.

What would you do differently if you had less pain? The key element here is the action-oriented word *do*. The information you are seeking here is some concept of the individual's goals in terms of function. Thus, "feel better" is the wrong answer. If a person struggles with this question, it may bode ill for the recovery, because it is difficult to rehabilitate a person to do nothing.

What are you willing to do to get better? This gives you some idea of the motivation and commitment that the person has to improve. I usually prod the patients a bit on this, because I want to assure myself that they mean it. It is very easy to answer this question with "anything," when, in fact, they might not be willing to do nearly as much as is asked of them.

The chronic pain patient presents with multiple problems that are not always immediately evident. These can range from undetected physical problems, to significant pain-induced emotional problems, to motivational or behavioral issues, any one of which, if left undiagnosed and untreated, may cause a treatment plan to fail. By familiarizing oneself with a different way of conceptualizing pain, one may gain a larger perspective on the presentation and construct or participate in a multifaceted management scheme that will have a greater chance of success for the patient, the practitioner, and society.

Treatment Issues

Placebo

One issue that frequently is discussed in the treatment of pain patients is the placebo response. This is defined as any nonspecific effect of the provider–patient interaction. The response may be beneficial or not. Some refer to undesirable placebo responses as "nocebo" effects. Bear in mind that placebo effects are not limited to drugs or injections but may occur in any therapeutic enterprise from massage to TENS to exercises to psychotherapy. This makes definitive evaluation of some of these methods difficult. Studies indicate that the placebo effect can occur from 15 to 100 percent of the time, depending on the nature of the endeavor, with an average of 20 to 30 percent. There is no foolproof way to detect if a treatment that you are doing on a particular patient is resulting in a placebo effect that is partially or wholly responsible for the beneficial effect. Because there is no readily discernable personality trait that accurately predicts placebo responsiveness, one should be very cautious in ascribing responses to placebo effect. The few trends that emerge from earlier research on the topic indicate that placebo responders tend to be more intelligent, more articulate, and more trusting of their physicians than nonresponders. When doing certain drug trials, it is accepted clinical practice to include a placebo phase to try to ascertain if there is any specific effect of the drug. Some clinicians use this technique as well.

Assessment of Pain

Because pain is entirely private, personal, and subjective, there is no objective way to determine whether a patient truly has pain. The question of whether a patient is suffering from "real" pain is frequently raised in consultations to me. The nature of this question is more revealing of the practitioner's bias than of the patient's presentation. To suggest that a patient who complains of pain is faking or imagining the pain, which is, therefore, not "real," is to fundamentally mistrust the patient. This implies a limited lack of understanding of some of the basic concepts put forth in this chapter. As mentioned earlier, malingering rarely occurs in this population, and individuals who have chronic pain, even if emotional overlay is a significant feature, suffer just as much as someone with an acute injury. Therefore, the most prudent approach to this apparent dilemma is to simply believe what the patient tells you. If it does not make as much sense as you would like, remember that there may be some missing elements to the history, or the history may be colored by the cognitive, behavioral, and affective factors in the experience, or, perhaps, you do not know everything there is to know about the patient or the problem. Remember that all pain is quite real to the person who experiences it. The most common diagnosis in patients who have been referred to this writer with a question of "real" pain is undiagnosed myofascial pain syndrome. This is a classic example of the referring physician not understanding the concept of myofascial pain, because it still is underdiagnosed and, therefore, undertreated, causing a great deal of needless suffering and impairment.

Chronic Muscle Pain Syndromes

Myofascial pain syndrome is first and foremost a clinical diagnosis. There is no imaging or electrodiagnostic test that will definitively rule out or diagnose this entity. The complaints are pain of a regional nature, often following trauma, which can be relatively minor, but usually includes the abrupt application of force to a muscle or muscle group that often has been out of shape and/or subjected to repeated microtrauma. There may be complaints of referred pain, usually in a pattern that is relatively characteristic of the involved muscle group. The pain is usually described as a deep aching that is diffuse and occasionally burning. Many patients describe it as sharp, especially during use of the affected muscle. Some describe tingling or numbness (a sensory deficit is only rarely discernable on examination). The pain is typically increased with effort and reduced, but rarely totally alleviated, with rest. It is quite common for the patient to report that weak to intermittent strength opioids "take the edge off" of the pain but do not relieve it.

The physical examination starts with inspection, which often reveals guarding and assymetry. Range of motion (ROM) is usually restricted but may be so minimally. Strength is often decreased, and formal muscle testing is characterized by "break away" weakness. Palpation of the muscles reveals the presence of taut bands within the substance of the muscle. These bands contain nodular areas, called trigger points, that are often well defined and exquisitely tender. The application of moderate pressure will cause the patient to complain of pain at the site and, often, in the referral zone. Snapping the trigger point out from under the finger may produce a local twitch response, which is an involuntary contraction of the taut band.

This is a commonly missed diagnosis in the chronic pain population, primarily because it is diagnosable only with thorough clinical evaluation and does not show up as an abnormality on electrodiagnostic or imaging studies. As such, it is quite common for the patient suffering from myofascial pain syndrome to enter the chronic phases before adequate diagnosis. This is unfortunate, because it means that a common and potentially benign condition is frequently allowed to become chronic, with all the previously addressed psychological factors becoming operant. The occurrence of these sequelae significantly complicates the management of myofascial syndrome.

Fibromyalgia is considered by many medical researchers, especially rheumatologists, to be an entity that is distinct from myofascial pain syndrome. It differs primarily in that the symptoms are generally more diffuse and the clinical examination includes both painful muscle nodules and areas of tenderness over some bony prominences, called *tender points*.

A sleep disturbance often accompanies the complaint of pain in both of these conditions. Many patients describe initial, middle, and terminal insomnia. Often they complain of only being able to catnap, stating that they may have only slept a few hours a day for months. They will report shifting positions, or changing between a bed and a chair all night, frequently interspersed with periods of pacing, television viewing, or reading as a distraction.

The treatment of chronic muscle pain syndromes involves several aspects, any of which may be the predominant focus with any given patient. The areas that need addressing are education, sleep restoration, instruction in body mechanics, instruction and monitoring of a daily program of gentle stretching of the involved muscles, a graded program of aerobic conditioning, and a relaxation or stress management program. Education is the most important of these, for if the patient is allowed to persist in unrealistic expectations of treatment or inappropriate notions of what is causing the pain, the treatment will likely be doomed to failure. The focus of the education of the patient should be to provide an understandable explanation of the condition, emphasizing that it is generally manageable, but only if the patient is enlisted as an active participant in the therapy. Many patients are unfamiliar with the concept of muscles causing pain that is different than that usually experienced as a "pulled muscle" and often have no notion of referred pain. It is common for patients to have been told by other providers that arthritis or a nerve impingement is the cause of the pain. It is often difficult to dissuade patients of these ideas. Another important concept is that, unlike with acute pain, the degree of hurt does not correlate with the severity of injury. Until patients learn this, they will naturally restrict their ROM to that which does not cause any increase in pain and will not participate fully in a physical therapy program.

The correction of sleep disturbance is of paramount importance in the treatment of chronic muscle pain syndromes, partly because rest enhances coping ability and partly because of the relationship between lack of restorative sleep (sleep that is not associated with rapid eye movement; non-REM sleep) and the perpetuation of chronic muscle pain syndromes. The patient should be questioned regarding sleep habits before injury, the nature of the sleep disturbance, and the use of stimulants such as caffeine. Many patients consume excessive amounts of caffeine in the form of soda drinks, coffee, tea, and chocolate. The notion that coffee consumed during the day has no effect on sleep is erroneous. The half-life of caffeine is in the range of 5 hours in the normal state, but excessive use allows accumulation of a metabolite that inhibits excretion, increasing half-life.

Initial sleep management begins with instruction in the principles of sleep hygiene. Simple protocols have been developed, such as being in bed only for sleep and sexual activity but not for television viewing, reading, resting, etc. This helps condition the person to associate going to bed with sleep and often can be useful in reversing a minor sleep disturbance. Another technique is to avoid any strenuous activity immediately before bedtime. When an individual has tried unsuccessfully to sleep for 20 minutes, he or she should get out of bed and engage in some other activity until sleepiness occurs.

The use of antidepressants can be of great value in facilitating restoration of a normal sleep–wake cycle. Unlike the treatment of depression, doses for sleep enhancement often are minimal, such as 10 to 25 mg each night of amitriptyline or equivalent. The antidepressants, used judiciously, are a safe and effective alternative to classical hypnotic agents such as barbiturates or benzodiazepines. They have commonly occurring side effects that usually constitute a nuisance to the patient rather than any serious health threat. These include somnolence, xerostomia, orthostatic hypotension, constipation, and weight gain. Most of these can be managed by careful attention to dosage or, if need be, changing drugs. Somnolence is quite common with the first few days of antidepressant therapy. This almost always resolves spontaneously after 2 or 3 days. If it persists, one should consider reduction of dosage or moving the daily dose to an earlier hour. Xerostomia is usually tolerated better with time and rarely is a cause for discontinuation of the drug. Orthostatic hypotension can generally be managed by instruction to the patient about precautions. It is of paramount importance to warn the elderly or the patient on antihypertensive medication to be alert to potential dizziness with rapid changes of posture. Constipation is more of a problem with the older antidepressants because of their strong antimuscarinic profiles. Regular consumption of a high-fiber diet is usually sufficient to correct irregularity. Weight gain occurs in about 25 percent of the patients taking first-generation antidepressants. This rarely exceeds 10 to 15 lb and generally stabilizes.

Although the effective dose varies with each patient, a workable scheme is to have the patient begin with 10 mg amitriptyline, doxepin, nortriptyline, or imipramine about 2 hours before bedtime. They should continue with this dose for 3 or 4 nights. If they are sleeping well, they should maintain that dose. If they are still having daytime somnolence or have developed other side effects, they should contact the prescribing practitioner. If they are free of side effects and not sleeping well, they should increase the dose to 20 mg each night. After another several days, the dose should be re-evaluated according to the same criteria and, if necessary, increased at intervals until a satisfactory result has been achieved.

Patients with chronic myofascial pain syndromes need instruction in body mechanics to avoid abrupt loading of affected muscles, which would serve to exacerbate or perpetuate their condition. Simple activities of daily living (ADL) such as housekeeping, hobbies, and work-related activities are frequently performed incorrectly, from a biomechanical perspective, by most of the population. When an individual has developed one of these pain syndromes, they no longer have the "muscular reserve" to do activities incorrectly and suffer no symptoms. Unless instruction is provided in how to pace activity and perform tasks in a manner that emphasizes good posture, gradual application of force, and proper use of appropriate muscles, the patient will be liable to suffer repeated setbacks and lose faith in the treatment plan.

Chronic myofascial pain syndrome involves shortened muscles, which result in decreased ROM. Instruction and monitoring in a graduated home program of passive stretch is useful. This may be more effective in some cases when combined with the "spray and stretch" technique, which, depending on the involved muscles and the skills of the patient and/or family, may be appropriate for a home program as well. Careful instruction and monitoring of this is critical. When a patient is simply handed a printed "stock" set of stretching instructions, they may not be appropriate for the involved muscles in that patient and he or she will inevitably under- or overdo the exercises, resulting in no benefit or exacerbation of the condition.

Most chronic pain patients, in addition to their primary pain diagnosis, suffer from a deconditioning syndrome. Analogous to the effect of prolonged space flight, this often is overlooked as a focus of treatment. It is characterized by loss of muscle mass, muscle stiffness, easy fatiguability, resting tachycardia with decreased cardiac reserve, listlessness, anxiety and depressive features, sympathetic nervous system predominance, and pooling of blood in the periphery, leading to dependent edema and sleep disturbance. In view of the information presented thus far, one can readily discern why attention to this generalized condition is important in the rehabilitation of the individual suffering from chronic myofascial pain syndrome. The services of a physical therapist or an exercise physiologist are needed to design and monitor a customized, graduated aerobic conditioning program that takes into account the prior athletic interests of the patient, any reversible and irreversible impairments, motivation, exercise tolerance, and previous attitudes toward exercise. As in the stretching protocols, a standard "one size fits all" approach will often be started too aggressively by the motivated patient, leading to a flare up of pain and noncompliance. By contrast, unmotivated or insecure patients may not advance the program fast enough and become stagnant at a level that they believe they cannot surpass. To many patients, the whole notion of a regular exercise program is, unfortunately, foreign (possibly contributing to the original injury), and they will need careful explanation of each aspect of a general program.

In the experience of this writer, strengthening should generally not be included in the rehabilitation plan until sleep has been restored, flexibility and ROM of the affected muscles have improved, and adherence to a regular schedule of exercises has been demonstrated. Too often people are more concerned with muscle bulk and subsequent appearance than they are with complete function. Although, according to some, muscle bulk is attractive, it often is pursued to the exclusion of complete ROM. Starling's law, which has been known for years, clearly demonstrates that skeletal muscle, while operating in a physiologic range, is able to exert more force if it contracts from a longer starting point up to a range of 33 percent beyond resting length. In other words, within reason, the longer a muscle is (i.e., the greater the ROM or the more flexible one becomes), the stronger it is. Notice the limited ROM frequently displayed by weight lifters in comparison with competitive swimmers. Although the weight lifters have more muscle mass, they often are not able to exert force throughout a complete ROM. Swimmers, however, although having somewhat less bulk, are able to take greater advantage of the strength they possess because they can generate force throughout a greater range. For most patients, this ability to apply force safely throughout a greater (normal) range is far more adaptive than sheer muscle mass. Recall that one of the cardinal features of myofascial pain syndrome is muscle shortening, which is also a result of the typical (improper) weight training that most of us see in our neighborhood health clubs.

Stress is a normal fact of life but can contribute to the maintenance or exacerbation of chronic muscle pain syndromes. People with such a condition may unconsciously make their painful muscles a focus or target organ for their stress. Recall how many times you have noticed someone who is angry clenching their teeth or how an anxious individual may furrow the brow. All this parafunctional activity as a result of emotional stress increases the demands on already painful muscles and typically works them within a narrow range, analogous to the improper strength training mentioned above. These behaviors frequently become habit and occur without conscious recognition. The stress management/relaxation/biofeedback approaches are too complex to detail in this chapter, but they do share some commonalities that can be discussed. All these approaches hinge on the theory that (1) parafunctional habits occur as a reaction to stress; (2) although usually these occur subconsciously, they can, through a variety of techniques, be brought to conscious awareness; and (3) once accessible to consciousness, they can be controlled by the individual. Some strategies, such as visual imagery, are fairly general, whereas others, such as trapezius EMG biofeedback of progressive muscle relaxation protocols, are quite specific for the muscular system or, in some cases, a particular muscle or functional group. Like the exercises mentioned above, these must be practiced and must be incorporated into a daily routine to have maximum benefit.

All these treatments for muscle pain syndromes may be overwhelming to the patient and, as such, are most effective when instituted sequentially as part of a comprehensive, multidisciplinary plan that has specific goals and time-frames, has specific aspects assigned to individual providers, is carried out with open lines of communication between the various providers, takes into account the patient's past experiences, fears, and wishes, and allows for periodic review and adjustment as conditions warrant.

CONCLUSION

To effectively manage the patient with a pain syndrome referred to the region of the TMJ, one must be cognizant of several factors in the history and physical examination. Patients with chronic pain are rarely amenable to a simplistic, unidimensional approach. Given this tenet of current pain management philosophy, one can argue that a unidimensional approach that focuses only on one aspect of the patient's presentation may, by its failure and subsequent prolongation of frustration with the health care system, contribute to the development and persistence of chronic pain.

Modern therapy for these patients must originate from a basic understanding of what is known about nervous system function and include a thoughtful and undirected history from the patient and a thorough pain-oriented physical examination by a knowledgable practitioner. Due consideration must be given to eliciting and formulating the influence of social, occupational, motivational, affective, behavioral, and cognitive factors in the origin and maintenance of the patient's symptoms.

As health care providers, we must continually serve as advocates for our patients. In the realm of chronic pain therapy, this often means that we must undertake to educate not only the patient and family, but third-party payors as well. Many payors are not yet familiar with the concept of treating chronic pain as a disease involving a whole person. They still focus on simple symptom-oriented approaches or exhaustive searches to find a cause for the patient's complaints. Unfortunately, this search is often conducted with purely a somatic focus and, according to the concepts put forth in Figure 13-1, is, therefore, fruitless.

Only by staying abreast of our own and related fields and expanding the manner in which we conceptualize, evaluate, and manage patients will we be able to restore maximal function and quality of life to the patients who seek relief from chronic pain.

SUGGESTED READINGS

Abram SE, Haddox JD, Kettler RE (eds): The Pain Clinic Manual. JB Lippincott, Philadelphia, 1990

Fields HL: Pain. McGraw-Hill, New York, 1987

Fields HL, Clanton CH, Anderson SD: Somatosensory properties of spinoreticular neurons in the cat. Brain Res 120:49, 1977

Mendell LM: Physiological properties of unmyelinated fiber projection to the spinal cord. Expl Neurol 16:316, 1966

Meyer RA, Campbell JN: Peripheral coding of pain sensation. Johns Hopkins APL Technical Digest 2:164, 1981

Wall PD, Melzack R (eds): Textbook of Pain. Churchill Livingstone, Edinburgh, 1989

White L, Tursky B, Schwartz GE (eds): Placebo Theory, Research and Mechanisms. Guilford Press, New York, 1985

Index

Page numbers followed by f *indicate figures; those followed by* t *indicate tables.*